Liberation from Allergies

**Recent Titles in
Complementary and Alternative Medicine**

Herbs and Nutrients for the Mind: A Guide to Natural Brain Enhancers
Chris Demetrios Meletis, N.D. and Jason E. Barker, N.D.

Asperger Syndrome: Natural Steps toward a Better Life
Suzanne C. Lawton, N.D.

Natural Treatments for Chronic Fatigue Syndrome
Daivati Bharadvaj, N.D.

His Change of Life: Male Menopause and Healthy Aging with Testosterone
Chris D. Meletis, N.D. and Sara G. Wood, N.D.

Liberation from Allergies

Natural Approaches to Freedom and Better Health

Chris D. Meletis, N.D.

Complementary and Alternative Medicine
Chris D. Meletis, N.D., Series Editor

PRAEGER
An Imprint of ABC-CLIO

A B C 🟊 C L I O

Santa Barbara, California • Denver, Colorado • Oxford, England

Library of Congress Cataloging-in-Publication Data

Meletis, Chris D.
    Liberation from allergies : natural approaches to freedom and better health /
Chris D. Meletis.
        p. cm. — (Recent titles in complementary and alternative medicine)
    Includes index.
    ISBN 978-0-313-35870-8 (alk. paper) — ISBN 978-0-313-35871-5 (ebook)
1. Allergy—Alternative treatment.   2. Naturopathy.   I. Title.
    RC584.M45 2009
    616.97—dc22   2009012774

13 12 11 10 9   1 2 3 4 5

This book is also available on the World Wide Web as an eBook.
Visit www.abc-clio.com for details.

ABC-CLIO, LLC
130 Cremona Drive, P.O. Box 1911
Santa Barbara, California 93116-1911

This book is printed on acid-free paper ∞

Manufactured in the United States of America

Information and advice published or made available by ABC-CLIO is not intended to
replace the services of a physician, nor does it constitute a doctor-patient relationship.
Information in this book and any related e-book, website, or database is provided for infor-
mational purposes only and is not a substitute for professional medical advice. You should
not use the information here for diagnosing or treating a medical or health condition. You
should consult a physician in all matters relating to your health, and particularly in respect
to any symptoms that may require diagnosis or medical attention. Any action on your part
in response to the information provided here is at the reader's discretion. Readers should
consult their own physicians concerning the information. ABC-CLIO will not be liable
for any direct, indirect, consequential, special, exemplary, or other damages arising from
use or misuse of the information in this book and related materials.

To all those who have educated me—professors, colleagues, and patients—on the importance of fueling the body properly and relieving the daily burden, I thank you.

Special thanks to my family: To my wife, for supporting my desire to be a perpetual advocate to help improve the quality of life of humanity. To my children, for inspiring me to achieve what can be imagined. To my parents, Demetrios and Madeleine, for instilling the desire to learn and ask the questions that most avoid.

Gratitude to God for providing insights that are indeed divine and for the Creation of all that we see and don't see.

Contents

Acknowledgments

I must thank all those who contributed to the manifestation of this book. I am deeply appreciative of the hard work and dedication of Dr. Shalima Gordon, Dr. Zia Robles Hernandez, and Dr. Nieske Zabriskie: Thank you for your tireless efforts and exuberant sharing.

Special thanks to USBioTek for providing me with the testing tools I have used extensively in my clinical practice to help my patients on their wellness journey over the many years. It is with great gratitude that I thank all the patients, all the doctors, and USBioTek for helping compile the amazing success stories of how testing for and eliminating allergies can unleash true wellness.

John Thoreson, thank you for your valiant efforts to tap into one of the world's leading experts in the field of immunology.

I thank all my patients who have demonstrated time and time again that when we all eat well, de-stress, become aware of our journey through life, and make proactive choices, wellness is most readily achieved.

Introduction

In a nutshell, this book provides you and your loved ones with the keys to a better life. You have one life to live, so it is essential that you enjoy peak performance and the ultimate potential you can achieve. Life is full of choices, including the choice about what you feed your body. This book is intended to help you appreciate the impact everyday foods may have on your health.

If you are like the average person, you probably take better care of your car than your body. When was the last time you considered fueling your car with a questionable quality gas? When was the last time you changed your car's oil and air filter? Being the owner of such a valuable and necessary possession, it would be irresponsible to not follow routine maintenance procedures to ensure an efficiently operating vehicle. After all, a car is expensive. Well, how about your body? You got it for free, and it doesn't come with a warranty system like your car. All the more reason to invest more in your health than your car, as it is supposed to last for an enjoyable lifetime.

Taking the time to read the following pages carefully and with an open mind may very well save your life from being lackluster and burdened with unnecessary symptoms. You probably remember the adage, "you are what you eat from your head to your toes." This is true. Eating foods that are the cause of your hidden food allergies may promote undue inflammation and damage that you may be unaware of as being caused by food allergies. Identifying and eliminating these foods from your diet is a simple and easy step to better health.

Knowledge is power, and you are in charge of your health. If you don't take care of yourself or your loved ones, who will? Giving this book to a friend or family member is giving the gift of health.

Remember, we all have a certain chronological age, the number of years we are old. This we have no control of. However, we are *fully* in charge of our biological age, the age our trillions of cells are in terms of quality and function. Continually eating foods we are allergic to creates inflammation in the body and causes our cells to function at "half-mast." A variety of ills can result when our cells are not working in their best form. Food allergies can affect any cell structure in the body: the joints, muscles, lungs, brain, and blood vessels. Basically, anywhere the blood flows, inflammation from food allergies follows, and symptoms may result.

Life is a buffet full of choices. Choose to invest in your health by identifying and eliminating your hidden food allergies.

ARE YOU EATING TO LIVE OR LIVING TO EAT?

Before you read another paragraph, ask yourself the following question. It may not be an easy question, but you know the answer. Sit quietly, think deeply, and wait until the answer becomes very clear: Why are you eating the foods you currently eat?

Stop reading until you write down your answer. An honest answer will give you valuable insight. What influences your choices? Where did those influences come from? You have the power to make daily "life and death" food choices. How much of that power have you given to outside influences? Are you willing to change who or what influences you?

You are *proactive* about your health if you are truly serious about pursuing a life that is full of the "Vs": vibrancy, vim, and vigor that yield true vitality and ultimate victory. This is in stark contrast to the person who is *reactive* and seeks medical attention after getting ill from eating indiscriminately. The latter is rather like intentionally running over a pile of nails with your car and then going in for a patch job on your tires.

Indiscriminate eating often follows illogical thought patterns such as:

- Wow, what a cool-looking package! It *must* be good!
- Everyone else is eating it, so I will, too.
- One more day won't matter; I'll start eating right tomorrow.
- Hmmm, that tastes good. Pass me some more.
- This is "my" brand; I belong to a special group.

CHOICES

You began making food choices even as a baby. You may believe your parents made these choices for you. However, does this sound familiar? A little tongue begins pushing, spit happens, the head turns, and the ever-so-powerful "I'll cry if you make me taste that food again" begins. Depending on how perceptive, creative, or persistent your parents were, your diet probably changed course a little bit with each protest. Those first opinions were determined by the mood you were in, the texture or taste of the food, or just some internal sense you had that "This food isn't for me."

When did you become an adult? Was it at a certain age? Was it a rite of passage determined by family tradition? Was it when you moved out on your own? Was it when you went off to college or got a job? Regardless of the defining moment, we have never once seen the rite of passage into adulthood defined as, "When I began making good health choices and eating a life-sustaining diet."

This may be the defining moment for you, right now, as you are reading these words. You might be asking yourself *big* questions: Why did I have that dinner last night? Will it improve my health or harm it? What are my health goals for the next 5, 10, or 20 years? Have I pursued financial goals, yet neglected my health goals? If so, why?

The reality is that "Today is the first day of the rest of your life." You are determining your health with each morsel you eat. If your choices are the same as those of the average North American, you may become a statistic and suffer from a preventable disease. However, your wise and moderate choices will have positive long-term results. You are already taking steps toward choosing wisely by reading this book. Congratulations!

This book is not designed to convert you into a health nut, because most health nuts either go nuts or all their friends think they are nuts. The key is moderation. The more you moderate your unhealthy habits, the healthier you can become. You may be amazed at how much better you feel in only a few weeks. Many of our patients report feeling significantly better when they begin to eat with intent instead of eating by habit.

Inaction is the active process of doing nothing.

—*Chris D. Meletis, N.D.*

IT IS NOT TOO LATE

Scientists have proven that even if you are 60 years or older, implementing a proactive diet and lifestyle can have a profound impact on your health. How can that be? Your body is continually replacing old cells with new at an amazing rate. When you eat with positive intent, those new cells will become resilient building blocks. Just like a remodeling job on the television series *This Old House*, it is never too late to restore and renovate your body.

Life is a buffet full of choices. Choose to invest in your health by identifying and eliminating your hidden food allergies.

CHAPTER 1

An Allergy Overview: Understanding the Task at Hand

WHAT IS AN ALLERGY?

In the 21st century, the word "allergy" seems to have become a household name. There are allergies to food, environmental toxins, and the environment in general. Those seeking to achieve health and survive in an increasingly hostile world must discover the answers to the following two critical questions: How are allergies acquired and why?

Throughout the ensuing discussions the consequences of out-of-control allergies that erode one's health throughout a lifetime, will be critically analyzed, and countless clinical success stories will be shared.

Strictly speaking, an allergic reaction is an overreaction of the immune system to a particular substance that is generally acquired over time. However, an allergy is not simply hay fever, hives, or anaphylactic reactions, but it encompasses a wide range of symptoms and pathways in the body generated by substances that escape the body's barriers and stray into the bloodstream.

Understanding the Body's Protective Processes

The human body is capable of differentiating self from nonself with the aid of the immune system. This is the how the body is able to identify and defend against invading bacteria, viruses, parasitic infections and even cancer. It is this innate mechanism by which the body is able to maintain nonself out and self in. These defenses include the following:

- The skin (integument)—skin cells form a protective barrier to prevent normal bacteria that live on the outer skin layer from entering the bloodstream. The integumentary system is the largest organ system. It distinguishes, separates, protects, and informs the body with regard to its surroundings.

- The lungs—epithelial cells that form the lining of the lungs secrete mucus and contain cilia—small hairlike structures—that move debris out of the lungs.
- The gastrointestinal system—the cells that make up the lining of the gastrointestinal walls tightly regulate what enters the micro-controlled inner world of the 75 trillion cells that make up the human body and the entropic unordered world outside the body. A healthy gastrointestinal tract allows nutrients to be absorbed and waste released. It is important to note that the low pH in the stomach acts as a barrier against bacterial and viral organisms, yet it also helps break down proteins in foods that could otherwise trigger a heightened allergic response.

The vast majority of the time, with rare exception, if these first-line defense mechanisms are intact and fully functioning, the body can enjoy a higher level of wellness and true health. However, when these mechanisms break down from wear and tear, stress, nutritional deficiencies, and environmental toxins, then the body is no longer able to protect itself from foreign substances.

Aside from their protective function, the skin, lungs, and gastrointestinal tract are also responsible for two other distinct functions:

1. Absorption
2. Excretion

These systems function as organs of detoxification. An important concept to remember is that when these systems are bogged down—that is, they are unable to excrete all the waste adequately, their function slows down. In other words, if environmental toxins were cars driving down a major roadway, and the roadway was the ability to eliminate some of its traffic burden, there would be a bottleneck along that roadway where exposure to more stress, a new allergy, a virus, or a higher level of chemical exposures would be factors that made the lanes on this roadway decrease. As a consequence, in any major city, there is more concentrated pollution in the particular area of bottlenecked traffic. In the same way, the system where toxins get stuck in the body—be it the skin, the lungs, or the gastrointestinal tract—becomes more overburdened with toxins and hence, more prone to disease.

It Is All about Total Burden

We live each day bombarded by stress, noise, electromagnetic pollution, radiation, chemical pollutants, smog, inadequate nutrition, and much more, depending on our lifestyle. All the different stimuli our body is exposed to increase the physiological demands on the body such that it needs more nutrients and needs to work harder to maintain a state of equilibrium, better known as homeostasis. Without homeostasis, the body is unable to function optimally; therefore, it becomes more prone to sluggish function of certain mechanisms and reactions. Amid all of these external influences, genetic predispositions also come into play. Deficiencies become exaggerated and our sense of well-being diminishes.

Furthermore, the excess of toxins that are not being able to be processed by the body also create a situation where the body is unable to accept the nutrition it requires from the food one eats. For example, if the lungs are inflamed, they will not be able to absorb as much of the oxygen that they need. The gastrointestinal tract would be taking in undigested proteins, and because of inflammation, it would also fail to transport essential nutrients into the body. Therefore, to improve or lessen the body's burden, it becomes crucial to reduce the total burden by removing offending agents from one's environment.

Each person has a certain tolerance for levels of stress. Certain people react to certain stressors more quickly than others. These people are said to carry a larger "burden," as their body is unable to handle much stress or changes in their lives. Every little exposure to stress; to a virus or bacteria; to new pollen, or even excessive pollen; to fumes; or to an extra smoggy day will produce a set of new symptoms and a sense of illness. For others, it takes a lot more to elicit an unfavorable response. These people, one could say, have a lighter burden. This could be because their body is genetically able to process toxins, chemicals and other noxious substances much more quickly, or perhaps their diet and lifestyle are such that they are not putting a lot of extra stress in those areas so they can overextend in others. Either way, their body is able to tolerate much more environmental abuse than someone whose body is already in a state of inflammation, toxicity, and/or malnutrition.

The best way to appreciate the reality of allergens, toxic burden, and the consequence on the human frame is to observe the actual effects as seen in actual clinical cases.

Case Studies

1. An 18-year-old woman was suffering from severe cystic acne. Her mother had spent hundreds of dollars on dermatologist appointments and prescriptions that worked only temporarily, if at all. The next step in their journey toward wellness was to have a blood sample collected to determine potential food allergies. The test results were positive for dairy, banana, and wheat allergies—foods the patient consumed almost on a daily basis, which explains why her acne never seemed to improve. When these items were removed from her diet, the patient noticed a remarkable improvement in her acne within *days*. She was then able to begin treatments to reduce the scars left from years of battling cystic acne.

2. A 10-year-old boy with autism presented with a positive stool culture for *Candida albicans*. Food allergy testing also revealed elevated antibody levels specific to dairy, egg, and gluten. The child was advised to avoid all allergenic foods and was given supplements with essential fatty acids (EFAs) and probiotics. After two months, great improvement was reported in this young boy's mental condition from strictly following the elimination and rotation diet guideline from the allergy testing lab.

3. A serious case of dermatitis, mainly on the arms, had tormented a 14-year-old girl for many years. She also complained of "heavy" headaches and a state of near constant fatigue. Dairy, cucumber, and strawberry were all associated with elevated antibody levels, as assessed through the food allergy testing laboratory. She was placed on a customized elimination and rotation diet guideline supplemented with EFAs. After two months, her headaches were completely gone. She began to feel strong and able again. After four months, the skin on her arms had become smooth and bright. She remarked that she has never had such beautiful skin before!

THE IMMUNE SYSTEM AND ALLERGIES

The immune system's response to foreign substances results in what is termed "sensitization"—or an alteration of the body's responsiveness to a foreign antigen, usually an allergen, such that on subsequent exposures to the allergen there is a heightened immune response. In other words, after the first exposure, subsequent exposures to that allergen result in a greater severity of symptoms. This often occurs, for example, when a person moves to a new area—generally the person will experience relief from hay fever symptoms if the pollens in that area are different enough; however, after several years of living in the new environment, a person begins to develop sensitivities to the local pollen. How does that happen? When the body's primary defense system—the skin, the lungs, and the gastrointestinal system are in a state of inflammation, they are rendered incapable of fully protecting the self, from the nonself.

The risk of allergic sensitization and the development of allergies varies with age, and young children are most at risk.[1] When the primary barriers are breached, the immune system then takes the lead in maintaining the body's integrity as best as possible. The sensitization process occurs through an imbalance in cytokine production. The body produces hormonal messengers called "cytokines," which signal the immune system when it needs to be active and when it needs to stand down. There are two basic types of cytokines: those that promote inflammation and those that promote allergic responses.

Cytokines are produced by immune cells called T helper cells. The T helper cells produce two types of cytokines: Th1 and Th2 cytokines. The Th1-type cytokines tend to produce the proinflammatory responses responsible for killing intracellular parasites. This type of response is useful for creating long-term immunity to a host of disease-causing organisms; however, when this immunity goes wild it can result in extensive tissue damage that can lead to autoimmune reactions. The Th2 cytokines decrease the inflammatory response and act as a balancing mechanism for the Th1 response. The Th2 cytokines promote IgE (immediate allergic reaction antibody) and decrease the inflammation caused by Th1. If this reaction is excessive, then the immune system is suppressed and the body develops an allergy, rather than an immunity, to the offending substance. The optimal scenario would therefore seem to be that humans should produce a well-balanced Th1 and Th2 response, suited to the immune challenge.[2]

An excess of Th2 then leads to four different types of hypersensitive reactions[3]:

- Type I: Immediate allergy. Mediated by IgE antibodies. Symptoms generally occur within 15 minutes of exposure. This type of allergy is recognized by conventional medicine. Examples of type I hypersensitivity reaction include atopy, anaphylaxis, and asthma.
- Type II: Cytotoxic reaction. Mediated by IgM, IgG antibodies or complement. Antibodies produced by the immune response bind to antigens found on the body's own cell surfaces. These "tagged" cells are then destroyed by other immune cells called macrophages. Symptoms generally occur minutes to hours after exposure. Examples of type II hypersensitivity reaction include rheumatic fever, Goodpasture's syndrome, and autoimmune hemolytic anemia.
- Type III: Immune complex reaction. Mediated by IgG antibodies. This reaction occurs when antigens and antibodies are present in roughly equal amounts and the antigens are not bound to the cells of the body. When the antibodies bind to the antigen, they form large immune complexes that essentially precipitate out of solution (the blood) and get stuck in a particular part of the body. The deposition of these large molecules create more local inflammation and tissue destruction. Examples of type III reaction include IgG-mediated food allergy, serum sickness, systemic lupus erythematosus, and subacute bacterial endocarditis.
- Type IV: Delayed-type hypersensitivity reaction. T-cell mediated immune memory response, antibody independent. The antigen is eaten by immune cells and taken to a T cell that recognizes this antigen. Pro-inflammatory markers are secreted by the immune cells which help destroy the foreign invader (the antigen). This reaction takes place when takes between three to five days to develop after the initial exposure. Examples of type IV reaction include contact dermatitis, tuberculin skin test, and chronic transplant rejection reaction.[4]

When it comes to food allergies, research has shown that a type III hypersensitivity reaction in combination with a delayed sensitivity reaction may be triggering symptoms that include chronic fatigue, arthritis, hives, eczema, headaches, water retention, irritable bowel, and many other symptoms. Real case examples provide excellent reflections of the reality and severity of overwhelming food allergies.

Case Studies

1. A 33-year-old woman suffered from four major complaints: fatigue, dark circles under her eyes, edema, and infertility. She was tested for food allergies, and blood sampling for IgG and IgE revealed significantly elevated antibody levels specific to dairy, egg, corn, pineapple, banana, and other foods. She was advised to avoid the allergenic foods and was given EFA supplements. Because of the seriousness of her complaints and the extent of her food allergies, she was also placed on an intestinal rebuilding protocol of supplements to strengthen the ability of her gastro-intestinal tract to filter out allergens. The dark circles under her eyes, edema, and fatigue all improved dramatically after two months. After five months she became a very happy mother-to-be.

2. An eight-year-old boy had, over the past several years, experienced several bouts of serous otitis media. Inflammation and fluid accumulation behind his eardrums was of such a chronic nature that he needed to be intubated at least twice per year. Use of IgG and IgE blood testing showed elevated antibodies specific to dairy, egg, sesame, sunflower seeds, blueberry, strawberry, cranberry, and other foods. He was advised to avoid the allergenic foods and supplemented with EFAs. Because of his many food allergies, he was also placed on an intestinal rebuilding formula and probiotics. After staying on the elimination and rotation diet guideline and supplements for three months, the boy's doctor found no abnormal fluid accumulation behind his ears. After six months, the child had not experienced another otitis media flare-up. He sprouted almost four inches within one year of being tested.

3. A 16-year-old male patient with a previous diagnosis of Tourette's syndrome presented with a complaint of neck pain and mild headaches. His neurological examination was within normal limits, and overall he was in excellent physical condition. He uncontrollably rotated his head to the right quickly and frequently. The patient's mother said he was on medication for the tics, but they had not noticed benefits from the medication. Allergy testing results showed that the patient was in the high-reactivity category to garlic. The patient noticed a significant improvement in the head movements once he started eliminating foods with garlic. His mother noted that he had definitely improved and that the dietary change was the first treatment to really have had an effect on his tics.

4. The mother of a six-year-old girl was concerned about her child's constantly congested nose, frequent yawning, and fatigue. As a piano teacher, she had observed that her daughter did not appear to be as healthy as any one of her seven-year-old students. Food allergy testing revealed that her daughter had strong allergies to dairy products, egg, cucumber, and mushroom. Implementing the customized elimination and rotation diet guideline provided by the lab company resulted in major symptom improvement in a matter of weeks.

TYPES OF ADVERSE FOOD REACTIONS

Food Allergies

The incidence of hidden, or delayed-onset, food allergies in the population is underestimated. In addition, the symptoms of delayed food allergies may be so diverse that it is virtually impossible to define the percentage of the population affected. Some argue that as many as 50 million people suffer from an allergy-based illness in America alone. Others say that food allergies affect up to *half* the American population.

A food allergy is an immune reaction to food proteins. During an immune reaction, the body makes antibodies to sequester these food proteins, which it recognizes as foreign invaders. One of the primary antibodies involved is IgG, of which four subclasses exist: IgG1, IgG2, IgG3, and IgG4. Think of the "G" in IgG as standing for "gradual," as in gradual or delayed-onset symptoms of a food allergy. Under certain circumstances an overzealous immune system may produce excessive quantities of these antibodies. Excess IgG antibodies may produce an excess reaction known as a hypersensitivity reaction. Hypersensitivity reactions can promote excess inflammation and symptoms anywhere in the body.

IgG-mediated food allergies can dramatically affect long-term health. IgG antibodies may remain active in the body for months at a time, which may promote a state of chronic inflammation and degeneration of tissues anywhere in the body. This process may be so gradual that a person may very well become accustomed to feeling less than optimal and may take aches and pains for granted or as part of getting older. Settling for feeling unwell does no one any good, and robs a person of the potential for optimal health.

Food antigen-antibody complexes may end up in tissues and organs and may trigger inflammatory reactions. Food allergies that take a while to hit are much more common than those that make a person sick right away. It can be argued that IgG-mediated food allergies may account for a variety of chronic health conditions that have been unresponsive to conventional medical care. Fatigue, irritability, aching joints, cognitive dysfunction, and chronic migraines are a few known complications that may be caused by delayed-onset food allergies.

There is a clear and definite relationship between what you eat and how you feel. The first order of business in promoting your health is to avoid the foods that are making you sick!

Food Poisoning

Food poisoning is an immediate toxic reaction from contaminants in the food. Perhaps you have experienced a case of food poisoning with stomach pains and diarrhea from eating potato salad that has been sitting out on the picnic table too long. Food poisoning can occur in anyone who has been exposed to contaminated food.

Food Intolerance

Food intolerance, unlike a food allergy, does not mount an immune reaction. Food intolerance may be caused by a number of factors, including an enzymatic defect inherent in a person or a chemical component—either an additive or a naturally occurring compound in the food that the body may be unable to handle.

A common food intolerance is lactose intolerance. People who are lactose intolerant are unable to digest milk products because they lack the enzyme lactase, which is usually present in the gut and is responsible for breaking down the milk sugar, lactose. An inability to break down lactose may cause cramping and diarrhea from eating milk products. What better way for your body to say, "I can't eat this. Don't give it to me!" As in the case of food allergies, your body may send you similar messages because of an immune reaction, which may include cramping, diarrhea, headache, fatigue, and aching joints, among others.

An adverse reaction to a food additive is also defined as food intolerance. Reactions to colorants, preservatives, fillers, stabilizers, and artificial sweeteners can wreak havoc in some people. These additives carry many names such as tartrazine (FD&C yellow No. 5), sodium benzoate, tragacanth, and aspartame. In a sensitive person, an additive may provoke a myriad of symptoms, including rash, headache, difficulty breathing, cognitive dysfunction, or fatigue through non–immune mediated mechanisms.

Some foods contain naturally occurring compounds that may mimic allergy inflammation and symptoms. Examples include histamine and tyramine, which are found in wine, fermented cheeses, certain fish, crustaceans, sauerkraut, tomatoes, and sausages. Tyramine in particular is found in beer, chocolate, and fermented and cured foods. In certain people, these compounds elicit what may otherwise be mistaken for a food allergy with symptoms such as sneezing, runny nose, headache, and wheezing.

Exorphins are another type of toxic food by-products. Exorphins are formed in the intestine from the improper digestion of gluten and casein in particular and yield the peptides gliadorphin and beta-casomorphin, respectively. Exorphins may affect neurotransmitter function in the brain of certain individuals. In one study, high levels of IgG antibodies to gluten were found in 87 percent of autistic patients and 86 percent of schizophrenic patients, and high levels of IgG antibodies to casein were found in 90 percent of autistic patients and 93 percent of schizophrenic patients. Within three months, a diet free of gluten and casein showed an improvement in symptoms in schizophrenic patients and an 81 percent improvement in autistic children.[5] Exorphin-like compounds have also been identified in corn and barley.

Psychosomatic Food Aversion

Some adverse food reactions are psychosomatic in nature. In such cases, your mind tricks you into thinking a food is bad for you. This most often results from a prior bad experience with the food. For example, ever since "Mark" became terribly ill immediately after eating pork-fried rice at a Chinese restaurant he has assumed that he is allergic to pork. However, when Mark does not know that the meat he is served at a dinner party is pork, he does not become sick. Ignorance can be bliss! Suffice to say, Mark has developed a psychosomatic adverse food reaction to pork from a prior bad experience, probably as a result of food poisoning.

Case Studies

1. A 33-year-old woman with a history of sinusitis, asthma, and allergic rhinitis was tested for food and inhalant allergies. Her inhalant panel revealed allergies to cat hair, mold, tree pollen, and dust. Her food allergy report showed an immediate hypersensitivity to dairy, mushroom, sesame, and beef. All symptoms resolved when the inhalants were eliminated from her environment and the foods were eliminated from her diet.

2. A two-year-old patient presented with a history of chronic vomiting that had occurred nearly on a daily basis all of his life. He also had chronic rhinorrhea, dysphagia, cough, and a tendency to aspirate thin fluids (i.e., water). He had seen a number of doctors and specialists, had undergone a swallow study and an adenoidectomy, and was recommended for an endoscopy, none of which provided an answer to his symptoms. An IgG antibody, however, revealed high reactions to dairy and egg, which were subsequently removed from his diet. In the eight weeks after he eliminated dairy and eggs from his diet, he only vomited four times: twice the first week and twice after accidental ingestion of dairy. His cough went away, the dysphagia resolved, and the rhinorrhea greatly improved.

3. A friendly, active, outgoing. nine-year-old boy, has experienced debilitating migraine headaches that occur weekly or more frequently ever since he was six years old. He takes Fenergan to control vomiting during the migraines. The frequency and severity of his migraines has had

a significant impact on his family. Family life revolves around his episodes, and planned events are tentative, ready to be called off at a moment's notice at first sign of a headache. Car travel frequently triggers a migraine and the family has to sit by the roadside waiting for him to feel better. His IgG results indicate a severe reaction to all dairy and a moderate response to eggs. The whole family decides to give up dairy products cold turkey. At his one-month follow-up, the boy reports that he has had two headaches, each lasting about 45 minutes, but he has not needed any medications.

ENVIRONMENTAL ALLERGIES

Environmental allergies also form part of the body's immune response to foreign substances that are able to pass through its first line of defense. In the case of environmental allergies, the barrier allergens are able to surpass is the respiratory tract. Hypersensitive reactions of the airway and lungs tend to be IgE-mediated reactions, meaning that the response to the allergen is immediate. There are several common allergic reactions to environmental allergens.

Allergic Rhinitis

Allergic rhinitis is an IgE-mediated hypersensitive reaction to substances such as plant pollens, fungi, animal dander, and dust mites. Allergic rhinitis consists of swelling of the nasal passages, red eyes and nose, and runny eyes and nose when exposed to the offending substance.

Asthma

Asthma routinely involves a chronic inflammation of the airways that causes recurrent episodes of wheezing, breathlessness, and chest tightness. Asthma is estimated to affect about 17 million people in the United States alone!

Asthma is typically a Th2-dominant condition, which consists of an allergic-type response of the immune system—IgE antibodies, macrophages, eosinophils, mast cells, neutrophils, and epithelial cells. All of these components are part of the inflammatory response. When these cells are called into action in the bloodstream, it results in a lot of congestion at the site of injury, as all these cells are trying to clean up the offender and take it into custody so to speak. Their eager response, though, creates a large traffic jam and results in inflammation of the airways. In many ways, asthma is a lot like a car crash—the entrance of the allergen into the respiratory tract represents the car crash. The ensuing traffic jam from the car crash and from the emergency responders blocking so many lanes in traffic is like the immune cells going to the site and trying to clear up the crash site.

Inflammation is thought to be the root cause of this high sensitivity to allergens in the bronchial passageways. There are three major causes for the development of asthma:

1. Genetic predisposition to type 1 hypersensitivity (atopy)/Th2 dominance.
2. Acute and chronic airway inflammation
3. Bronchial hyperresponsiveness

In addition to the inflammation, the airway is also remodeled into thicker smooth muscle and collagen, which results in a more restricted airway.

There are four types of asthma:

1. Atopic asthma—This is the most common type of asthma, particularly in childhood. It is an IgE-mediated disorder (type 1) that is generally triggered by environmental allergens, such as dust, pollen, animal dander, and foods. There is often a family history of asthma or atopy (such as eczema, allergic rhinitis, allergic conjunctivitis, and asthma).
2. Nonatopic asthma—This type of asthma is generally triggered by an upper respiratory viral infection and is not an antibody-mediated illness. Those with nonatopic asthma typically have no other associated allergies, and there is generally no family history of asthma.
3. Occupational asthma—This asthma is triggered by chemical fumes, dusts, gases, and other chemicals.
4. Drug-induced asthma—This type of asthma is triggered by drugs, particularly aspirin. It is seen in people who suffer from recurrent rhinitis and nasal polyps. The mechanism of action varies in this type of asthma, but it can include a type I hypersensitivity reaction.

Case Studies

1. An 11-year-old girl complains of difficulty hearing and chronic mouth breathing. She cannot breathe through her nose but denies having nasal or sinus congestion and headaches. Chronic mouth breathing is a common symptom with food allergies or sensitivities. After eliminating her moderate and highly reactive foods for three months, this patient notices significant improvement in hearing and can hear her ears popping for the first time. Currently, she is on a rotation diet and symptom free.

2. A patient has suffered from sinus headaches for more than 10 years. Her food allergy panel shows an allergy to whey, casein, kidney beans, black

beans, cane sugar, sesame, and eggs. After removing the offending foods, she is clear of sinus headaches.

3. A 48-year-old woman with a 10-year history of chronic cough, which has not improved despite a variety of treatments, seeks intervention through food allergy assessment via enzyme-linked immunosorbent assay (ELISA) testing. Her food allergy panel reveals elevated antibodies to dairy products, shrimp, corn, barley, oat, sesame, and rice. Among the fruits she reacts strongly to are banana, grape, and pear. She also shows a moderate reaction to egg white. By following the customized elimination and rotation diet guideline provided with her lab report from US BioTek, she improves dramatically and has complete remission of her symptoms.

ALLERGIC EXPOSURES

How is the body exposed to allergens? Think of the digestive tract as a tube that begins at the mouth and extends to the anus. The inside of the tube is in effect the *outside* of your body. This tube is heavily guarded—more than 60 percent of the immune system lives in the tissues that line the gut wall, and only specific nutrients and substances recognized by the body as essential are allowed through. However, when the body is exposed to stress, inadequate diet, genetic predisposition, infections and inflammation, chemicals, drugs, environmental pollutants, and toxins, the barrier between the outside and the inside becomes compromised and is no longer efficient at keeping foreign particles and organisms at bay. It is at this point where, for example, partially undigested proteins are able to enter the bloodstream. When this occurs, the immune cells circulating in the blood mount a response to clear the foreign invader out of the body. When enough foreign proteins are able to enter the bloodstream, the immune system mounts a response that leads to the symptoms related to food allergy. Once the body mounts a response to these allergens, the immune system remembers the offender, so that each time the offender is encountered, the same or a greater response is mounted against it. This is why the more frequently a food is eaten, the greater the symptoms and vice versa. To successfully manage a delayed hypersensitivity reaction to food, it then becomes extremely important to eat a diet as varied as possible to minimize overexposure to one type of food.

PREDISPOSING FACTORS TO ALLERGIES

Genetic Factors

Studies have shown that food allergies can have a genetic component.[6] It has been established that family history of allergies is one of the predisposing factors for an individual having food allergies. Allergic diseases are strongly familial: identical twins are likely to have the same allergic diseases about 70 percent of the time; the same allergy occurs about 40 percent of the time in nonidentical twins.[7] As new research comes to light, however, it has been recognized that environmental influences are significant. Therefore, given the appropriate information, food allergies can be managed successfully with a change in the environmental factors in a person's lifestyle.

Stress

Studies have found that increased stress hormones reduce immunity in the body,[8] which means that if you eat an offending food, it will take more time to mount an immune response to that food; however, it does not mean damage is not occurring. When there is exposure to chronic stress, chronic high levels of cortisol induce a state of chronic inflammation in the body.[9] When the gastrointestinal tract is inflamed, the cells no longer form an effective barrier to foreign matter. The more foreign matter that is able to enter the bloodstream, the more likely it is to develop an allergy to that foreign substance. Recent studies have shown that stress may be one of the primary causes for the development of food allergies, as the intestine is more permeable to antigens during periods of chronic stress, which allows for sensitization to that antigen.[10]

More often than not, in today's society people eat meals on the run. We wake up in the morning, run out the door, drive furiously to work and stop at a nearby drive-thru to pick up a bite to eat. We eat while we drive, full of adrenalin to make sure no one hits us and we get to our destination safely and on time. We eat our meals in a state of fight or flight, which inevitably, affects how we process our foods—because even though it takes a few hours to digest what we ate, the way we started to eat that meal sets the stage for how we finish digesting the meal. This high-stress mode of eating meals maximizes our chances of developing a food allergy over time. To make matters more complicated, because today's meals are made with such variety of ingredients, we are even more at risk of developing a host of food allergies in a short period of time.

Environmental Exposure

The hygiene hypothesis was developed to explain the observation that hay fever and eczema, both allergic diseases, we re less common in children from larger families, who were presumably exposed to more infectious agents through their siblings than were children from families with only one child. The hypothesis states that a lack of early childhood exposure to infectious agents, symbiotic microorganisms (e.g., gut flora), and parasites increases susceptibility to allergic diseases by modulating immune system development.[11] Exposure to different types of stimuli (from infectious agents, symbiotic bacteria, or parasites) is thought to allow the immune system to adequately develop regulatory T cells. If the stimulus is lacking, the organism is more likely to be susceptible to autoimmune diseases and allergic diseases because of insufficiently repressed Th1 and Th2 responses, respectively.[12]

Allergies and asthma have been linked to an excessive Th2 response, which occurs because the permeability of the cells allows foreign substances into the blood stream. The Th2 response shuts down response, which further promotes allergies in adults.

Aside from inadequate exposure to natural stimuli in early childhood, increasing exposure to artificial toxins also increases the likelihood of developing allergies. Studies have found that exposure to certain toxins, such as pesticides and herbicides as well as genetically modified foods can trigger the development of food allergies.[13] This may be due in part to the alteration of function of the gastrointestinal system as well as an increased stress response of the body to these foreign substances.

Case Studies

1. Constant migraine headaches have plagued a 55-year-old woman and have been the bane of her life. When she was 31 years old she had to quit her job because of the debilitating pain. At age 50, she became suicidal and was diagnosed by a psychologist as melancholic. Her food allergy test results reveal elevated antibody levels specific to dairy, gluten, honey, and coffee. She is advised to avoid the allergenic foods and is given EFA supplements along with probiotics and a hypoallergenic gastrointestinal restoration product. After one month, her debilitating migraines cease and have not recurred since. Her psychologist has also noted a much improved mental status and outlook on life.

2. After eliminating offending foods (dairy products, egg, banana) from her diet, a 33-year-old woman reports, "Three to four weeks later, I've noticed significant improvement in my sleep pattern. I've been a 'light sleeper' all my life. I have difficulties falling asleep, I'm easily awoken in the middle of the night, and have difficulty falling back to sleep. But since I've stayed off the 'offending' foods, I'm able to sleep through the night, every single night. Even my husband, the 'sound' sleeper has woken up several times (due to thunderstorms and the baby) and [has been] amazed to find that I'm still sound asleep! I thought being a 'light sleeper' was just part of my personality. I had no idea that food sensitivities were behind my sleep problems. For all those people that have sleep problems, they may identify with me saying that being able to have a good night sleep is 'priceless.' In addition, I've also lost 7–8 lbs since I've stopped eating my reactive foods. I have been trying to lose five pounds post the baby for over two years, without any success. In the last two months, I was able to lose the weight without eating less or increasing the amount of exercise. So, I think it must be related to the type of food I'm eating. While being able to sleep is priceless and the top benefit,

being able to lose the added pounds from the pregnancy is definitely a nice bonus.

Thank you so much for introducing me to this test. I think it's the best thing that has happened to me, and I hope that many of our friends/family who have taken this test will find it equally beneficial."

3. A 35-year-old gentleman suffers from constipation, muscle pain, lingering infections, nasosinusitis, and chronic fatigue. A blood test through US BioTek Laboratories reveals elevated antibody levels specific to egg. After two months of avoiding eggs, and following the dietary guidelines from the laboratory, he reports considerable improvement and relief from his symptoms.

The human body is a wonderful and complete organism unto itself; however, it is intricately interrelated to the environment in which it lives. Many of the cues we receive from our environment shape our susceptibilities and allergic burden as well as our capability to deal with these stressors. The body adapts to a certain extent in order to maximize its state of well-being or health. However, with such great changes occurring in today's world, the body has become more and more bogged down and thus unable to fully adapt to the new environment. Because of this new challenge, it becomes increasingly important to take the steps necessary to remove the stressors that so strongly affect our health and well-being in order to more fully adapt to the changing environment in which we now live.

NOTES

1. Croner S. Prediction and detection of allergy development: influence of genetic and environmental factors. *J Pediatr*. 1992;121(5 Pt 2):S58–S63.

2. Berge A. Th1 and Th2 responses: what are they? *Br Med J*. 2000;32:424. 321 (7258): 424.

3. Doan T, Melvold R, Waltenbaugh C, Viselli S. *Immunology* (Lippincott's Illustrated Reviews Series). Philadelphia: Lippincott Williams & Wilkins; 2007.

4. Ghaffar A. Seventeen hypersensitivity reactions. Available at: http://pathmicro. med.sc.edu/ghaffar/hyper00.htm. Accessed October 20, 2008.

5. Cade R, et al. Autism and schizophrenia: Intestinal disorders. *Nutritional Neuroscience*, March 2000. Available at: http://www.feingold.org/Research/cade.html. Accessed April 10, 2009.

6. Dreskin S. Genetics of food allergy. *Curr Allergy Asthma Rep*. 2006;6:58–64.

7. Galli SJ. Allergy. *Curr Biol*. 2000;10(3):R93–R5.

8. Gleeson M. Exercise, nutrition and immune function. *J Sports Sci*. 2004; 22:115–125.

9. Collins SM. Stress and the gastrointestinal tract. IV. Modulation of intestinal inflammation by stress: basic mechanisms and clinical relevance. *Am J Physiol*. 2001;280:G315–G318.

10. Yang PC, Jury J, Soderholm JD, Sherman PM, McKay DM, Perdue MH. Chronic psychological stress in rats induces intestinal sensitization to luminal antigens. *Am J Pathol*. 2005;168:104–114.

11. Strachan DP. Family size, infection and atopy: the first decade of the "hygiene hypothesis." *Thorax*. 2000;55(suppl 1):S2–S10.

12. Guarner F, Bourdet-Sicard R, Brandtzaeg P, et al. Mechanisms of disease: the hygiene hypothesis revisited. *Natl Clin Pract Gastroenterol Hepatol*. 2006;3:275–284.

13. Smith JM. Genetically Engineered Foods May Cause Rising Food Allergies. Part 2: Genetically Engineered Corn. Available at: AmericanwellnessRadio.com. Accessed October 20, 2008.

CHAPTER 2

The Gut and Immune System: Allergic Burden Handling

The immune system is responsible for protecting the body. However, immune system dysregulation may lead to overstimulation and immune responses to generally nonharmful agents such as foods and pollens. It also important to understand that the immune and gastrointestinal systems are interconnected and that the health of both systems is necessary to combat allergies.

THE IMMUNE SYSTEM

Having a basic knowledge of the immune system and how it functions is vital for understanding allergies. The primary function of the immune system is to protect the body from foreign agents such as bacteria, viruses, parasites, and other pathogens. The immune system has two main components: innate and acquired immunity.

Innate immunity is a nonspecific immune response that is present at birth. It includes such barriers as skin and mucous membranes, fever, stomach acid, and chemical mediators that induce inflammation and activate the acquired immune response. The white blood cells (leukocytes) of the innate response function to identify and eliminate pathogens. These leukocytes include natural killer cells, mast cells, eosinophils, basophils, neutrophils, macrophages, and dendritic cells. Macrophages, neutrophils, and dendritic cells function by engulfing and destroying pathogens, particles, or cellular debris, a process known as phagocytosis. Basophils, neutrophils, and eosinophils are specialized white blood cells known as granulocytes or polymorphonuclear leukocytes; they contain enzymes, proteins, and chemicals that kill and digest pathogens and cellular debris.

The acquired immune response is highly specialized and functions to recognize and remember specific pathogens. This allows for faster and stronger immune responses each time a particular pathogen is encountered. The acquired immune response has specialized cells that respond to antigens. An antigen is any substance, usually a protein or polysaccharide (sugar), that causes your immune system to produce antibodies to it or elicit an immune response. An antigen may be a foreign substance from the environment such as bacteria, viruses, other microorganisms, or pollen. Harmless antigens include food proteins, pollens, and resident intestinal microflora. There are two major types of acquired immunity responses; humoral and cell-mediated.

Humoral responses are mediated by antibodies, also known as immunoglobulins (Igs), which are proteins made by B lymphocytes (white blood cells that mature in the bone marrow), and are used by the immune system to identify and neutralize foreign agents, such as bacteria and viruses. Each antibody has an area called the hypervariable region, which allows it to identify and bind to a specific antigen. Humans produce an estimated 10 billion different antibodies, each capable of binding a distinct epitope, the unique area on an antigen recognized by the antibodies.[1] There are five main types of immunoglobulins: IgA, IgD, IgE, IgM, and IgG. IgA is primarily found on mucous membranes, but it is also found in saliva, tears, and breast milk. IgG is the most abundant antibody, and IgG, IgM, and IgA respond primarily to bacteria, viruses, and toxins. IgE is involved with parasitic infections and immediate-type hypersensitivity reactions, such as anaphylaxis. Although the immune system is designed to respond to specific antigens, it will often respond to agents with similar structure. This is known as cross-reactivity. Many foods and pollens have structurally similar epitopes, causing cross-reactive immune responses.

The cell-mediated immune response involves white blood cells that mature in the thymus called T lymphocytes (T cells). The T cells recognize infectious agents that have entered cells of the body, unlike B cells and antibodies that interact with agents in the circulation. T cells are processed in the thymus to recognize and interact with a specific antigen. When an antigen binds a receptor on a lymphocyte, the cell is activated and releases chemical messengers known as lymphokines or cytokines. The release of these chemical messengers induces activity by other white blood cells, causing inflammation, and cytotoxic and regulatory activity. T cells are also involved with delayed-type hypersensitivity inflammatory reactions. There are several types of T cells. The main groups include the following:

- *Helper T cells* (also known as T helper cells, Th cells or T4 cells) direct the immune response. They secrete cytokines that stimulate B and cytotoxic T cells. Helper T cells become activated by interacting with antigen-presenting cells.
- *Killer T cells* (also known as cytotoxic T cells, Tc cells, or T8 cells) directly kill cells that pose a threat, such as cells containing a pathogen or cancerous cells.
- *Memory T cells* (T8 cell) are long-living cells programmed to recognize and respond to a pathogen once it has invaded.
- *Suppressor T cells* inhibit the production of cytotoxic T cellsonce they are no longer necessary.

T cells have receptors on their surface that interact with antigens as well as molecules on their surface that interact with the cells that present antigens, known as antigen presenting cells, to the T cells. CD4 and CD8 are two of these molecules. They bind with the major histocompatability complex (MHC) molecules on antigen presenting cells. Once a T helper cell recognizes an antigen, lymphocytes migrate to lymphoid tissues, such as Peyer's patches, and divide into memory cells and killer T cells.

T helper cells are generally categorized as Th1 or Th2, depending on the types of chemical mediators they secrete. Th1 cells secrete the cytokines interleukin (IL)-2, interferon-gamma, and tumor necrosis factor-beta. Th2 cells secrete IL-4, IL-5, IL-6, IL-9, IL-10, and IL-13. The Th1 cells function to stimulate cytotoxic T cells and macrophages; thus, they predominate in viral and bacterial infections. Th2 cells stimulate the production of antibodies by B cells and predominate in allergic and parasitic infections. Interestingly, Th1 cells secrete cytokines that inhibits the synthesis of Th2 cells, and vice versa. Therefore, some disease states can actually suppress activity of the immune response against other pathogens. Excessive Th2 activity can lead to atopy. Some scientists believe the increase in allergic and autoimmune diseases is attributable to the "hygiene hypothesis," which suggests that the eradication of many infectious diseases had led to an immunological imbalance in the intestine and a predominately Th2 state.[2] Inflammation is also part of the immune response. Inflammation includes vasodilation of local blood vessels, increased permeability of capillaries, migration of monocytes and granulocytes, and localized swelling. These reactions are often initiated by the chemical mediators released from white blood cells, including histamine, prostaglandins, and leukotrienes. Clotting also occurs in the surrounding tissue, which acts to wall off the injured area and decrease the spread of the microorganisms or toxins. Macrophages will also migrate to the area of injury and cause localized tissue damage. In addition, neutrophils and monocytes move to the inflamed area to directly attack any microorganisms, and the production of circulating granulocytes and monocytes from the bone marrow increases.

THE GASTROINTESTINAL AND IMMUNE SYSTEM CONNECTION

When addressing allergies, it is imperative to understand the connection between the immune system and the gastrointestinal system. The gastrointestinal system plays a central role in immune system homeostasis, or the state of equilibrium. The mucosa is the tissue that lines the hollow organs of the digestive tract. Scattered along mucosal linings is lymphoid (immune) tissue known as mucosa-associated lymphoid tissue (MALT). A major part of MALT, and of the entire immune system, is gut-associated lymphoid tissue (GALT). In fact, 70 percent of the immune system is located in the gut. The immune system of the intestine has the task of discriminating between pathogens and harmless antigens and responding accordingly. The development of normal immune function of the intestine is vital for survival. One of the main functions of GALT is to decipher whether an antigen requires an immune response. When GALT receives a signal from a food antigen, for example, it induces a state of nonresponsiveness, known as tolerance. However, when pathogenic bacteria invade the intestinal mucosa, it is necessary to elicit a strong immune response. Thus, GALT has the immensely important role of determining which type of response to generate in each case, which is key to preventing immune dysregulation and tissue damage. GALT is located throughout the gastrointestinal tract. It includes the tonsils, adenoids, Peyer's patches, and lymphoid tissue in the appendix, large intestine, and esophagus; it is also diffusely distributed throughout the lamina propria, which is part of the mucosal lining of the gut. Peyer's patches are large, complex aggregates of lymphoid tissue in the small intestines. They contain epithelial cells known as M cells, named for microfolds in their surface. These cells play an important role in the transfer of antigens from the gut lumen to the Peyer's patch. M cells are believed to function as an antigen sampling system with rapid uptake and presentation of antigens and microorganisms to the immune cells of the lymphoid tissues to induce an appropriate immune response. The Peyer's patches then facilitate an immune response within the mucosa. GALT also has distinct B-cell follicles and T-cell areas, as well as antigen presenting accessory cells. Moreover, about 80 percent of plasma cells, mainly immunoglobulin A (IgA)-bearing cells, reside in GALT. The number of eosinophils (a white blood cell that plays an important role in allergies) is also substantially higher in the gastrointestinal tract than in other tissues. During healthy conditions, most of the eosinophils reside in the lamina propria in the stomach and intestine. However, during a Th2-associated inflammatory response, such as with allergies, there is a notable increase in eosinophils in the lamina propria as well as in the Peyer's patches.[3] GALT also plays a role in increasing intestinal permeability.[4]

The Intestinal Barrier

The gastrointestinal system functions as a semipermeable barrier. This means that it actively selects which molecules can pass through into the bloodstream, and which stay in the intestines. The digestive system has the enormous task of breaking down food into usable nutrients, selectively absorbing these molecules, and removing waste products. In addition, it has to do this without provoking an immune response to all harmless antigens, such as dietary proteins and beneficial colonic bacteria, while simultaneously maintaining an immune defense against pathogenic microorganisms. Gastric acid and digestive enzymes, such as amylase, lipase, proteases, bile, and pepsin secreted from the mouth, stomach, pancreas, or liver, aid in the breakdown of food into smaller, absorbable molecules. Trypsin is a particularly important digestive enzyme in regards to allergic sensitization. It is a protease, meaning it breaks down proteins. Proteins are cleaved into smaller units, called peptides, and then further into amino acids. This is necessary for normal absorption. However, if the proteins are not broken down completely, they may pass through a faulty intestinal barrier and trigger an immune response, as the immune system responds to proteins, not amino acids.

Most nutrients are absorbed in the small intestines. However, the overall health of the intestines affects nutrient absorption. Infection or inflammation can compromise the semipermeable barrier, thus allowing molecules usually too large to pass through the intestinal wall to pass into the bloodstream. Additionally, pathogenic microbes may also pass through the barrier. The immune system does not recognize these larger molecules and responds to them as foreign antigens, which can lead to numerous symptoms, ranging from local digestive complaints to systemic reactions, such as headaches or inflammation. The increase in intestinal permeability is also associated with numerous diseases, such as food allergies, irritable bowel syndrome (IBS), ulcerative colitis, Crohn's disease, chronic fatigue syndrome, psoriasis, autoimmune disease, arthritis, and heart disease. The M cells found in the intestinal mucosa play a direct role in intestinal barrier function. M cells increase in number and in programmed cell death (apoptosis) during chronic intestinal inflammatory states. These changes in M cells appear to be responsible for the increase of the uptake of microorganisms that is observed during intestinal inflammatory conditions; thus, M cells affect the breakdown in the intestinal epithelial barrier with inflammation.[5]

Increased intestinal permeability can be induced by numerous causes. Intestinal infections, inflammation, trauma, abnormal microflora, parasites, medications, poor diet, psychological stress,[6] and low levels of hydrochloric acid and digestive enzymes may affect the integrity of the barrier. Maintaining proper intestinal microflora is important to maintaining the barrier. There are more than 400 strains of bacteria found in the intestines. Probiotics are beneficial bacteria, such as *Lactobacillus acidophilus* and *Bifidobacterium bifidum*, that compete with pathogenic bacteria and yeast for space and resources, aid in the absorption of food, and help maintain intestinal integrity; some strains produce vitamins. Medications such as antibiotics, steroids, and chemotherapy can decrease the amount of beneficial bacteria. Also, digestive disorders such as constipation or diarrhea or a poor diet may also inhibit the microflora, thus leading to an increase in intestinal permeability. Parasites, such as *Giardia* spp, *Cryptosporidium*, *Entamoeba histolytica*, and *Blastocystis hominis* cause inflammation and may also increase intestinal permeability. Additionally, decreased levels of hydrochloric acid or digestive enzymes lead to improper breakdown of food and increased risk of infection. Hydrochloric acid is very strong and kills many of the microorganisms present in the ingested food; however, low levels of this acid may allow pathogens to enter the intestines. Gastric acid also activates the digestive enzymes in the stomach, without which ingested food would not be broken down completely. Incomplete breakdown of food can combine with increased intestinal permeability resulting in large molecules that can lead to immune system activation passing through the intestinal barrier.

Researchers have demonstrated that patients with food allergies or food hypersensitivities who were on allergen-free diets were found to have statistically significant differences in intestinal permeability compared with control patients. In fact, the researchers showed that the worse the intestinal permeability, the more serious the clinical symptoms in patients with food allergy and hypersensitivity. This study also showed that impaired intestinal permeability function was present in all subjects studied with adverse food reactions.[7] Other researchers suggest that intestinal permeability is so predictable that testing for intestinal permeability is a reliable test for diagnosing food allergies among children.[8]

Secretory Immunoglobulin A

Secretory immunoglobulin A (sIgA) also plays an important role in providing a protective barrier in the intestines and is the main immunoglobulin found in mucous secretions, such as tears, saliva, colostrum, intestinal fluids, vaginal fluids, and secretions from the prostate and the respiratory tract. In these fluids, sIgA provides protection against microorganisms along the moist surfaces of the body that have contact with the external environment. In the digestive tract, sIgA depends on the function of the M cells. An antigen is taken up by the M cells, transported to dendritic cells, and then transported to antigen-specific precursors for IgA-secreting plasma cells. This results in activation of a strong sIgA response and suppression of a systemic IgG, IgE, and delayed-type hypersensitivity reaction to the antigen.[9] Also, sIgA induces eosinophils and neutrophils, the white blood cells important in the allergic response, more strongly then the serum IgA counterpart, which suggests that sIgA plays a role in allergic inflammation in the intestines.[10]

Oral Tolerance

Oral tolerance, a control mechanism of immense immunological importance, refers to the suppression of the immune response to an antigen acquired from the oral route. Tolerance to antigens results from the lack of a T-lymphocyte response.[11] Developing oral tolerance is crucial so the body does not react to harmless antigens such as food proteins and resident intestinal microflora. In general, only a small percentage of people experience adverse immunological reactions to food as a result of the induction of oral tolerance. However, when there is a dysfunction in the process of oral tolerance, food hypersensitivity, autoimmune diseases, and mucosal inflammation can develop.[12] Common autoimmune diseases include multiple sclerosis, rheumatoid arthritis, systemic lupus erythematosus, scleroderma and vitiligo. In addition, other conditions, such as inflammatory bowel diseases, are associated with failure of oral tolerance. Some researchers believe the development of the immune system in infancy plays a role in the development of oral tolerance. During this time, there is an expansion of GALT as well as changes in the presence of colonic bacteria, which some researchers believe causes the increase in IgE-mediated and non–IgE-mediated food allergy seen during this period.[13] Other researchers propose that the increased incidence of allergic and inflammatory diseases may be attributable to an increase in formula-feeding versus breast-feeding.[14] Overall gastrointestinal health is also an important factor in the development of oral tolerance.[15]

Additional Immune Reactions to Foods

The immune system can respond to foods without the typical interaction with antibodies and antigens that is seen with food allergies. The immune system responds to lectins and some proteins with a non–antibody-mediated response. Lectins are protein molecules that bind to carbohydrates (sugars) present on the surface of cells, and they function in cell recognition and signaling. This reaction causes the molecules to stick together in agglutination reactions. Lectins are found in many foods, but are particularly high in seeds and tubers like cereals, potatoes, and beans. They are not degraded by stomach acid or digestive enzymes, which makes them virtually resistant to breakdown in the digestive process. Lectins are also found in the body as well as on some microorganisms. Lectins, present in much of our food, can cause toxic or inflammatory reactions by binding to carbohydrates on the surfaces of cells in the body.[16] Genetics influence which dietary lectins will cause symptoms, although some lectins are toxic and can cause severe reactions if ingested regardless of one's genetic makeup. In the intestinal tract, lectins can affect the turnover and loss of gut epithelial cells, damage the epithelial lining, interfere with nutrient digestion and absorption, stimulate changes in the colonic bacterial flora, and modulate the immune state of the digestive tract. When lectins are absorbed, they may disrupt lipid, carbohydrate, and protein metabolism, affect distant internal organs and tissues, and modulate hormones and immunological functions.[17] Lectins that do not bind to the intestinal mucosa do not generally have harmful effects. In addition, lectins can act as metabolic signals, altering the state of glycosylation (sugar residues) on the gut epithelium, which may further amplify their physiological activity.[18]

Dietary lectins bind to the microvilli, the fingerlike projections that increase surface area for absorption of nutrients in the small intestines. Interestingly, lectins can pass through the intestinal barrier and deposit themselves in other organs.[19] Lectins are believed to play a role in numerous diseases, such as intestinal disorders and autoimmune diseases. Commonly, grain/cereal lectins, dairy lectins, and legume lectins, such as peanut and soybean, are reported to cause increased inflammatory responses. Research also suggests that dietary lectins interact with intestinal microflora and that an imbalance in healthy gut bacteria may lead to intestinal injury and autoimmune disease. For example, rheumatoid arthritis is a relatively common autoimmune condition. Researchers suggest that dietary lectins interact with the enterocytes and lymphocytes that facilitate the translocation of dietary and gut-derived pathogenic antigens to peripheral tissues. This causes persistent peripheral antigenic stimulation and, in genetically susceptible persons, leads to a cross-reaction with endogenous "self" proteins.[20]

Celiac Disease: A Special Case

Celiac disease, also known as nontropical sprue or gluten-sensitive enteropathy, is a digestive condition caused by an autoimmune reaction, which is unlike typical food allergies. Patients with celiac disease react to the gliadin portion of the protein gluten, which is found in wheat and all of its varieties, rye, barley, triticale, and oats (if processed with gluten containing grains). Gluten is also added to numerous other food products, cosmetics, supplements, and medicines. Celiac disease is caused by an immune reaction to gliadin, which causes white blood cells to accumulate in the lining of the intestines, which in turn, damages the villi and microvilli in the intestines. This causes severe malabsorption of nutrients. More specifically, plasma cells produce IgA and IgG antibodies against several antigens, such as transglutaminase, endomysium (a connective tissue sheath that surrounds muscle fibers), gliadin, and reticulin. Chemical messengers are released, which leads to a local inflammatory response, and then causes the damage to the villi and microvilli. It is suggested that gliadin binds with the cellular enzyme transglutaminase in the enterocytes when ingested. The transglutaminase enzyme then modifies the gliadin, which increases the immunogenicity by making it appear foreign and not recognized by the immune response. Researchers have also shown that antigliadin antibodies cross-react with molecules on the enterocytes such as calreticulin. The reactivity of the antigliadin antibodies has been shown to be significantly higher with human enterocytes and human calreticulin than with other antigens tested.[21] Currently, blood tests to measure anti-tissue transglutaminase antibodies, anti-endomysium antibodies, and antigliadin antibodies are used in the diagnosis of celiac disease. In addition, researchers suggest that lectins such as the mannose-binding lectin also play a role in the pathophysiology of celiac disease.[22]

Persons with celiac disease may have a variety of symptoms, including chronic diarrhea, constipation, bloating, abdominal pain, vomiting, fatty stools, weight loss, fatigue, arthritis, unexplained iron-deficiency anemia, osteoporosis or bone loss, infertility, irregular menstrual cycles, skin rash, mouth sores, depression, or anxiety. Symptoms and associated conditions vary from patient to patient, likely because of variations in the extent of intestinal damage, age of onset, and exposure to gluten before diagnosis. In addition, persons with celiac disease are at increased risk for autoimmune diseases such as type 1 diabetes, rheumatoid arthritis, Sjögren's syndrome, and autoimmune thyroid or liver diseases. Many of the associated conditions are believed to be caused by long-term malnutrition. However, increased serum antigliadin IgA has been demonstrated in such other conditions as Crohn's disease, ulcerative colitis, rheumatoid arthritis, Bergers' disease, and Sjögren's syndrome, which may reflect an underlying commonality, whether cause or effect, to these conditions. Celiac disease runs in families, thus showing a genetic component. It is estimated that 1 in 133 people in the U.S. general population have celiac disease, and the prevalence is as high as 1 in 22 people who have a first-degree relative with the condition, and 1 in 39 if a second-degree relative has the disease.[23] In addition, based on the fact that newborn infant have increased intestinal permeability in order to absorb complete immune proteins from breast milk, researchers have investigated early introduction of gluten as a risk factor for celiac disease. Studies have shown that infants given gluten-containing foods such as wheat, barley, or rye during the first three months of life have had a fivefold increased risk of celiac disease autoimmunity compared with children exposed to gluten-containing foods at the age of four to six months.[24]

Probiotics, Immune Function, and Allergies

Numerous strains of bacteria reside in the intestines and are important for optimal intestinal health. Particular strains, such as *Lactobacillus* and *Bifidobacterium*, have been well-studied and have been shown to provide several health benefits. Most importantly, probiotics can improve the integrity of the intestinal barrier. They can also compete with and suppress the growth of pathogenic bacteria, modulate or stimulate the immune response,[25] and aid in nutrient and enzyme synthesis and absorption. Levels of beneficial bacteria can be adversely affected by several factors, such as drinking chlorinated water, consuming a low-fiber diet, or using antibiotics or other medications. Any imbalance of the intestinal microflora can result in immune system dysfunctions such as allergies or inflammation.

Studies have shown that immune regulation in the intestinal mucosa–associated lymphoid tissue plays an important role in allergic sensitization and is influenced by the intestinal microflora. Probiotics may provide maturational signals for the gut-associated lymphoid tissue, balance the production of pro- and anti-inflammatory cytokines, reduce the dietary antigen load by degrading and modifying large molecules, normalize the gut microecology, and reverse increased intestinal permeability. In children with allergies, probiotics have been shown to not only decrease intestinal permeability but also enhance the deficient IgA responses.[26] Probiotics are also important in the development of the intestinal immune response in infancy. Evidence suggests that the gut must first be exposed to colonizing bacteria before the development of a protective immune response. Colonization with diverse intestinal flora is necessary for the development of important gut defenses such as the synthesis and secretion of sIgA to protect the intestinal surface and the generation of a balanced T helper cell response to prevent chronic inflammation by induction of oral tolerance to resident bacteria and food proteins.

Lactobacillus and *Bifidobacteria* are both gram-positive colonic bacteria that produce lactic acid. Various species are found in the gut, including *Lactobacillus acidophilus*, *Lactobacillus rhamnosus*, *Lactobacillus reuteri*, *Lactobacillus sporogenes*, *Lactobacillus fermentum*, *Bifidobacterium bifidum*, *Bifidobacterium breve*, *Bifidobacterium longum*, and *Bifidobacterium infantis*. These bacteria bind to the mucosal lining in the intestines where they suppress pathogenic bacteria by producing lactic acid and hydrogen peroxide, increase epithelial mucous production, and compete for mucosal binding sites.[27] They also support the intestinal barrier and suppress bacterial translocation through the intestinal lining and into the circulation.[28] *Bifidobacterium* also produce antimicrobial substances that are active against many pathogenic organisms.

Prebiotics are dietary fibers that pass through the small intestines undigested and are fermented in the colon by the resident microflora where they selectively promote the growth and activity of beneficial bacteria.[29] Prebiotics provide beneficial effects, such as increased fecal mass, decreased pH, production of short-chain fatty acids (SCFAs), and decreased intestinal inflammation.[30] There is increasing evidence that prebiotics can modulate various properties of the immune system, including those of the GALT. Researchers suggest that the changes in the intestinal microflora that occur with the consumption of prebiotics may mediate immune changes because of the direct contact of lactic acid bacteria or bacterial products with immune cells in the intestine, the production of SCFAs, or changes in mucin production.[31]

Beneficial Health Effects of Probiotics

Numerous studies demonstrate the positive health effects of probiotics. Probiotics have been shown to benefit many conditions, including allergies, infections, inflammatory conditions, and gastrointestinal disorders, likely because of its ability to modulate the immune and inflammatory processes. Interestingly, researchers have shown that *Lactobacillus* stimulates the immune system in healthy people while suppressing the immune response in hypersensitive people with overactive immune responses.[32]

Various studies support the use of probiotics in allergies and atopic conditions, including food allergies, allergic rhinitis, and atopic eczema.[33] In fact, both *Lactobacillus* and *Bifidobacterium* affect the sensitization to dietary antigens in infants and have been shown to significantly decrease the extent and severity of atopic eczema in these patients. Decreased levels of lactic-acid producing intestinal microflora in children, such as *Lactobacillus* and *Bifidobacterium*, increase the incidence of allergies and atopy. Researchers have shown that *Lactobacillus* can decrease levels of IgE and IgG1 antibodies as well as decrease systemic anaphylactic food allergy reactions in animal models.[34]

Autoimmune diseases demonstrate immune dysfunctions similar to those of allergic disorders, and *Lactobacillus* supplementation has been shown to protect against rheumatoid arthritis progression and reduce swelling, cartilage destruction, and proinflammatory mediators using animal models.[35] Probiotics apparently modulate the immune response other than the allergic cascade, as studies also show that supplementation with *Lactobacillus* decreases the number and severity of respiratory infections and absenteeism is children that attend day care,[36] as well as decrease cell proliferation and other cancer markers in patients with colon cancer while stimulating the immune response.[37] Probiotic supplementation also benefits several digestive disorders such as diarrhea, chronic inflammatory bowel diseases, IBS, and pouchitis (inflammation of the pouch surgically created for the management of ulcerative colitis).[38] For example, one study showed that *Lactobacillus* and *Bifidobacterium* supplementation in the treatment of IBS had an efficacy rate of 56.8 percent by the second week of treatment and 74.3 percent during the fourth week.[39] Another study demonstrated that probiotic and prebiotic supplementation decreased nausea, indigestion, flatulence and marginal colitis in patients with IBS after two weeks of treatment. After 52 weeks of treatment, the rate of IBS remissions was 81.5 to 100 percent.[40]

Eczema and Probiotics

Eczema, or atopic dermatitis, is an allergic skin condition that is most common in infants, although it can affect individuals of any age. Ninety percent of cases occur before the age of 5, versus six percent of cases in 6- to 10-year-olds and two percent of cases those older than 10 years. Overall, it is estimated that 20 percent of children and one to two percent of adults have eczema. Eczema presents as a dry, flaky, red rash that may itch or burn. The rash typically occurs on the face, neck, and the insides of the elbows, knees, and ankles in adults. In infants, eczema typically occurs on the forehead, cheeks, forearms, legs, scalp, and neck. Any number of allergens can cause eczema. Interestingly, 40 percent of children with atopic dermatitis have food allergies.[41] Although eczema is a skin condition, evidence supports the role of abnormal intestinal function and intestinal commensal bacteria in the development of this condition. It is proposed that supplementation with probiotics provides a microbial challenge for the maturation of the gut-associated lymphoid tissue, normalizes the increased intestinal permeability, reestablishes beneficial gut microorganisms, improves the immunological defense barrier (IgA) of the intestines, decreases intestinal inflammation, and down-regulates the proinflammatory cytokines seen with allergic inflammation. In a double-blind placebo-controlled crossover study, *Lactobacillus* probiotics were given for six weeks to 1- to 13-year-old children with eczema. Eczema symptoms improved in 56 percent of the patients. In addition, the response to treatment was more pronounced in patients with allergies who had at least one positive skin-prick test response and elevated IgE levels.[42] In another study, very young children with eczema were supplemented with probiotics for eight weeks to evaluate the efficacy of probiotics as a therapeutic agent. Probiotic supplementation increased the levels of Th1 cytokines directly proportional to the decrease in the severity of the atopic dermatitis. Additionally, after eight weeks, cytokines in response to allergens such as egg ovalbumin were significantly reduced in children receiving probiotics.[43] Additional research has shown that a *Lactobacillus* and *Bifidobacterium* probiotic supplement in children with atopic dermatitis is effective in improving symptoms, particularly in the children with food allergies.[44]

CONCLUSION

It is imperative to remember that the gastrointestinal tract is the interface between the well-ordered approximately 75 trillion cells that make up your body and the chaotic, less-ordered world that surrounds each person. It is absolutely essential to ensure gastrointestinal integrity to minimize excess immune challenge and burden.

The immune system functions to protect the body from foreign agents. However, immune system dysfunction can lead to overstimulation and immune responses to harmless antigens such as food and pollen. The gastrointestinal system plays an important role in healthy immune function. At the level of the intestinal mucosa, the gastrointestinal and immune systems have the enormous task of presenting antigens and coordinating proper responses, whether inducing oral tolerance or stimulating the immune responses to a pathogen or other foreign agent. To make this relationship even more complex, some food reactions are mediated by lectins or autoimmune responses. Intestinal health, including proper levels of beneficial microflora, is critical to optimal immune system function, and thus, decrease the allergic response.

NOTES

1. Fanning LJ, Connor AM, Wu GE. Development of the immunoglobulin repertoire. *Clin Immunol Immunopathol*. 1996;79(1):1–14.

2. Shi HN, Walker A. Bacterial colonization and the development of intestinal defences. *Can J Gastroenterol*. 2004;18:493–500.

3. Rothenberg ME, Mishra A, Brandt EB, et al. Gastrointestinal eosinophils. *Immunol Rev*. 2001;179:139–155.

4. Vighi G, Marcucci F, Sensi L, et al. Allergy and the gastrointestinal system. *Clin Exp Immunol*. 2008;153(suppl 1):3–6.

5. Kucharzik T, Lügering N, Rautenberg K, et al. Role of M cells in intestinal barrier function. *Ann N Y Acad Sci*. 2000;915:171–183.

6. Zareie M, Johnson-Henry K, Jury J, et al. Probiotics prevent bacterial translocation and improve intestinal barrier function in rats following chronic psychological stress. *Gut*. 2006;55:1553–1560.

7. Ventura MT, Polimeno L, Amoruso AC, et al. Intestinal permeability in patients with adverse reactions to food. *Dig Liver Dis*. 2006;38:732–736.

8. Laudat A, Arnaud P, Napoly A, et al. The intestinal permeability test applied to the diagnosis of food allergy in paediatrics. *West Indian Med J*. 1994;43(3):87–88.

9. Keren DF. Antigen processing in the mucosal immune system. *Semin Immunol*. 1992;4(4):217–226.

10. Motegi Y, Kita H, Kato M, et al. Role of secretory IgA, secretory component, and eosinophils in mucosal inflammation. *Int Arch Allergy Immunol*. 2000;122:25–27.

11. Grethlein S, Perez JA. Mucosa-associated lymphoid tissue. Available at: http://www.emedicine.com/med/topic3204.htm. Accessed December 2, 2008.

12. Shanahan F. Nutrient tasting and signaling mechanisms in the gut V. Mechanisms of immunologic sensation of intestinal contents. *Am J Physiol Gastrointest Liver Physiol*. 2000;278:G191–G196.

13. Jyonouchi H. Non-IgE mediated food allergy. *Inflamm Allergy Drug Targets*. 2008;7(3):173–180.

14. Kelly D, Coutts AG. Early nutrition and the development of immune function in the neonate. *Proc Nutr Soc*. 2000;59(2).177–185.

15. Bjorksten B. Effects of intestinal microflora and the environment on the development of asthma and allergy. *Springer Semin Immunopathol*. 2004;25(3–4):257–270.

16. Van Damme EJM, Peumans WJ, Pusztai A, et al. *Handbook of Plant Lectins: Properties and Biomedical Applications*. London: Wiley; 1998:31–50.

17. Vasconcelos IM, Oliveira JT. Antinutritional properties of plant lectins. *Toxicon*. 2004;44:385–403.

18. Pusztai A. Characteristics and consequences of interactions of lectins with the intestinal mucosa. *Arch Latinoam Nutr*. 1996;44(4 suppl 1):10S–15S.

19. Pusztai A, Greer F, Grant G. Specific uptake of dietary lectins into the systemic circulation of rats. *Biochem Soc Trans*. 1989;17:481–482; Wang Q, Yu L-G, Campbell BJ, et al. Identification of intact peanut lectinin peripheral venous blood. *Lancet*. 1998; 352:1831–1832.

20. Cordain L, Toohey L, Smith MJ, et al. Modulation of immune function by dietary lectins in rheumatoid arthritis. *Br J Nutr.* 2000;83:207–217.

21. Tucková L, Karská K, Walters JR, et al. Anti-gliadin antibodies in patients with celiac disease cross-react with enterocytes and human calreticulin. *Clin Immunol Immunopathol.* 1997;85:289–296.

22. Boniotto M, Braida L, Spanò A, et al. Variant mannose-binding lectin alleles are associated with celiac disease. *Immunogenetics.* 2002;54:596–598.

23. Fasano A, Berti I, Gerarduzzi T, et al. Prevalence of celiac disease in at-risk and not-at-risk groups in the United States. *Arch Intern Med.* 2003;163:268–292.

24. Norris JM, Barriga K, Hoffenberg EJ, et al. Risk of celiac disease autoimmunity and timing of gluten introduction in the diet of infants at increased risk of disease. *JAMA.* 2005;293:2343–2351.

25. Fedorak RN, Madsen KL. Probiotics and the management of inflammatory bowel disease. *Inflamm Bowel Dis.* 2004;10:286–299.

26. Laitinen K, Isolauri E. Management of food allergy: vitamins, fatty acids or probiotics? *Eur J Gastroenterol Hepatol.* 2005;17:1305–1311.

27. deRoos NM, Katan MB. Effects of probiotic bacteria on diarrhea, lipid metabolism, and carcinogenesis: a review of papers published between 1988 and 1998. *Am J Clin Nutr.* 2000;71:405–11; Mack DR, Michail S, et al. Probiotics inhibit enteropathogenic E. coli adherence in vitro by inducing intestinal mucin gene expression. *Am J Physiol Gastrointest Liver Physiol.* 1999;276: G941–G950; McGroarty JA. Probiotic use of lactobacilli in the human female urogenital tract. *FEMS Immunol Med Microbiol.* 1993;6:251–264.

28. Madsen KL, Doyle JS, Jewell LD, et al. Lactobacillus species prevents colitis in interleukin 10 gene-deficient mice. *Gastroenterology.* 1999;116:1107–1114.

29. Bouhnik Y, Vahedi K et al. Short-chain fructo-oligosaccharide administration dose-dependently increases fecal bifidobacteria in healthy humans. *J Nutr.* 1999;129:113–116.

30. Lara-Villoslada F, de Haro O, Camuesco D, et al. Short-chain fructooligosaccharides, in spite of being fermented in the upper part of the large intestine, have anti-inflammatory activity in the TNBS model of colitis. *Eur J Nutr.* 2006;45:418–425.

31. Schley PD, Field CJ. The immune-enhancing effects of dietary fibres and prebiotics. *Br J Nutr.* 2002;87(suppl 2):S221–S230.

32. Pelto L, Isolauri E, Lilius EM, et al. Probiotic bacteria down-regulate the milk-induced inflammatory response in milk-hypersensitive subjects but have an immunostimulatory effect in healthy subjects. *Clin Exp Allergy.* 1998;28:1474–1479.

33. Savilahti E, Kuitunen M, Vaarala O. Pre and probiotics in the prevention and treatment of food allergy. *Curr Opin Allergy Clin Immunol.* 2008;8:243–248; Giovannini M, Agostoni C, Riva E, et al. A randomized prospective double blind controlled trial on effects of long-term consumption of fermented milk containing Lactobacillus casei in pre-school children with allergic asthma and/or rhinitis. *Pediatr Res.* 2007;62:215–220; Isolauri E, Arvola T, Sütas Y, et al. Probiotics in the management of atopic eczema. *Clin Exp Allergy.* 2000;30:1604–1610.

34. Shida K, Takahashi R, Iwadate E, et al. Lactobacillus casei strain Shirota suppresses serum immunoglobulin E and immunoglobulin G1 responses and systemic anaphylaxis in a food allergy model. *Clin Exp Allergy.* 2002;32:563–570.

35. So JS, Kwon HK, Lee CG, et al. Lactobacillus casei suppresses experimental arthritis by down-regulating T helper 1 effector functions. *Mol Immunol.* 2008;45:2690–2699.

36. Hatakka K, Savilahti E, Pönkä A, et al. Effect of long term consumption of probiotic milk on infections in children attending day care centres: double blind, randomised trial. *BMJ.* 2001;322:1327.

37. Rafter J, Bennett M, Caderni G, et al. Dietary synbiotics reduce cancer risk factors in polypectomized and colon cancer patients. *Am J Clin Nutr.* 2007;85:488–496.

38. Schultz M, Sartor RB. Probiotics and inflammatory bowel diseases. *Am J Gastroenterol.* 2000;95(1 suppl):S19–S21; Nobaek S, Johansson ML, Molin G, et al. Alteration of intestinal microflora is associated with reduction in abdominal bloating and pain in patients with irritable bowel syndrome. *Am J Gastroenterol.* 2000;95:1231–1238.

39. Fan YJ, Chen SJ, Yu YC, et al. A probiotic treatment containing Lactobacillus, Bifidobacterium and Enterococcus improves IBS symptoms in an open label trial. *J Zhejiang Univ Sci B.* 2006;7:987–991.

40. Bittner AC, Croffut RM, Stranahan MC, et al. Prescript-assist probiotic-prebiotic treatment for irritable bowel syndrome: an open-label, partially controlled, 1-year extension of a previously published controlled clinical trial. *Clin Ther.* 2007;29:1153–1160.

41. Miraglia del Giudice M Jr, De Luca MG, Capristo C. Probiotics and atopic dermatitis. A new strategy in atopic dermatitis. *Dig Liver Dis.* 2002;34(suppl 2):S68–S71.

42. Rosenfeldt V, Benfeldt E, Nielsen SD, et al. Effect of probiotic Lactobacillus strains in children with atopic dermatitis. *J Allergy Clin Immunol.* 2003;111:389–395.

43. Prescott SL, Dunstan JA, Hale J, et al. Clinical effects of probiotics are associated with increased interferon-gamma responses in very young children with atopic dermatitis. *Clin Exp Allergy.* 2005;35:1557–1564.

44. Sistek D, Kelly R, Wickens K, et al. Is the effect of probiotics on atopic dermatitis confined to food sensitized children? *Clin Exp Allergy.* 2006;36:629–633.

CHAPTER 3

Eating Right for Your Body's Unique Chemistry

Allergies and food sensitivities are two greatly debated subjects both in the medical community and the mainstream media. There is more consciousness about how the environment in which we live affects our health—and the environment also includes our foods.

Nowadays, foods are no longer as straightforward as they were even 50 years ago, let alone 100 years ago. All one has to do is look at the ingredient list for a loaf of bread. It used to read: flour, yeast, sugar/honey, and water. Now the list goes on for an entire paragraph, and most of the words are unfamiliar even to the most educated consumer. To find a loaf of bread that actually only has real food for ingredients, you have to look in special stores that carry what is now called "natural foods." Since when have foods not been "natural"? The beginning of the Industrial Revolution marked the end of unprocessed foods. As industry moved in, foods became more processed. People moved in to the city, so food had to be brought in, preserved, and stored in such a way that it would last longer on the shelves. People were no longer getting their food directly from the farm. Food had to be refrigerated and stored. With more people living in the city, farms had to get bigger to feed all the folk in the city. With the enlargement of farm size also came the use of farm machines to till and harvest. Consequently, the earth began to lose its ability to produce. Nutrients were no longer being put back, so fertilizers came into the picture. With crops receiving only partial nutrients, they became less effective at warding off pests, so pesticides became a matter of fact in conventional farming.

Genetic engineering has now made it so that the plants themselves produce pesticides. The U.S. Environmental Protection Agency estimates that in 2000–2001, the world community used more than five *billion* pounds of pesticide, and the United States was responsible for almost 25 percent of that total.[1] Evidence suggests that the effects of pesticides, particularly in children, increase the risk of immune dysfunction and asthma, among other adverse reactions.[2] The disruption these chemicals cause in the human body invariably harms the digestive process. The altered immune function can lead to an abnormal response to foods—or perhaps, it is an appropriate response. If we are eating food that is no longer just food, then it only stands to reason that the body would want to mount an immune response when it encounters so many different foreign substances in the food. When considering food allergies, one must also keep in mind the radical alterations our food sources have undergone in just over 50 years—a drop in the bucket when it comes to our ability to adapt to new environments and situations. Until the recent past, the human body had only food substances to deal with—now we have added other stressors that are ingested throughout the day, every day without end. Perhaps the body's reaction is simply a response to these radical changes, and a radical call to action to remove it from our daily existence.

So where do we stand? The integrity of our foods has largely disappeared from the face of the earth. The variety of foods at our table has shrunk. All this is in addition to the new stressors we currently live in as a matter of course: radiation; electromagnetic, noise, and air pollution; heavy metals, and the list goes on and on. All of these factors add up in such a manner that our bodies now have to multitask 24 hours per day, seven days a week—and even doing that, it is running behind on daily repair and maintenance. Out of the many thousands and thousands of years the human race has been around, it has only been in the past 100 years that the human body has been exposed to this multitude of stressors.

Why is the amount of stress important? Well, when the human body experiences stress, levels of a hormone called cortisol increase in the body. On a short-term basis, cortisol suppresses digestion, inflammation, and the immune system and frees up glucose so that we can escape danger. On a long-term basis, however, this suppression of the immune system and inflammation, leaves the mucous membranes in the body particularly vulnerable to outside influences. The next thing you know, poorly undigested food particles are free to wreak havoc in the blood, where this type of insult should never be found. Once the immune system in the blood mounts a reaction to this food—you have now developed a food allergy.

Once a food allergy has developed, it affects the body in different ways. Everyone is born with strengths and weaknesses. This is what makes us unique. It not only applies to our mental/emotional sphere but also to our physiology. As the saying goes "one man's treasure is another man's poison." This is why you can take any two individuals, feed them the same foods at the same time, cooked the same way—and one will flourish and radiate health, and the other will become ill. With a food allergy, when we continue to provide the allergen on a daily basis, symptoms will begin to develop. Depending on your genetic strengths and vulnerability, you may start with hay fever symptoms, rashes, eczema, and acne. It may show up as headaches, muscular tension, or perhaps irritability and anxiety. The symptoms are as wide and varied as there are people. Most of the time, the longer one is exposed to these foods, the more insidious the symptoms will become. Often, there will be fatigue or aching joints—in short, the body begins to accumulate inflammatory by-products.

Inflammation in the body is like a traffic jam or a bottleneck on the commute to work. Wastes and nutrients do not travel to where they have to go, so certain organs will begin to deteriorate—first in function and then physically—if the inflammation is not addressed. The organs and functions that deteriorate first depend largely on what elements are causing the inflammation and where the body first responds to these elements. Inflammation is generally a protective mechanism in the body. It serves as a red flag or an alarm for the body to pay attention to that particular area of the body. When foreign substances/toxins are in the body, the body makes inflammatory substances to alert the nervous system, the immune system, and the brain that something is wrong. As with smoke alarms, we do want to get rid of the smoke, but we also want to find out what caused the smoke in the first place, put out the fire, and take safety precautions so that a fire is much less likely to occur there. In terms of our health, we want to find out why we have inflammation in the body, we want to remove the inflammation, and most importantly, we want to make lifestyle changes that prevent the inflammation from happening in the first place.

BASIC DIETARY HYGIENE

Before going much further, you can make some important lifestyle choices to decrease inflammation in your body. These simple steps will bring you a bit closer to maintaining good health and moving away from chronic illness.

- Remove refined carbohydrates from daily consumption

  - Refined carbohydrates are digested into glucose and absorbed into the bloodstream quickly, which elevates blood sugar levels quickly. When red blood cells are exposed to high levels of glucose, they become glycated, which is a haphazard process that impairs the functioning of biomolecules via oxidation. Glycation leads to the formation of advanced glycation endproducts (AGEs), which have been implicated in many age-related chronic diseases, such as type 2 diabetes mellitus (beta-cell damage), cardiovascular diseases (the endothelium, fibrinogen, and collagen are damaged), Alzheimer's disease (amyloid proteins are a side products of the reactions progressing to AGEs), cancer (acrylamide and other side products are released), peripheral neuropathy (the myelin is attacked), and other sensory losses, such as deafness (due to demyelination) and blindness (mostly due to microvascular damage in the retina).[3]
  - AGEs are also found in foods, where they have been added as flavor enhancers and colorants to improve appearance.[4] Research has found that these AGEs are highly proinflammatory and are implicated in the initiation of retinal dysfunction, cardiovascular diseases, type 2 diabetes, and many other age-related chronic diseases.

- Some of the most highly exogenous AGEs include doughnuts, barbecued meats, cake, and dark-colored soft drinks,[5] all refined carbohydrates.
- Another recent study found that eating a high-carbohydrate diet increases inflammation and the levels of lipids in the blood.[6]

- Add organic and locally grown (when possible) fruits and vegetables

  - Organic produce is grown without the use of chemical pesticides or fertilizers. The organic agricultural method enriches the soil by the use of crop rotation, natural pest management, and natural fertilizers (such as manure, bone meal). Though organic produce may seem more costly, the consumption of conventionally grown foods has a higher cost when the repercussions of the pesticides and fertilizers are factored in.
  - Research suggests that pesticide exposure affects male reproductive function, resulting in decreased fertilizing ability of the sperm and reduced fertilization rates.[7]
  - In another study, sperm concentration was 43.1 percent higher among men eating organically produced food.[8]
  - A literature review of 41 studies and 1,240 comparisons between organic and conventional vegetables found statistically significant differences in the nutrient content of organic and conventional crops. Organic crops contained significantly more nutrients—such as vitamin C, iron, magnesium, and phosphorus—and significantly less nitrates (a toxic compound) than conventional crops.[9]
  - Once produce is harvested or taken off the vine, its nutritional content begins decreasing. Opting for locally grown organic produce increases the likelihood of the maximum nutritional benefit because the produce has not been on the road or on the shelf as long as produce that has travelled halfway across the world and was picked when it was not quite ripe to maintain freshness.

- Drink plenty of filtered water (half one's body weight in ounces is recommended)

  - The human body is made up of about 75 percent water.
  - *Every* function in the body takes place in water.
  - Water acts as a solvent to move nutrients, hormones, antibodies, and oxygen through the blood and lymph.
  - Water removes wastes from the body.
  - Chronic dehydration can result in increased inflammation, joint pain and lack of energy, as well as decreased resiliency to illness.

- Limit consumption of saturated fats and animal products

  - Animal fats are rich in omega-6 fatty acids, which are easily converted to arachidonic acid, a major proinflammatory fatty acid in the body.

- Arachidonic acid is oxidized into prostaglandins, which produce inflammation in the body.
- Decreasing saturated animal fats will decrease the amount of circulating prostaglandins in the body, thus, reducing inflammation.

- Limit or remove the use of stimulants, such as caffeine, nicotine, and alcohol

  - Research shows that ingesting caffeine-containing products increases inflammatory markers in the body.[10]
  - Alcohol has been also shown to inhibit the body's ability to recuperate from the effects of inflammation. If the body is already in a state of inflammation, adding alcohol ensures continual degeneration of the organs affected by the inflammation.[11]
  - Studies have shown that tobacco use increases low-grade inflammation, atherogenic dyslipidemia, and hypercoagulability.[12]

- Eat in a relaxed, joyful manner

  - The way in which we eat our meals affects the way in which we are able to digest. The digestive function depends on parasympathetic influence. The parasympathetic system is dominant when we are not under stress or under any imminent threat or danger. When we eat in a rush, in the car (making sure other drivers don't run into us) or while watching the evening news, discussing stressful things around the table, we stimulate our sympathetic nervous system. When this occurs, digestive juices dry up, circulation decreases to the digestive organs, and the body does not stimulate intestinal movements.

- Remove food allergies and food sensitivities

  - Of all the different steps to improve the body's state of inflammation, this last step seems to be the most challenging. After all, many diets claim to be the best diet for your health, but which should you choose? Amidst the plethora of available diets and tests, you can make an informed choice about which follow. Ultimately, your bodies will tell you if you've hit the jackpot or not. In the past two decades, different methods to evaluate what food is good for your particular body have gained popularity. Some have been around longer than others and are backed by more research and clinical results. These include the elimination challenge, blood type diet, EAV (electroacupuncture according to Voll) test, radioallergosorbent test (RAST), and enzyme-linked immunosorbent assay (ELISA) IgG and IgE Food Antibody Assessment. All of these tests look at different aspects of health and must be compared based on what they test.

    1. Elimination challenge—the elimination challenge is considered the gold standard to determine adverse reactions to foods. It consists of removing all possible allergenic foods from the diet for six

weeks. After the six weeks, the individual reintroduces the food, waits three days to look for any emerging symptoms. If symptoms arise, then that food is removed indefinitely, if no symptoms arise, that food can become part of the diet once more. A new food is tested every three to five days. This method of testing is reliable and cost-effective; however, it is very limiting in terms of the food a person can eat and it requires a long period of time to resume a more normal diet.

2. RAST—The RAST was introduced in the 1970s. It uses a person's extracted blood to detect the amount of immunoglobulin that reacts specifically with suspected or known allergens. The advantage of this particular test is that the individual does not need to eliminate the use of allergy medicines to have a valid test. This test is also useful when a skin condition makes a skin prick test inconvenient because of the extent of the skin problem. A RAST is often limited to measuring a limited number of foods, and it does not provide the full breadth of clinical findings. Also, keep in mind that, practically speaking, looking at IgE alone is not sufficient to uncover the full array of foods that are burdening the body; IgG Food Antibody Assessment should always be included when seeking the broadest look at potential food triggers.

3. Skin-prick test—Skin-prick testing is easy to do and results are available in minutes. Different allergists may use different devices for skin-prick testing. Some use a "bifurcated needle," which looks like a fork with two prongs. Others use a "multi-test," which may look like a small board with several pins sticking out of it. In these tests, a tiny amount of the suspected allergen is put onto the skin or into a testing device, and the device is placed on the skin to prick, or break through, the top layer of skin. This puts a small amount of the allergen under the skin. A hive will form at any spot where the person is allergic. This test generally yields a positive or negative result. It is good for quickly learning if a person is allergic to a particular food or not, because it detects allergic antibodies known as IgE. Skin tests cannot predict if a reaction will occur or what kind of reaction might occur if a person ingests that particular allergen. They can, however, confirm an allergy in light of a patient's history of reactions to a particular food. Non–IgE-mediated allergies *cannot* be detected by this method.

4. Blood-type diet—The blood-type diet is based on the idea that different blood groups react differently to particular types of food depending on the evolution of human nutrition. According to this theory, four different red blood cell antigens are taken into consideration, including the basic ABO antigens, Rh A1/A2 subgroup, Lewis blood group system, and secretor status. The basic premise of this diet is that O blood type is the oldest blood type, when our

ancestors' diet consisted of mainly meat and vegetables; therefore, modern O blood types should adhere to these food choices to be more in line with ancestral digestive capabilities. Type A and B are thought to be newer blood types that correspond more to an agricultural lifestyle, consisting of more grains and vegetables diet (type A) and a balanced diet for type B blood type consisting of some meat, dairy, vegetables, and grain. Another factor that is looked at in this diet is what is termed as the secretor status of the person. Secretors have a greater secretory immunoglobulin A production by the mucous membranes, which provide greater protection against any infection entering through the respiratory and/or gastrointestional tract. The secretor status concept depends only on genetics based on the Lewis blood groups. Lewis blood groups are either A or B. Group A individuals are found to be nonsecretors, and group B individuals are found to be secretors. It is estimated that about 75 percent of individuals secrete substances in their saliva with ABO antigen specificity. To find out all the different subgroups to determine this blood type requires laboratory testing. The full merits of this dietary approach is based in common sense, as the foods that sustained one's ancestors. At this time there is insufficient scientific studies yet to fully validate this approach. Given that most people are a genetic composite of various cultures, adherence to a traditional ancestral diet can be less precise than needed.

5. EAV test—The EAV test was developed by Dr. Rheinhold Voll in 1953. His methods were later refined by Dr. Helmut Schimmel, which resulted in what is now known as EAV/VEGA testing. This type of test requires no blood sample. It is a bioenergetic system that tests for food sensitivities and quantifies reactions to particular foods that measurably lower an individual's energy. Food sensitivities are mainly related to gastrointestinal health rather than actual allergies. The test is performed by using an instrument that measures skin resistance. The individual being tested holds a negative electrode in one hand, the practitioner tests an acupuncture point corresponding to digestion with the positive electrode on the fingers of the opposite hands. The test begins by using water and benzene as controls. Skin resistance increases between the electrodes when a food sensitivity is placed in the circuit. There have been experiments in controlled experiments that show a high degree of correlation with food-challenge testing, skin-prick testing, RAST, and IgE test results; however, the number of foods tested is more limited than a typical panel of IgG Food Antibody Assessments.

6. ELISA IgG Food Antibody Assessment Panels—Enzyme-linked immunosorbent assay, also called ELISA, enzyme immunoassay or EIA, is a biochemical technique used mainly in immunology to

detect the presence of an antibody or an antigen in a sample. The ELISA has been used as a diagnostic tool in medicine and plant pathology as well as a quality-control check in various industries. In simple terms, in ELISA an unknown amount of antigen is affixed to a surface, and then a specific antibody is washed over the surface so that it can bind to the antigen. This antibody is linked to an enzyme, and in the final step a substance is added that the enzyme can convert to some detectable signal. Thus, in the case of fluorescence ELISA, when light of the appropriate wavelength is shone on the sample, any antigen/antibody complexes will fluoresce so that the amount of antigen in the sample can be inferred through the magnitude of the fluorescence. This test is an accurate and very reliable way to identify IgG and IgE food-antigen-specific antibodies in blood. ELISA is a semiquantitative analysis designed to assess for immediate (IgE) and delayed (IgG) immune reactivity to food antigens. Through this testing method, a multi-well plate is coated with purified, lyophilized (powdered) food proteins at a specific concentration. The patient's blood sample is then added to the plate. If the patient's blood sample contains specific antibodies to any of the food proteins on the plate, a binding reaction will occur. The degree of antibody-antigen binding is dependent on the concentration of antibodies in the individual's blood sample. This reaction is detected through a color change and measured using an optical density reader. The color intensity correlates to the amount of antibody-food antigen binding. Testing for IgG levels rather than IgE levels allows for detection of delayed type sensitivity reactions to foods. In general, high IgG levels are directed against specific foods that are eaten often and have passed through the gastrointestinal barrier and into the blood stream. The difference between IgE and IgE is that IgG antibodies have a circulation half-life of 21 days, and a binding time on mast cells (cells that release inflammatory products) of two to three months, therefore, testing for IgG antibodies will identify foods that have been eaten at least over the last 20 days that have elicited a reaction. IgE tests do not go back that far since IgE antibodies only have a half-life in circulation of about one to two days and only bind with mast cells for a maximum of two weeks. A typical food allergy panel consists of 96 to 100 foods that are tested for individual reactions. The turnaround period is approximately one to two weeks and there is no need to remove any foods from the diet until results are given. Thanks to advances in technology a small pinprick and small sample of blood is necessary to run this test, so it is convenient and mostly painless. This is a primary tool for many holistic practitioners because of cost, efficiency, accuracy, and breadth of testing available.

ELISA IgG Food Antibody Assessment Panel has been successfully and consistently used by many practitioners. This method of testing has proven to be a life-turning event in people's lives as shown in the following case studies.

Case Studies

1. One young man has experienced chronic headaches since the age of 6, at least three or four times a week. He suffers severe stomach pain and vomiting that last up to 12 hours per episode. As a child his headaches were so incapacitating that his mother had to homeschool him. He always feels very tired and has a very rapid pulse. After seeing multiple physicians, being given conventional medications to try, receiving chiropractic treatments, and undergoing neurological workups, there has been no change in his condition. Finally, one physician recommends that he be tested for food allergies. The IgG Food Antibody Assessment Panel shows that he is strongly allergic to three foods and has both IgE and IgG reactions to them. Once he eliminates these foods, the headaches stop completely, the nausea and vomiting occurs only twice the first month and never thereafter. His energy improves and he has no more nosebleeds.

2. A two-year-old child is covered with eczema from head to toe. He has cracks and bleeding on the inside of the elbows and the backside of the knees. He scratches so much that his skin bleeds. The lesions never heal because he scratches day and night. His medication does not help alleviate the itchiness or inflammation of his skin. His parents take him to several doctors and he is treated at a national skin center by dermatologists, but there is no improvement. Finally, one doctor suggests IgG Food Antibody Assessment Panel, which shows a very high reaction to most fish. The parents had been feeding him fish on a daily basis, so they now understood why the eczema never improved. Once fish was removed from his diet, the skin conditioned improved greatly.

3. A 40-year-old woman has been suffering from esophageal reflux and nausea. The nausea is often so bad that it leads to vomiting. She has seen different gastroenterologists, with no results. They cannot diagnose the cause of her condition. Along with esophageal reflux, she tends to suffer from constipation with loose stools, multiple chemical sensitivities, upper respiratory infections, fatigue, anxiety, low libido, and rosacea. Her doctor suggests an IgG Food Antibody Assessment Panel and finds that she has high antibody levels specific to dairy and egg. When she stops consuming these two foods, her reflux and nausea fully resolve within two days. She is also less anxious and no longer has bouts of constipation with loose stools. Her energy level and libido also improve—all

within two days. After a few months of following the new diet, she also notices that her chemical sensitivities and rosacea are also diminished.

These case studies show how simple changes can drastically change someone's health and lifestyle. The medical community at large is beginning to have a greater appreciation for how important the gastrointestinal tract's integrity is to overall health and wellness. Rather than using medication to continually suppress the symptoms caused by these food allergies, simply removing the allergen is enough to restore people to better health. The reason for this is simple. When the allergens are no longer circulating in the bloodstream, the body no longer needs to mount an immune reaction to try and clean up and remove these foreign substances. This drastically lowers the inflammatory state in the body. Any time inflammation decreases in the body, it gives one a sense of better well-being. Energy returns because the body is no longer spending all its resources controlling the inflammation. Other functions that also suffer from this inordinate amount of energy spent by the immune system will return to balance—insomnia, hormonal imbalances, and digestive disturbances, among others. On the other hand, if the inflammation is not checked, then the organs continue to deteriorate. People become much more sensitive to their environment—chemical sensitivities and environmental allergies all grow worse as the barriers to the environment break down in the body. The more inflammation in the body, the less integrity the body has in the gastrointestinal and respiratory tracts. Hence, asthma and leaky gut syndrome becomes more prevalent.

ASTHMA

Hay fever and asthma are thought to be the predominant allergic conditions in the population at large. Asthma is considered the most common inflammatory disorder of the airways. About 40 percent of children of parents with asthma also develop asthma,[13] and more than 70 percent of people with asthma suffer from allergies.[14] Asthma is a chronic lung condition characterized by episodes of inflammation and narrowing of the small airways in response to various triggers. Common allergic triggers include pollen, house-dust mite excreta, and pet dander. According to the American Lung Association, approximately 20 million Americans have asthma, of which nine million are children under the age of 18.[15] Asthma-related deaths account for about 5,000 annually.[16] From an epidemiological perspective, experts agree that the burden of allergy and the presence of atopic disorders, such as asthma, atopic dermatitis, and allergic rhinitis have increased in epidemic proportions in industrialized countries over the past two decades. According to the Centers for Disease Control and Prevention, asthma rates in children under the age of five increased more than 160 percent from 1980 to 1994 with little change observed during 2000–2004. Atopy is a genetic predisposition to allergic conditions that tend to cluster in families, including hay fever, asthma, eczema, and most notably, common environmental allergens. This trend is typically found in industrialized countries and points to the general state of inflammation to which the industrialized lifestyle lends itself.

LEAKY GUT SYNDROME/INTESTINAL PERMEABILITY

Leaky gut syndrome is generally not recognized by mainstream medicine. Some studies have supported the theory that the body becomes more susceptible to developing food allergies and sensitivities when the lining of the gastro-intestinal tract has lost its integrity.[17] Over the past 20 years, the medical community has developed reliable methods to determine intestinal permeability[18]; however, research is lagging behind clinical experience because the syndrome is not recognized in mainstream medicine. In general, intestinal permeability refers to the integrity of the mucosal layer of the digestive tract that prevents bacteria, antigens, and undigested food proteins from seeping through the gastrointestinal barrier and into the systemic circulation. Increased permeability in the digestive tract can result in a chronically overreactive immune system in constant battle with toxins and allergens normally kept outside the bloodstream. The small intestine has the paradoxical dual function of being a digestive/absorptive organ as well as a barrier to permeation of toxic compounds and macromolecules. When this barrier loses its integrity, through inflammation for example, the nutrients it is supposed to absorb decrease, and the substances it is supposed to take out are able to seep inside. The disruption of the function of the small intestine inevitably leads to systemic problems, such as delayed sensitivity food allergies, arthritis, and inflammatory bowel diseases, among others. The distal portion of the intestine (colon) is the habitat for a great number of bacteria. It also contains a number of dietary and bacterial by-products that can be toxic to the system, hence, the importance of bowel regularity. Any type of dysfunction of the immune or mechanical barriers in the colon can lead to increased uptake of inflammatory and toxic substances as well as an increase in pathogenic bacteria because of the disruption of the ecology in the colon. If the intestine does not function properly, the amount of normally excluded substances that are absorbed through the mucosal lining increases dramatically. Intestinal permeability then becomes a gateway for more chronic disorders in the body. Today, intestinal permeability can be assessed by a physician through a study called an intestinal permeability assessment, in which a patient drinks a substance containing two sugars the body does not metabolize: mannitol and lactulose. These sugars are then measured in the urine to see how well the intestine absorbs these substances. Mannitol is an easily absorbed sugar and serves as a marker of transcellular uptake in the intestine. Lactulose, on the other hand, is generally not well absorbed and elevated amounts should not be found in the urine.

CONCLUSION

The immune system is a vast subject of study. New discoveries are being made rapidly and our understanding of how the body functions can change quickly;

however, clinically, doctors have found a strong correlation between the foods we eat and our health. It is extremely important to understand the role of allergy in our general well-being. Having a food allergy does not stop at the immediate or delayed symptoms—but they form a complete barrier on the road to wellness. Delayed food allergies have a *huge* impact on health. Fortunately, with today's technology, they are easy to detect. The first step is finding out what foods are making you sick. The next step is doing something about it. Health does not come to those who wait. Health is a journey that lasts a lifetime, and it takes a commitment to give your body exactly what it needs to the best of your ability so that it can function optimally and help you lead a more satisfying life. It may seem impossible to give up a few foods that have become a staple in your diet; however, when the benefits are weighed against the inconveniences, the benefits of modifying your lifestyle far outweigh the inconveniences. Many lives have been radically changed by what may seem to be a small change—it is time to start taking your health into your own hands—you are responsible for what you put in your mouths. Although it may be challenging to figure out the details of what to eat and not to eat, the rewards are enormous. There will always be more than one diet that claims to have the ultimate answer to your body's needs; however, only your body can tell you what it does and does not need. Follow a few sensible guidelines to maximize health—and this will take you part of the way. The rest of the way consists in knowing what foods your body recognizes as friend and foe. With diligence, consistency, and the help of additional supplementation, the gastrointestinal tract can be healed and returned to a state of greater integrity and strength. Of course, some allergies are genetic; however, those that develop from intestinal permeability problems will likely resolve with time and diligence. Most importantly, aspects of health that you thought were lost to you will return.

NOTES

1. Shea KM. *Reducing Low-Dose Pesticide Exposures in Infants and Children: A Clinicians' Guide from PSR*, Physicians for Social Responsibility. Available at: http://www.psr.org/site/DocServer/Reducing_Low-Dose_Pesticide_Exposures.pdf?docID=663. Accessed March 20, 2009.

2. Salam MT, Li YF, Langholz B, Gilliland FD. Early-life environmental risk factors for asthma: findings from the children's health study. *Environ Health Perspect.* 2004;112:760–765.

3. Vlassara H. Advanced glycation in health and disease: role of the modern environment. *Ann N Y Acad Sci.* 2005;1043:452–460.

4. Peppa M, Uribarri J, Vlassara H. Glucose, advanced glycation end products, and diabetes complications: what is new and what works. *Clin Diabetes.* 2003;21(4):186–187.

5. Koschinsky T, He CJ, Mitsuhashi T, et al. Orally absorbed reactive glycation products: an environmental risk factor in diabetic nephropathy. *Proc Natl Acad Sci USA.* 1997;94:6474–6479.

6. Forsythe CE, Phinney SD, Fernandez ML, et al. Comparison of low fat and low carbohydrate diets on circulating fatty acid composition and markers of inflammation. *Lipids.* 2008;43(1):65–77. Epub November 29, 2007.

7. Tielemans E, van Kooij E, te Velde ER, Burdorf A, Heederik D. Pesticide exposure and decreased fertilisation rates in vitro. *Lancet.* 1999;354:484–485.

8. Jensen TK, Giwercman A, Carlsen E, Scheike T, Skakkebaek NE. Semen quality among members of organic food associations in Zealand, Denmark. *Lancet.* 1996;347:1844.

9. Worthington V. Nutritional quality of organic versus conventional fruits, vegetables, and grains. *J Alternative Complementary Med.* 2001;7(2):161–173.

10. Naderali EK, Poyser NL. The effect of caffeine on prostaglandin output from the guinea-pig uterus. *Br J Pharmacol.* 1994;113(1):103–110.

11. Fortunato F, Deng X, Gates LK, McClain CJ, Bimmler D, Graf R, Whitcomb DC. Pancreatic response to endotoxin after chronic alcohol exposure: switch from apoptosis to necrosis? *Am J Physiol Gastrointest Liver Physiol.* 2006;290:G232–G241.

12. Yasue H, Hirai N, Mizuno Y, Harada E, Itoh T, Yoshimura M, Kugiyama K, Ogawa H. Low-grade inflammation, thrombogenicity, and atherogenic lipid profile in cigarette smokers. *Circulation J.* 2006;70(1):8–13.

13. Martinez FD, Wright AL, Taussig LM, et al. Asthma and wheezing in the first six years of life. *N Engl J Med.* 1995;332:133–138.

14. Gershwin ME, Albertson TE. *Bronchial asthma: A guide for practical understanding and treatment.* Totowa, NJ: Humana Press. 2006.

15. Dey AN, Schiller JS, Tai DA. Summary Health Statistics for U.S. Children: National Health Interview Survey, 2002. *Vital Health Stat.* 2004;10 (221):1–78.

16. Richardson L, Jagoda A. Management of life-threatening asthma in the emergency department. *Mt Sinai J Med.* 1997;64:275–282.

17. Forbes EE, Groschwitz K, Abonia JP, et al. IL-9– and mast cell–mediated intestinal permeability predisposes to oral antigen hypersensitivity. *J Exp Med.* 2008;205:897–913.

18. Bjarnason I, MacPherson A, Hollander D. Intestinal permeability: an overview. *Gastroenterology.* 1995;108:1566–1581.

CHAPTER 4

The Clinical Impact of Food Allergy

According to general surveys, adverse reactions to foods have been reported in up to 25 to 30 percent of the population, with the highest prevalence observed in infants and children. Controlled scientific studies, however, show an estimated prevalence of food allergies in about six percent in infants and children and about four percent in adults. Clearly, there is a huge apparent difference in these two sets of percentages. The reason for this discrepancy lies in how "allergy" is defined by conventional medicine. In conventional medicine, a food allergy is defined as an IgE (immediate) reaction, such as asthma, immediate rashes, anaphylaxis, and other immediate reactions. Yet, by the time you are reading this chapter you already have a greater appreciation of the broad and diverse the list of overt and delayed food allergies.

The following list demonstrates the variety of symptoms or conditions that may be associated with delayed food allergies and sensitivities. These symptoms and conditions can indicate other medical problems, so you should consult your doctor for any symptom you may have to help discern underlying causes.

The Digestive System

Includes symptoms in the mouth, esophagus, stomach, pancreas, small intestine, large intestine, liver, and gallbladder

Abdominal cramping
Abdominal pain
Anal itching
Bloating after meals
Colitis
Constipation

Crohn's disease
Diarrhea
Feeling of fullness in the stomach
Flatulence
Irritable bowel syndrome
Mucus in stools
Ulcerative colitis
Undigested food in stools
Aphthous ulcers/canker sores
Bad breath
Belching
Coated tongue
Itching on roof of the mouth
Failure to thrive
Infantile colic
Gagging
Gallbladder disease
Vomiting

Nervous System

Includes symptoms related to brain, brainstem, spinal cord, nerves, and nervous tissue function

Aggressive behavior
Anxiety
Confusion
Depression
Excessive daydreaming
Hyperactivity
Inability to concentrate
Indifference
Irritability
Learning disabilities
Mental dullness
Mental lethargy
Numbness
Poor work habits
Restlessness
Slurred speech
Stuttering

Musculoskeletal System

Includes symptoms relating to muscle, bone, and cartilaginous tissues

Arthritis
Growing pains

Joint aches and pains
Muscle aches and pains
Osteoarthritis
Rheumatoid arthritis
Weakness

Genitourinary System

Includes symptoms relating to the kidneys, urethra, bladder, urethra, vagina, uterus, ovaries, penis, testicles, and adjoining structures

Bed wetting
Premenstrual syndrome
Frequent urination frequency
Urinary urgency
Vaginal discharge
Vaginal itching

Respiratory System

Includes symptoms relating to the nose, trachea, larynx, bronchi, and lungs

Asthma
Chest congestion
Chronic cough
Chronic nasal congestion
Excessive mucus formation
Exercise-induced anaphylaxis
Exercise-induced asthma
Gagging
Hoarseness
Horizontal crease across the nose
Persistent nose picking
Postnasal drip
Recurrent sinusitis
Runny nose
Sore throat
Stuffy nose

Cardiovascular System

Includes symptoms relating to the heart, veins, arteries, and capillaries

Angina
Arrhythmias
High blood pressure
Palpitations

Rapid heart rate
Vascular headaches

Integumentary System

Includes symptoms relating to the hair, nails, and skin

Acne
Brittle nails and hair
Dandruff
Dark circles under eyes
Dermatitis herpetiformis
Dry skin
Eczema
Hives
Paleness
Psoriasis
Rashes
Swelling and wrinkles under eyes

Ears and Eyes

Includes internal and external symptoms of eyes and ears

Blurry vision
Ear drainage
Earache
Fluid in the middle ear
Fullness in the ears
Hearing loss
Itchy ears
Meniere's disease
Motion sickness
Recurrent ear infections
Tinnitus
Watery eyes

Miscellaneous

Includes symptoms that affect multiple systems

Chronic fatigue
Dizziness
Excessive drowsiness after eating
Faintness

Fatigue
Feeling of fullness in the head
Frequent awakenings during the night
Food cravings
Headaches
Insomnia
Nausea
Nightmares
Obesity
Rapid weight fluctuation
Swelling of hands, feet, and ankles
Teeth grinding
Water retention

If you have any of these symptoms, a food allergy test panel may be beneficial for you to discern the root cause of your symptoms. You may be feeding your body the wrong fuel and compromising your health unknowingly.

The preceding list does not include every conceivable ache and pain. In fact, nearly all symptoms known to humankind may be related to or aggravated by food allergies. Even if your specific symptoms do not appear on the list, you may still be affected by food allergies. Have yourself tested today and discover your relationship with food.

If food allergies were suspected for the previously listed symptoms, the percentage of Americans reported to be affected by food allergies would be significantly higher.

The issue of underreporting food-triggered reactions can be circumvented by being vigilant and having a broad perspective on exactly how an allergen can present in the body. It is important to remember that a reaction can take a couple of days to manifest after an exposure, and a reaction can occur at a sufficiently removed period of time from the food insult that may not be able to make the correlation. An adverse food reaction is defined as *any* new symptom that arises after the intake of a particular food. A reaction can range from mood changes, skin quality, to how one feels and functions, to more overt symptoms like achy joints or fatigue. These reactions are classified into three subgroups:

1. Toxic
2. Psychological
3. Nontoxic reactions
   a. Immune mediated (food allergy)
   b. Nonimmune mediated (food intolerance)

Figure 4.1 is a simple diagram to put the many types of adverse food reactions into visual perspective.

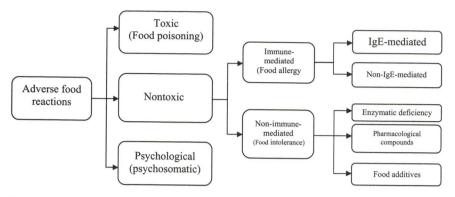

Figure 4.1: Types of adverse food reactions. Adapted in part from the European Academy of Allergy and Clinical Immunology (EAACI).

TOXIC REACTIONS

A toxic food reaction is commonly known as food poisoning and is the result of contaminants in food. These contaminants may be an infectious agent, such as a bacterium or parasite, or a toxic agent, such as a pesticide or poisonous mushroom. Accounting for up to 76 million illnesses a year in the United States, food-borne illness is an immediate reaction that usually occurs within 48-hours after eating the contaminated food or drink and may occur in any individual; all age groups; both sexes; exposed to the agent. Typical symptoms include nausea, vomiting, abdominal cramping and diarrhea. More severe reactions may include fever, chills, bloody stools and dehydration. According to the Centers for Disease Control and Prevention (CDC), food poisoning accounts for up to 5,000 deaths a year in the United States. One of the most common causes of food poisoning is *Salmonella*, a bacterium carried in poultry, eggs, unprocessed milk, meat, and water. Mild *Salmonella* infections clear up in about a week without any treatment other than rest and plenty of liquids. More severe cases may require intervention with antibiotics.

PSYCHOLOGICAL

A second type of adverse food reaction is known as a psychological reaction, or food aversion. This type of reaction is most often related to a former unpleasant experience with a particular food and is largely psychosomatic in nature. This is an interesting phenomenon in the field of psychosomatic medicine. Food aversion is complex and multifactorial. Pairing food and illness typically results in a powerful taste aversion. This is a conditioned response and, in many cases, the affected person is aware that the illness was caused by something absolutely unrelated to the food. A common example is the food aversion experienced by cancer patients. Cancer treatments are well known to cause food aversions to normal dietary items and are presumed to develop via conditioning processes. The nausea and vomiting induced by chemotherapy treatments, in addition to changes in perceived tastes, are believed to be a major causative factor to the development of food aversion and consequent appetite problems in cancer patients.[1] Another example is the food aversions experienced during pregnancy. An estimated 85 percent of expectant mothers experience some kind of food aversion during the course of their pregnancy, most often in the first trimester. It is speculated that the food aversions are due to the tremendous hormonal changes that take place in the body during this time. Some women may find themselves nauseated by the smell or even the sight of certain foods throughout their pregnancy. Experts speculate that this could be from an outdated biological mechanism that protected the mother and child from foods that were most likely contaminated or potentially harmful.

NONTOXIC FOOD REACTION

A third type of adverse food reaction is defined as nontoxic. These reactions are further subdivided into immune, and non–immune-mediated groups.

Non–Immune-Mediated Reactions

Non–immune-mediated reactions are commonly known as food intolerances. Food intolerance can be the results of an enzymatic deficiency—when the body is genetically unable to make the enzyme required to break down a particular molecule that is ingested. The most common food intolerance is lactose intolerance, which is caused by a deficiency in the enzyme lactase. Lactase is naturally found in the lining of the small intestine and is involved in the breakdown of the milk sugar lactose, which is found in dairy products. Without lactase, the unprocessed lactose can cause gas, bloating, and diarrhea as the bacteria in the large intestine contend with it. The causes of lactose intolerance are many. As babies, most humans produce enough lactase to break down breast milk; however, as we age and become less dependent on milk as our primary source of nutrition, the body makes less and less lactase; therefore, lactose intolerance is relatively common in adults. This type of lactose intolerance occurs gradually over the years and usually manifests in young adulthood. Another cause of lactose intolerance is illness; for example, acute gastroenteritis, Crohn's disease, or celiac disease may damage the cells of the small intestine, reducing lactase activity. Congenital lactose intolerance, although rare, is a metabolic disorder that causes vomiting, diarrhea, dehydration, and failure to thrive from birth because of intolerance to lactose from the mother's breast milk.

Pharmacological food reactions are another form of food intolerance. Some naturally occurring chemicals found in food are capable of producing a clinical reaction. Caffeine, for example, which is found in tea, coffee, chocolate, and soft drinks, in a large enough dose, may cause migraine headaches and heart palpitations. Other pharmacologically active substances found in food include histamine, tyramine, glutamate, phenylethylamine, and serotonin, which are found in such foods as red wine, aged cheese, soy sauce, chocolate, avocados, and bananas. In susceptible people, these food substances can trigger rash, nausea, diarrhea, flushing, sweating, and headaches.

Food intolerance to food additives—food dyes and colorings, preservatives, flavorings, taste enhancers, and the like—is assumed to be relatively rare at less than one percent of the general population.[2] These reactions may involve an allergic component and therefore cover the spectrum of nontoxic reactions; immune mediated and non–immune-mediated. Restaurant syndrome, which is tied to sulfite allergy or sensitivity, is a typical example. Banned for it use in restaurants in the 1980s by the Food and Drug Administration because of deaths, sulfites (sodium bisulfite, sodium metabisulfite, potassium bisulfite, and potassium metabisulfite) were a common preservative used in salad bars to inhibit browning and discoloration. Chinese restaurant syndrome, which was first described in the late 1960s, was attributed to liberal usage of the flavor enhancer, monosodium glutamate (MSG). Effects of MSG can range from a mild headache, flushing, and urticaria to severe, life-threatening swelling of the throat, shortness of breath, and chest pains that may ensue in the sensitive person two hours after consuming MSG-laden food. Because of conflicting data on this cause-and-effect relationship, however, MSG is still in use. Symptoms such as anaphylaxis, urticaria, angioedema, bronchospasm, and death have been attributed to adverse reactions from food additives. Although this type of reaction is most likely when symptoms occur soon after contact with a particular food or beverage, this type of non–immune-mediated reaction should not be ruled out if it occurs in a more delayed fashion. Both immune-mediated and non–immune-mediated food reactions can be severe and life threatening.

Immune-Mediated Reactions

Immune-mediated adverse food reactions are roughly divided into classes I through IV. This classification system dates back to 1963 when Philip George Houthem Gell (1914–2001) and Robert Royston Amos Coombs (1921–2006), outlined four basic types of hypersensitivity reactions under what became known as Gell and Coombs's classification of immunologic reactions. It is important to keep in mind that immune-mediated adverse food reactions are a heterogeneous group and that more than one immunological mechanism may exist, including those yet to be identified.

The classic type I, IgE-mediated, reaction is the most thoroughly studied for its close association to asthma, hay fever, perennial rhinitis, atopic dermatitis, and food allergies. Elevated serum IgE levels against several allergens has been demonstrated in many of these instances. An allergy of this type develops when food or environmental allergen-specific IgE antibodies bound to tissue mast cells and basophils that are present in the skin, gut, and respiratory tract come into contact with and bind the circulating allergen. This binding activates these cells to release inflammatory mediators, including histamine, prostaglandins, leukotrienes, and cytokines. Exposure to a small amount of allergen can provoke a reaction. For this reason tolerance is low to none. Vasodilatation, local edema, mucus secretion, and smooth muscle contraction are some of the effects of these mediators released into the neighboring tissues. IgE hypersensitivity affects an estimated six percent of young children and about four percent of adults in the United States,[3] a prevalence that is much higher than recognized in the past. IgE hypersensitivity is important because it can cause potentially life-threatening anaphylactic reactions in some people. Although U.S. estimates of food-related anaphylaxis are less than one percent,[4] the percentage of those with IgE-mediated food allergies who are at risk of anaphylaxis is not known. Nevertheless, those with a history of anaphylaxis are at increased risk of a subsequent attack. Food allergens are a frequent cause of severe anaphylaxis, particularly in persons with concomitant asthma and nut or seafood allergy,[5] and they are the leading cause of anaphylactic reactions treated at hospital emergency departments. Estimates suggest that 30,000 anaphylactic food reactions are treated in U.S. emergency departments annually, 150 to 200 of which result in death. Peanuts, tree nuts, fish, and shellfish account for most severe food anaphylactic reactions.[6] These are significant numbers. Combined with somewhat clouded mechanistic details and the fact that the prevalence of allergies are much higher today than in the past, clear guidelines for the recognition and treatment are aggressively sought by health care providers.

Type II and III hypersensitivity reactions are generally not due to food-related reactions; however type II and III hypersensitivity reactions have not been fully studied. Type II hypersensitivity reaction occurs when there are antigens on a person's cells and antibodies bind to these antigens. The result of this reaction results in autoimmune-type reactions like autoimmune hemolytic anemia, Goodpasture's syndrome, myasthenia gravis, Grave's disease, or acute rheumatic fever. Type III hypersensitivity reactions generally occur when antigens floating in the blood bind to antibodies and form very large immune complexes that the body cannot clear. These types of reactions generally cause damage in whatever area they precipitate; for example, post-streptococcal reaction, serum sickness, reactive arthritis, or systemic lupus erythematosus.[7]

Non–IgE-mediated food allergies cover a spectrum of immune reactions involving cell-mediated reactions, immunoglobulins other than IgE, and immune complexes. A cell-mediated reaction is commonly known as type IV, or delayed-type hypersensitivity reaction. These reactions are instigated by T lymphocytes, monocytes, and macrophages rather than antibodies. The term "delayed" is used because the cellular response occurs about 48 to 72 hours after antigen exposure; in contrast, a type I immediate hypersensitivity response occurs about 12 minutes after antigen exposure.[8]

A classic example of a cell-mediated hypersensitivity is celiac disease, or gluten-sensitive enteropathy. Celiac disease is a permanent intolerance to wheat gluten and related proteins from gluten-containing grain such as wheat, rye and barley. The disease develops from an abnormal T cell–initiated immune response to gluten. This abnormal response is influenced by molecules that present gluten peptides to T cells found in the small intestine. These molecules are products of what is known as human leukocyte antigen–linked genes.[9] A local immune and inflammatory response ensues in the small intestine from the presentation of the gluten to the T cells. If gluten-containing food is continually ingested, the inflammation becomes chronic. This chronic inflammation causes a wasting and flattening of the intestinal lining, called villi. Individuals with celiac disease have increased levels of serum antibodies to gluten and the autoantigen tissue transglutaminase. The presence of these antibodies and the devastating effects on the small intestinal mucosa are strictly dependent on dietary exposure to gluten. Traditionally considered uncommon, this disease was simply thought of as a gastrointestinal disorder recognized, if at all, in early childhood when cereals are typically introduced into the diet. With the growing awareness of the diverse manifestations of celiac disease, it is now understood to be a relatively common disease that affects approximately one percent of the general U.S. population. Interestingly, only 20 to 50 percent of affected individuals have subjective symptoms.[10] Celiac disease is a multisystem disorder and presentation may occur at any age in both sexes under a wide variety of clinical circumstances that can be roughly divided into the following four groups:

1. **Classic Celiac Disease Presentation**
   Gastrointestinal symptoms—Pain; diarrhea/constipation, steatorrhea (fat in the stool), flatulence, vomiting, distention, and weight loss. Manifestations of malabsorption may include anemia from iron, folate and vitamin B-12 deficiencies, coagulopathy from vitamin K deficiency, and hypocalcemia (low blood calcium levels) from vitamin D deficiency.

2. **Celiac Disease with Atypical Symptoms**
   Extraintestinal manifestations may predominate with little or no gastrointestinal symptoms. A key example is dermatitis herpetiformis, a skin disorder characterized by itchy, blistering lesions on the extensor surfaces of the extremities (back of the arms and legs) and trunk. Other examples of atypical symptoms include iron deficiency anemia that is unresponsive to treatment with iron supplementation, persistent aphthous ulcers (canker sores), arthritis, delayed puberty, and infertility to name a few. Affected children may present with behavioral problems, including depression, irritability, and impaired scholastic performance.

3. **Silent Celiac Disease**
   Persons with silent celiac disease are asymptomatic but have positive serologic results (blood test results) and villous atrophy (wasting of intestinal villi) on biopsy of intestinal mucosa. Diagnosis in these cases most often comes from a routine screening of high-risk persons or biopsy performed for another reason. High-risk people include the following:

   • First- and second-degree relatives of persons with celiac disease. Silent celiac disease is 24–48 times more frequent in the siblings of celiac patients than in the general population.[11]
   • People with type 1 diabetes mellitus or another autoimmune disorder.

- Persons with Down syndrome and other genetic disorders. Prevalence of silent celiac disease is higher among children with idiopathic epilepsy.[12]
- Persons with selective IgA deficiency.

4. Latent Celiac Disease
Asymptomatic persons with positive serology but no villous atrophy on biopsy. Over time these patients may develop symptoms and/or histological changes.

Considerable morbidity and mortality are associated with celiac disease because of chronic gastrointestinal complaints and resulting malabsorption, poor diet compliance, and the number of cases that go undiagnosed. Long-term complications include an increased risk of certain malignancies, especially of the small bowel, but they may manifest elsewhere in the gastrointestinal tract. Management of celiac disease consists of adopting a completely gluten-free diet for life.

Immunoglobulins other than IgE and immune complexes have also been incriminated in food allergic disorders and disorders that have not otherwise been universally recognized as having a food allergy component. The current field of allergy research and the current definitions in this field has evolved rapidly over a few decades and continue to grow as knowledge about immunological mechanisms grow and understanding improves.

Antibodies are part of the body's natural immune defense. Elevated levels, however, may suggest an up-regulated gastrointestinal mucosal immune response from damage due to a variety of reasons. A local IgE-mediated reaction, for example, may act as an initial trigger that alters the permeability of the gut mucosa. Loss of integrity in the lining allows entry of antigens and the formation of an elaborate immune response involving other antibodies, such as IgG antibodies. Other factors, such as infections and medications, can hinder the competency of the gut barrier and may also play a part in the development and perpetuation of food allergies.

An increase in antigliadin IgA (IgA hyperglobulinemia) blood levels has been demonstrated in celiac disease, Crohn's disease, ulcerative colitis, rheumatoid arthritis, Bergers' disease, Sjögren's syndrome and Henoch-Schönlein purpura (HSP). This commonality in all these diseases may reflect an underlying occult inflammation of the small intestine from a runaway immune system combined with compromised intestinal integrity. The food-specific antibodies magnify the multiple hypersensitivity reactions that drive these diseases. It has been suggested that increased intestinal permeability plays a central role in the development of a number of diseases, but it remains unclear what comes first, intestinal permeability or the inflammation that promotes dysfunction of the intestinal barrier.

HENOCH-SCHÖNLEIN PUPURA

IgA hyperglobulinemia is commonly observed in the blood of persons with HSP, which is also known as purpura. HSP is a systemic autoimmune inflammation of the blood vessels that develops in childhood and affects the skin, gastrointestinal tract, and joints. A bruise-like rash occurs on the lower extremities and is accompanied by abdominal pain, headache, fatigue, diarrhea, and arthritis. The classic triad includes rash, gastrointestinal complaints/hematuria, and arthritis. In about 22 to 70 percent of patients there is also kidney involvement. Medications; immunizations; insect bites; exposure to cold; infectious agents such as Group A streptococci, *Mycoplasma*, varicella virus; and exposure to allergens in foods have all been reported associated factors. Twenty-five percent of patients have a family history of allergy. Of these, food allergies have been reported to result in bouts of acute nephrotic syndrome, a kidney disease. A characteristic feature of HSP is the deposition of IgA-dominant immune complexes in smaller venules, capillaries, and arterioles, including that of the mesangium of the kidney. Although the precise cause of HSP is unknown, the presence of elevated serum IgA is thought to represent a disturbance of the gut mucosal immune system. In addition, increased intestinal permeability from vascular lesions, elevated secretory IgA of mucosal origin in the blood, and the presence of elevated food-specific IgA immune complexes (for example, gluten, gliadin, bovine, casein) in the blood have been suggested as possible causes. Renal failure may occur in a small percentage of patients. Generally, the disease is self-limiting but deserves close follow-up. There is a tendency to relapse, and successive episodes may be accompanied by kidney complications.

IRRITABLE BOWEL SYNDROME

An example of a chronic disease that may involve a food-related component is irritable bowel syndrome (IBS). IBS is a chronic gastrointestinal disorder characterized by abdominal pains, bloating, gassiness, and altered bowel habits (diarrhea and/or constipation). The exact cause is not known but may involve a dysregulation in the communication between the nervous system of the gastrointestinal tract and the brain. Some persons with IBS appear to have a low-grade inflammatory process occurring in the gut mucosa, which had been formerly attributed to gastrointestinal infection. It has been suggested that food allergies may play a role in this disorder and food hypersensitivity is a common perception among patients with IBS. The presence of food-specific IgG antibodies as an immunological basis is a distinct possibility in some IBS patients. Atkinson and colleagues examined IgG antibodies to foods to guide an elimination diet in a randomized, double blind, controlled, parallel design trial. Food elimination based on IgG antibodies was shown to be effective in reducing IBS symptom severity during the study period.[13] Zar et al.[14] examined food-specific IgG antibodies in patients with IBS, specifically IgG4 subclass. They found increased titers of IgG4 to common foods, including wheat, beef, pork, and lamb compared with titers for controls. In a follow-up study, this group designed food-specific IgG4 antibody-exclusion diets and found significant overall improvement in symptoms of IBS.[15] Drisko et al.[16] also used an elimination diet based on food-specific IgG. Their results showed a sustained clinical response with a positive impact on overall well- being and quality of life in patients with IBS. A number of laboratories offer food-specific IgG Food Antibody Assessment Panel. The assays may measure IgG4 alone or all four subclasses (IgG1, IgG2, IgG3, and IgG4) reported as IgG total for any particular food item. Some laboratories also offer a suggested rotation diet guideline based on the patient's test results. In my clinical practice I find this particular form of testing essential when establishing a strong health and wellness foundation from which to work when it comes to all health conditions. If the body is not fueled properly, let alone fueled improperly with notably burdens to health, these obstacles to wellness must be identified and eliminated.

RHEUMATOID ARTHRITIS

Rheumatoid arthritis (RA) is another condition that may be benefited by food-specific IgG testing. RA is a chronic inflammatory autoimmune disease of unknown cause. The notion that dietary factors may influence this disease dates as far back as the disease itself. Although relatively few studies have tested the effect of diet therapy on disease activity in RA, they have all focused on some form of dietary elimination and have had promising results. Several studies support the concept that food sensitivity may contribute significantly to symptoms. Darlington et al.[17] showed significant improvement in more than 35 percent of patients studied with RA in both objective and subjective variables in a single-blinded, placebo-controlled six-week study of dietary manipulation. During the first week of the study, the only foods allowed in the diet were those to which the patient was unlikely to be intolerant. Other foods were then reintroduced one at a time to see whether any symptoms were produced by dietary challenge. Foods producing symptoms were then excluded from the diet. Similar results were found by Kjeldsen-Kragh et al.[18] This single-blinded controlled trial studied the effect of dietary elimination followed by one year of a vegetarian diet. Of the total patients studied, 44 percent responded well in all measured indices, most of which gave positive reactions to food challenges. A two-year follow-up study of these patients showed sustained improvement in all measured indices.[19] Brostoff and Gamlin[20] support these findings noting that a significant percentage (30–40 percent) of patients with RA from most double-blind placebo-controlled trials can see substantial improvement to the point of discontinuing drug treatment by using an elimination diet to identify foods that precipitate symptoms, followed by their elimination. Although the mechanism by which food reactions aggravate RA remains controversial, possible changes in immune parameters provide a promising line of investigation. In the extensive but short study by Van de Laar et al.[21] a small group of food intolerant and seropositive patients with RA, showed partial or total remission during allergen-free feeding over a four-month study period. Intolerant foods were defined by the presence of specific food antibodies (IgE, IgG1, IgG4), skin reactions, or subjective history intake from a diet dairy, all of which were confirmed by double-blind, placebo-controlled rechallenges. A subset of these patients had a concomitant clinical reduction of inflammatory parameters of the synovial membrane and proximal portion of the small intestine on the allergen-free diet as expressed histolgically. Ratner et al.[22] describes a 14-year-old girl of European ancestry who had suffered from seronegative juvenile RA for six years. She was lactase deficient and had a family history of milk allergy. Her joint symptoms were provoked by milk, and she showed high levels of antibodies IgG and IgM specific for milk using enzyme-linked immunosorbent assay (ELISA) technique. Four positive provocation tests (two inadvertent blind challenges) strongly indicated a connection between the milk-free diet that she was placed on and the clinical remissions seen in this patient. Ratner provides an interesting point:

- Slow response to dietary elimination (three weeks) as seen in this patient is not typical for IgE-mediated food allergies and therefore belongs to a different category.

Ratner concludes that identifying milk-specific IgG and IgM antibodies in this patient in addition to the clinical response to elimination and subsequent positive challenge demonstrate the diagnosis of milk allergy. A case of seronegative RA and milk allergy was also reported by Parke and Hughes[23]: a 38-year-old woman reported similar improvements three weeks after starting dairy elimination. The improvement was maintained apart from when she advertently or inadvertently consumed dairy—after which symptoms returned within 12 hours. Although IgE antibodies to milk and cheese protein became positive during the food challenge, radioallergosorbent test (RAST) tests performed on the synovial fluid remained negative throughout the challenge. Panush et al.[24] studied a patient with inflammatory arthritis in a prospective, blinded, controlled fashion to assess the association with an immunologic hypersensitivity to milk. This 52-year-old white woman had an 11-year history of inflammatory arthritis that was allegedly exacerbated by certain foods (meat, milk, and beans), so the patient limited the intake. The patient also had a history of urticaria from shellfish ingestion and cold-related vasospasm. Open unblinded and blinded food challenge produced notable deterioration in subjective and objective measures. Immunological studies revealed negative elevated IgE antibodies to foods, including milk. The patient did have mildly increased amounts of IgG anti-milk and large amounts of IgG4 anti-milk. In addition, IgG-containing and milk-containing circulating immune complexes were elevated, though marginally, 48 hours after one of the milk challenges, which was concomitant to symptom aggravation. In a controlled clinical trial, Hafström et al.[25] showed a significant reduction in serum IgG anti-gliadin and anti-b-lactoglobulin levels over a one-year period from baseline in all patients who responded positively to a vegan diet (40 percent) compared with a nonvegan group. He concludes that dietary modification may be of clinical benefit for certain patients with RA.

ADD/ADHD

There is increasing evidence that many children with behavioral problems such as attention-deficit disorder (ADD) and attention-deficit hyperactive disorder (ADHD) are sensitive to one or more food components that can negatively affect their behavior. The idea that foods can have a behavioral effect is slowly gaining acceptance in the scientific community. Individual response is an important factor for determining the proper approach in treating children and adults with ADHD. In general, diet modification plays a major role in the management of ADHD and should be considered as part of the treatment protocol.[26]

Some initial evidence suggests that fatty acids may influence hyperactivity in children with specific learning disabilities. The findings also suggest that some food additives (colorings, flavorings, and preservatives) may increase hyperactivity in children with behavior problems. For children showing behavior problems such as hyperactivity the use of dietary manipulation tends to be a more acceptable approach to treatment than the use of drugs.[27] ADHD is a disorder where patients have difficulty maintaining an attention span and maintaining focus on relevant stimuli and focus too intensely on nonrelevant stimuli. Inattention and distractibility appear to be related to low levels of norepinephrine. The impulse and behavior problems appear related to low levels of dopamine in the brain.[28] Both of these neurotransmitters are made from amino acids—both essential and nonessential. The question is then, how do we acquire the necessary amino acids to make the necessary neurotransmitters? The body acquires these nutrients through the process of digestion; however, when digestion is compromised because of, for example, delayed food allergies, the proteins ingested may not be broken down and/or the immune system can use the amino acids absorbed to produce inflammatory markers rather than building blocks. The end result remains a deficiency in essential amino acids for the brain. The food allergy connection with ADHD has not been strongly established because conventional medicine does not fully recognize the tie between gastrointestinal health and neurotransmitter production. However, study after study has showed the relationship between digestion and neurotransmitter health. For example:

- Boys diagnosed with ADHD had lower levels of the omega-3 essential fatty acid docosahexaenoic acid (DHA).[29] Ninety-five percent of children with ADHD tested found to have magnesium deficiency.[30]
- Children with ADHD had zinc levels that were only two-thirds the level of children without ADHD.[31]

What these studies demonstrate is the nutritional deficiencies inherent in this disorder. Nutritional deficiencies indicate that either the child does not receive adequate nutrition, or—more likely—the child is unable to absorb nutrients that are essential to brain function because of the inflammation brought on by non–IgE-mediated food allergies. The fact remains that, clinically, food allergy eliminations in children and adults suffering from ADHD have resulted in a decrease in symptoms and an increase in cognitive capabilities.

Many recent studies have suggested that IgG-food immune complexes are a component in low-grade chronic allergic inflammation. One study defined these effects in the development of early atherosclerotic lesions in obese youth. The study found a significant increase and tight correlation in intima media layer thickness of the carotid arteries, elevated C-reactive protein (CRP) values, and anti-food IgG antibody concentrations in a group of 30 obese youth compared with a group of 30 healthy-weight children. The authors speculate a low-level absorption of food molecules from the gut with the production of anti-food IgG or food intolerance is linked to low-grade chronic inflammation. The tight correlation of the acute-phase protein CRP (an inflammation marker) with anti-food IgG raise the possibility, as suggested by the authors, that anti-food IgG elements are involved in the development of obesity and early atherosclerosis. CRP is a marker that is elevated in the presence of systemic inflammation. It has been consistently related to obesity and is used as one of the markers to assess cardiovascular disease risk.

All of the aforementioned conditions show how an improper immune response—characterized by inflammatory responses to antigens—can cause reactions throughout the body that produce disease. The immune system in the intestinal walls loses its ability to distinguish between disease-causing antigens and those that do not. The overreaction of the intestinal immune system is influenced by the intestinal environment—which includes the interaction between the intestinal walls and the resident microflora and with the immune system to determine subsequent reactions. The compromise of the integrity of oral tolerance has both gastrointestinal and systemic consequences, such as IgE food allergy; inflammatory bowel disease, including ulcerative colitis and Crohn's disease; atherogenesis, and autoimmune disease, such as celiac disease. All of these diseases have a diverse clinical presentation and represent the heterogeneity of a whole spectrum of imbalanced immune responses. Risk of systemic consequences may be associated with loss of protective barrier function and an increase in intestinal permeability because of the inflammation.

The inherent value in IgG Food Antibody Assessment Panels is evident in certain chronic conditions. Foods that create an immune reaction in the body necessarily create inflammation in the body. How the inflammation manifests is different for every person. The common denominator in these chronic conditions remains the same: the inflammatory response brought about by the immune system. When the offending foods are eliminated, steps can be taken to repair the integrity of the gut to heal it, tighten up the junctions, and prevent further immune reactions. Patients often find that after a certain amount of time, certain foods can be reintroduced into the diet without adverse effects.

Case Studies

1. A patient presents with back pain, chronic headaches, depression, fatigue, and a prior diagnoses of reactive arthritis, IBS, and fibromyalgia. An IgG Food Antibody Assessment Panel is ordered and the results of the test are discussed with the patient. After eliminating the reactive

foods as identified on her dietary report, implementing the rotation diet, and implementing other nutritional interventions, she now feels and looks fantastic. The transformation was phenomenal.

2. A patient presents with severe belching and IBS of 30 years' duration, unresponsive to any treatments. After removing the reactive foods identified on an IgG Food Antibody Assessment Panel from her diet, the IBS clears and belching is reduced by 75 percent. The patient also lost 25 pounds of excess weight.

3. A 6-year-old girl is brought in by her mother. She has a had a hard time sitting and focusing for long periods of time. She also could not control her bladder at night. Her doctor recommends an IgG Food Antibody Assessment Panel and within 24 hours of removing wheat, dairy, and eggs she reports finding it easier to think and to sit in class. She can follow directions and feels calmer and happier over all. Bedwetting is no longer an issue for her and she enjoys feeling better now.

CONCLUSION

The medical field and society in general need to look beyond the blinders of previous definitions of allergies and realize that the medical and scientific literature continues to validate the true significance of previously held nontraditional types of allergies and their clinical manifestation. A lifetime of suffering can often be mitigated when the body is fueled as it was designed relative to an individual's unique biochemistry and immunological sensitivities. It is far better to test than to guess when it comes to identifying potential obstacles to wellness, and when it comes to delayed allergic responses, guessing at the existence of specific allergens is virtually impossible.

NOTES

1. Holmes S. Food avoidance in patients undergoing cancer chemotherapy. *Supportive Care Cancer.* 1993;1:326–330; Bernstein I. Aversion conditioning in response to cancer and cancer treatment. *Clin Psychol Rev.* 1991;11:185–191.

2. Wuthrich B. Adverse reactions to food additives. *Ann Allergy.* 1993;71:379–384.

3. Sicherer SH, Muñoz-Furlong A, Sampson HA. Prevalence of seafood allergy in the United States determined by a random telephone survey. *J Allergy Clin Immunol.* 2004;114:159–165; Sampson HA. Update on food allergy. *J Allergy Clin Immunol.* 2004;113:805–819.

4. Neugut AI, Ghatak AT, Miller RL. Anaphylaxis in the United States: an investigation into its epidemiology. *Arch Intern Med.* 2001;161:15–21; Bohlke K, Davis RL, DeStefano F, et al. Epidemiology of anaphylaxis among children and adolescents enrolled in a health maintenance organization. *J Allergy Clin Immunol.* 2004;113:536–542; Simons FE, Peterson S, Black CD. Epinephrine dispensing patterns for an out-of-hospita population: a novel approach to studying the epidemiology of anaphylaxis. *J Allergy Clin Immunol* 2002;110:647–651; Sicherer SH, Muñoz-Furlong A, Burks AW, Sampson HA. Prevalence

of peanut and tree nut allergy in the US determined by a random digit dial telephone survey. *J Allergy Clin Immunol.* 1999;103:559–562.

5. Food allergy: a practice parameter. *Ann Allergy Asthma Immunol.* 2006;96 (3 suppl 2):S1–S68.

6. Sampson HA. Anaphylaxis and emergency treatment. *Pediatrics.* 2003;111; 1601–1608.

7. Ghaffar A. Hypersensitivity reactions. *Microbiology and Immunology On-Line.* University of South Carolina School of Medicine. Available at: http://pathmicro.med. sc.edu/ghaffar/hyper00.htm. Accessed April 12, 2009.

8. Hinshaw WD, Neyman GP, Olmstead SM. Hypersensitivity Reactions, Delayed. 2005. Available at: http://www.emedicine.com/MED/topic1100.htm. Accessed March 21, 2009.

9. Sollid LM. Coeliac disease: dissecting a complex inflammatory disorder. *Nature Rev.* 2002;2:647–655.

10. Fasano A, Catassi C. Current approaches to diagnosis and treatment of celiac disease: an evolving spectrum. *Gastroenterology.* 2001;120:636–651.

11. Bardella MT, Elli L, Velio P, Fredella C, Prampolini L, Cesana B. Silent celiac disease is frequent in the siblings of newly diagnosed celiac patients. *Digestion.* 2007;75:182–187.

12. Antigoni M. Increased prevalence of silent celiac disease among Greek epileptic children. *Pediatr Neurol.* 2007;36(3):165–169.

13. Atkinson W, Sheldon TA, Shaath N, Whorwell PJ. Food elimination based on IgG antibodies in irritable bowel syndrome: a randomised controlled trial. *Gut.* 2004;53:1459–1464.

14. Zar S, Benson MJ, Kumar D. Food-specific serum IgG4 and IgE titers to common food antigens in irritable bowel syndrome. *Am J Gastroenterol.* 2005;100:1550–1557.

15. Zar S, Mincher L, Benson MJ, Kumar D. Food-specifc IgG4 antibody-guided exclusion duet improves symptoms of rectal compliance in irritable bowel syndrome. *Scand J Gastroenterol.* 2005;40:800–807.

16. Drisko J, Bischoff B, Hall M, McCallum R. Treating irritable bowel syndrome with a food elimination diet followed by food challenge and probiotics. *J Am Coll Nutr.* 2006;25:514–522.

17. Darlington LG, Ramsey NW, Mansfield JR. Placebo-controlled, blind study of dietary manipulation therapy in rheumatoid arthritis. *Lancet.* 1986;1:236–238.

18. Kjeldsen-Kragh J, Haugen M, Borchgrevink CF, et al. Controlled trial of fasting and one-year vegetarian diet in rheumatoid arthritis. *Lancet.* 1991;338:899–902.

19. Kjeldsen-Kragh J, Haugen M, Borchgrevink CF, Forre O. Vegetarian diet for patients with rheumatoid arthritis—status: two years after introduction of the diet. *Clin Rheumatol.* 1994;13:475–482.

20. Brostoff J, Gamlin L. Food sensitivity and rheumatoid arthritis. *Environ Toxicol Pharmacol.* 1996;4:43–49.

21. Van de Laar MAF, Aalbers M, Bruins FG, van Dinther-Janssen AC, van der Korst JK, Meijer CJ. Food intolerance in rheumatoid arthritis. II. Clinical and histological aspects. *Ann Rheum Dis.* 1992;51:303–306.

22. Ratner D, Eshel E, Vigder K. Juvenile rheumatoid arthritis and milk allergy. *J Royal Soc Med.* 1985;78:410–413.

23. Parke AL, Hughes GR. Rheumatoid arthritis and food: a case study. *BMJ.* 1981;282:2027–2029.

24. Panush RS, Stroud RM, Webster EM. Food-induced (allergic) arthritis. Inflammatory arthritis exacerbated by milk. *Arthritis Rheum.* 1986;29(2):220–226.

25. Hafström I, Ringertz B, Spånberg A, et al. A vegan diet free of gluten improves the signs and symptoms of rheumatoid arthritis: the effects on arthritis correlate with a reduction in antibodies to food antigens. *Rheumatology.* 2001;40:1175–1179.

26. Schnoll R, Burshteyn D, Cea-Aravena J. Nutrition in the treatment of attention-deficit hyperactivity disorder: a neglected but important aspect. *J Appl Psychophysiol Biofeedback.* 2003;28(1):63–75.

27. Stevenson J. Dietary influences on cognitive development and behaviour in children. *Proc Nutr Soc.* 2006;65:361–365.

28. Nora D, Volkow MD, Gene-Jack Wang MD, et al. Depressed dopamine activity in caudate and preliminary evidence of limbic involvement in adults with Attention-Deficit/Hyperactivity Disorder. *Arch Gen Psychiatry.* 2007;64(8):932–940.

29. Harding KL, Judah RD, Gant C. Outcome-based comparison of Ritalin versus food-supplement treated children with AD/HD. *Altern Med Rev.* 2003;8(3):319–330.

30. Kozielec T, Starobrat-Hermelin B. Assessment of magnesium levels in children with attention deficit hyperactivity disorder (ADHD). *Magnesium Res.* 1997;10:143–148.

31. Toren P, et al. Zinc deficiency in attention deficit hyperactivity disorder. *Bio Psychiatry.* 1996;40:1308–1310.

CHAPTER 5

Food Allergy Testing

When it comes to food allergy testing the many techniques and immune considerations often lead to confusion. Testing methods include enzyme-linked immunosorbent assay (ELISA), radioallergosobent test (RAST), skin-prick testing, EAV/VEGA testing, blood-type testing, and Carroll Food Intolerance Testing. Specific immune approaches include but are not limited to IgE, IgG, IgM, and IgA. The latter tests measure different aspects of immune responsiveness to particular allergens. For example:

- IgE—Testing measures immediate or anaphylactic responses associated with the most commonly appreciated emergency-type reactions, hives, asthma, and so on.
- IgG—Testing measures more long-term responses that are activated by proinflammatory cytokines. Reactions to this type of response are varied, and research is still being done to better understand this type of reaction.
- IgM—This type of reaction is seen mainly in primary infections. IgM reactions in the body tend to be in response to an infectious pathogen rather than an allergic response.
- Serum IgA—This immunoglobulin mainly functions as a second line of defense mediating elimination of pathogens that have breached the mucosal surface.[1]
- Secretory IgA (sIgA)—Levels of this immunoglobulin mark the state of health of mucosa. Its function is to exclude potential pathogens and allergens from entering the body.[2] Low levels of sIgA have been correlated with inflammatory diseases, such as celiac disease and ankylosing spondylitis.

A wide spectrum of adverse reactions may occur from ingestion of food or beverage. These include such symptoms as irritability, poor appetite, constipation or loose stools, or chronic upper respiratory congestion. The double-blind, placebo-controlled trial has been considered the gold standard in the diagnosis of food hypersensitivity. This means a patient would go on an elimination diet and would challenge foods at specific times. This method of evaluation, however, is typically not realistic for clinicians. The effectiveness of an open dietary elimination and challenge is usually poor because of the time-consuming nature of the procedure and poor patient compliance. The clinician must use other tools to evaluate the potential for food allergy.

There remains great debate in the medical community as to what the real gold standard should be for the evaluation of allergies. When it comes to environmental allergies many still believe the skin-prick test is the best approach. It has been the leading approach used by the allopathic medical community. Yet in clinical practice this test can sometimes miss allergic burdens contributed via other immunological pathways, as this test only looks for IgE-mediated allergic responses to foods. Delayed hypersensitivities can also cause symptoms severe enough to be considered an IgE reaction; however, when tested in this manner, the results often leave the patients thinking it's all in their head.

For clinicians, taking a thorough medical history and performing a thorough physical exam help in the diagnosis of food allergies; It is also important to use such tests as skin-prick testing, ELISA, and non–IgE-mediated allergy testing to distinguish between the different reactions the body is having from the different foods ingested on a daily basis. Clinicians are faced with many choices regarding the diagnosis of a patient's symptoms; therefore, it is important to use the tools available wisely in order to help the patient feel better about appropriate treatment, which can only be arrived at with the judicious use of testing.

Although the medical history and physical examination are the mainstay for diagnosis, corroborating evidence can come from skin testing or from a test for circulating IgE antibodies such as ELISA. Testing for non–IgE-mediated food allergies, where possible, through serum or skin can prove essential in distinguishing allergic reaction due to late-phase IgE and delayed reaction from a non–IgE-mediated food allergy such as types II, III or IV Gell and Coombs immunologic reactions. The onset of symptoms may overlap to a degree. Both may manifest some hours after exposure to the food allergen. Symptoms of non–IgE-mediated allergy can be quite variable in their time of onset and may not occur for 24 hours or more and persist for days involving any organ system. Late-phase IgE, on the other hand, may persist for 24 to 48 hours, and symptoms are primarily localized to the skin, nose, and lungs. Reoccurring late-phase IgE reactions, non-IgE delayed reactions, or a mixture of both confounded by complaints of symptoms that are not well defined, symptoms that do not obviously have a possible food allergic component, or a history that does not reveal a culpable food can create a clouded picture for the clinician.

IgE ALLERGY EVALUATION

It is well established in the medical literature that IgE (type I) hypersensitivity is often inherited, but it does not manifest the same in all family members. The risk of a child developing a type I hypersensitivity is 40 to 60 percent if both parents have a type I hypersensitivity, compared with a 5 to 10 percent risk if neither parent is atopic (type I hypersensitivity).[3] How can we tell whether we are dealing with a type I hypersensitivity? The following are general guidelines; however, as stated previously, other types of allergic reactions can manifest similarly:

- Reaction is usually immediate, from 15 to 30 minutes after exposure to the allergen. A delayed reaction may occur 10 to 12 hours afterwards and lasts generally for 24 to 48 hours.
- Reaction is usually precipitated by a *minimal* amount of food that is usually eaten infrequently.
- Reaction is persistent irrespective of the frequency or dose of allergen exposure.
- Reaction increases in intensity and rapidity with each subsequent exposure.
- Because of the immediate and explosive nature of the reaction to a food that is eaten infrequently, the cause is usually self-evident.
- Diagnostic testing includes identification of allergen-specific IgE antibodies via in vivo or in vitro methods.

Symptoms of an IgE-associated allergy may be localized or generalized in many organ systems, such as the cardiovascular system, respiratory tract, skin, gastrointestinal system, or central nervous system. Examples of this type of reaction may be mild to severe and include the following:

- Angioedema—Rapid swelling of a body part under the skin, rather than on the surface. When food is the culprit, the tongue, throat, and lips generally become extremely swollen.
- Asthma—Narrowing of the bronchial passages, which make breathing very difficult during an episode.
- Wheezing—Another pulmonary symptom, similar to asthma though not as severe. There may be shortness of breath and a definitive wheezing sound when breathing in or out.
- Rhinoconjunctivitis—Inflammation of the nose and the eyes, which generally results in weepy eyes and runny nose.
- Urticaria—Generalized itching over a part of the body or over the entire body. The skin can form welts in affected parts.
- Acute gastrointestinal distress—Diarrhea, nausea, vomiting, abdominal pain; these reactions are more rare than the rest.

- Oral allergy syndrome (OAS)—Discussed in more detail later. OAS is generally attributable to cross-reactivity between food antigens and environmental (pollen usually) antigens. The reactions are similar to systemic anaphylaxis but vary in degree of intensity.
- Systemic anaphylaxis—This is the most severe reaction that can be elicited from an IgE allergic reaction. It is a life-threatening event that will occur within minutes from contact. Initial symptoms include itching of the lips, tongue, and mouth followed by skin itching, angioedema, flushing, airway obstruction, and fainting. This type of reaction often requires the use of epinephrine (usually in the form of EpiPens) to subdue the allergic reaction and stabilize the patient.

The incidence of anaphylactic symptoms is as follows[4]:

Anaphylactic Symptom	Incidence
Skin reactions	90%
Urticaria, angioedema	85–90%
Upper airway edema	50–60%
Respiratory reactions	40–60%
Flushing	45–55%
Difficult or labored breathing, wheezing	45–50%
Syncope, dizziness, hypotension	30–35%
Gastrointestinal reactions: Nausea, vomiting, diarrhea, pain	25–30%
Headache	5–8%
Chest pain	4–6%
Seizure	1–2%

Foods that are most associated with severe IgE-mediated reactions are somewhat different in children than adults. Although peanuts, tree nuts (walnuts, pecans, and so on), milk, and eggs are the usual culprits in children, fish, shellfish (shrimp, lobster, crab, scallops, oyster), and peanuts are the usual offenders in adults in the United States. Other foods that are known to induce IgE-mediated reactions include some fruit (kiwi) and seeds (cottonseed, sesame, psyllium).

A single anaphylactic event is sufficient to diagnose an IgE reaction of this magnitude and no further testing is necessary nor medically indicated. If skin test is considered to officially diagnose an IgE allergy, it must be done under the supervision of an experienced physician with the appropriate rescue equipment and medication.[5] Complete avoidance of the allergen and education regarding exposure is indicated for this type of allergy.

Among the IgE reactions, OAS is a common immediate allergy in adults. Four distinguishing features of OAS that are commonly reported among patients include the following:

1. Reactions mainly from fresh or raw fruits and/or vegetables and spices, but shellfish, fish, and eggs may be play a role in triggering this event.[6]
2. Symptoms occur immediately after eating the raw food. The patient usually identifies a causative relationship and subsequently avoids the food. There is a common observation that cooked or canned varieties of the inciting food do not elicit symptoms.
3. Symptoms of OAS are generally confined to the head and neck, occur within minutes after contact with the food, and resolve fairly rapidly. Symptoms include itching/tingling and angioedema of the lips, mouth, tongue, and throat; itching and watering eyes; nasal congestion; sneezing; and throat tightness but not upper respiratory obstruction. Abdominal pain, nausea, vomiting, and diarrhea may result from swallowing the inciting food. Anaphylaxis may occur in about two percent of affected individuals.
4. Generally, individuals affected have a personal and family history of atopic symptoms: hay fever, asthma, eczema, urticaria, or allergic rhinitis. There is a frequent association between pollen allergy and this syndrome.[7]

OAS is caused by cross-reactivity between certain proteins found in the raw food and pollens due to shared allergenic epitopes—regions that can bind to antibodies to create an immune reaction. For example many patients with birch pollen allergy report oral allergy symptoms from eating fresh apples. The major birch pollen allergen Bet v 1 is very similar to that of the apple allergen Mal d 1. In a person with allergies, IgE antibodies synthesized and bound to mast cells in response to pollen exposure may bind to a similar antigen from a raw fruit or vegetable that is botanically related, as in the case of birch pollen and apples. It is thought that sensitization first occurs to the pollen aeroallergen, which leads to the production of pollen-specific IgE antibodies that cross-react to various botanically related fruit and vegetable antigens that in turn produce symptoms of OAS. Clusters of botanically related fruits, vegetables, and pollens that have been implicated in OAS are listed in the table:[8]

Pollen Allergy	Associated Foods in Oral Allergy Syndrome
Ragweed	Melons (cantaloupe, watermelon, honeydew), banana, cucumbers, zucchini
Birch	Apple, almond, apricot, carrot, celery, cherry, fennel, hazelnut, kiwi, nectarine, parsley, parsnip, peach, pear, potato, plum, prune, walnut
Mugwort	Melons, apple, celery, carrot, coriander, fennel, pepper
Grasses	Tomato, melons, fennel, celery, kiwi

Diagnosis of OAS is supported by a history of seasonal allergies. The prick-prick skin test remains a simple method of choice in the allergy work up. The skin-testing lancet is first pricked into the flesh of the incriminating raw fruit or vegetable and then immediately pricked onto the patient's skin, usually on the forearm so any redness and swelling can be easily seen. Treatment involves avoiding trigger and cross-reactive foods. Because of the small possibility for a severe reaction, many patients are prescribed an epinephrine pen with instruction on its use. Immunotherapy remains a possibility as reported by some studies.[9]

Types of IgE Symptoms

Symptoms of the upper and lower airways (rhinoconjunctivitis, laryngeal edema, bronchospasm), cutaneous reactions (urticaria, angioedema), and/or gastrointestinal symptoms (postprandial nausea, abdominal pain, vomiting, and diarrhea) can be part of an IgE-mediated systemic allergy as in anaphylaxis, or can present only on the exposed body part without other IgE-mediated symptoms. Acute skin reactions are among the most common IgE allergy manifestations. Topical contact with an allergen can result in urticaria and angioedema.[10] Shellfish, raw meats, raw fruits and vegetables, milk, and eggs, for example, have been implicated in these circumstances.

Chronic urticaria and angioedema, which relate to symptoms lasting longer than six weeks, is rarely attributable to IgE allergy and will seldom cause or trigger atopic dermatitis in adults. On the other hand, IgE-mediated food allergy has been implicated in about one-third of children with atopic dermatitis. Food allergies can play an integral role in the development of atopic dermatitis in children. Generally, children with atopic dermatitis develop red and itchy lesions as early as three months old. These lesions most often affect the scalp, cheeks, and ears. The rash may evolve into eczematous and crusty lesions around the eyes, at the bend of the wrist and elbow, behind the knees, and on the hands and feet. Early exposure to ingested food allergens in children who are at high risk for atopy will increase their risk of developing atopic dermatitis in the future. The most common food allergens in children include milk, egg, wheat, soy, peanut, and fish according to double-blind, placebo-controlled food challenge.[11] Typical symptoms of allergy to these foods can include diarrhea, bloody stools, or other gastrointestinal disturbances and/or eczema.

IgE food allergies are not the main type of food allergy found in the U.S. population. However, even though the symptoms are easily recognized and attributed to a particular food, a person with allergies may suffer from chronic illnesses such as asthma, migraines, or gastrointestinal complaints, which can obscure the immediate nature of IgE food allergies. When a patient consumes a mixed diet, no one food can be identified as the culprit without further testing. Oftentimes, more than one offending food is responsible for a patient's symptom picture. In this case, a low-grade, chronic IgE symptomatology can be involved.[12]

IgG ALLERGY EVALUATION

Although not absolutely characterized, delayed food reactions are mixed immune reactions; they tend to be classified as hypersensitivities types II, III or IV and involve other classes of antibodies, such as IgG. Distinguishing features of these immune reactions include the following:

- Reaction is delayed. Symptoms may occur several hours to days after the inciting food is ingested and may persist after the food is omitted.
- The more often a food is eaten the less it is tolerated. Symptoms are triggered by foods that are consumed frequently and eaten liberally.
- Symptoms are chronic or recurrent and may involve many organ systems. Many affected persons develop symptoms not usually associated with a food allergy.
- A temporal relationship between the inciting food and the symptoms produced does not exist. As such, a relationship between the food and reaction is rarely suspected.

As discussed in Chapter 1, ELISA IgG allergy testing is now a reliable and accurate method of testing delayed hypersensitive reactions. Because IgG antibodies remain in circulation for long periods of time (months), they can cause more damage in the long term through inflammatory reactions in the body. The reactions can occur anywhere and everywhere in the body, and symptoms tend to worsen over time if the offending foods are not removed and steps are not taken to heal the permeability of the gut. Remember that due to the gradual accumulation of symptoms, the body is much affected like a frog in a pot of warming water. Before it knows it's dying, it's already dead. Fortunately, an ELISA IgG Food Antibody Assessment Panel can serve as a tool to "turn off the heat" for our body and allow us to regain our health.

IgG Food Antibody Assessment Panels present a great advantage to our health here. Numerous studies have shown that eliminating foods decreases the amounts of food-specific IgG concentrations in the blood. For example, in a single-blind prospective study, 22 children (aged 3 to 14 years) suffering from asthma were divided into two groups, one in which either dairy and eggs were eliminated from their die or another in which subjects consumed their normal diets. After eight weeks, the children on the elimination diet had greater peak expiratory flow rate (22 percent better). The control group remained unchanged. Scientists also noted that food-specific IgG concentrations decreased in the children who eliminated eggs and dairy and their overall well-being improved.[13]

The exact mechanisms by which IgG antibodies are produced against dietary antigens has not been yet studied in full; however, it is speculated that intestinal permeability and intestinal inflammation play a role in the formation of IgG food allergies.

One aspect of IgG testing that has been greatly debated is the variability in test results. Currently, some labs will only test one type of IgG, whereas others will test all four subtypes of IgG antibodies. Because of this difference in testing, results from one lab cannot be compared to results from another lab. It is important to find a lab that will test all four IgG subtypes to obtain the most accurate IgG food-allergy test results. Ideally, your personal health care provider will order this testing as part of your workup to identify if you are indeed fueling your body optimally, if you wish to pursue this testing directly as a consumer, CP Medical is a professional company that offers the test directly to consumers (www.CPMedical.net, pin No. 587556). When you get your results for the 96 foods tested, make sure to discuss the results with your health care provider.

Types of IgG Symptoms

Because IgG delayed food hypersensitivity reactions have only recently been studied, the types of symptoms attributed to IgG reactions are varied and mostly based on what clinicians see as their patients improve when they eliminate IgG-reactive foods from their diets. Refer to chapter 4, which has a comprehensive list of symptoms that have been correlated to IgG food allergies.

IgA EVALUATION

So where does IgA come into play with all these tests? First, it must be clarified that IgA exists both in the mucosal barriers of the body—where it is most prevalent—as well as in the blood. The results for each type of IgA mean different things, so it is important to know what is being tested and the implications of each test. Serum IgA responses in the body were discussed in chapter 4; however, secretory IgA (sIgA) and its role in food allergies remains to be discussed.

Secretory IgA is an antibody that is found in the saliva and throughout the gastrointestinal tract; it is not destroyed by enzymes in the gastrointestinal tract. Unlike the other immunoglobulins, the function of sIgA is to suppress immune response. Research has shown that when there is a deficiency of sIgA, there is a greater incidence of serum antibodies to food allergens.[14] In the case of sIgA, the greater the number, the better—it is equivalent to a highly functioning gastrointestinal immunity. Where there are low levels of sIgA, then, it is more likely that antigens will actually penetrate the gastrointestinal lining and produce an inflammatory immune response to that food. When we are born, our first exposure to sIgA is from breast milk, which is prophylactic against allergies and is thought to be protective throughout adulthood.[15] Exclusive and prolonged breast-feeding of at least 6 months is highly recommended both by the American Academy of Pediatrics and the European Society for Pediatric Allergology and Clinical Immunology/European Society for Pediatric Gastroenterology, Hepatology, and Nutrition for food allergy prevention.[16] Breast milk supplies a number of natural factors that supplement the infant's physiologically immature and developing immune system of the gastrointestinal tract. It transfers protective sIgA antibodies to the baby for first-line mucosal immune defense. As previously mentioned, sIgA acts by immune exclusion, inhibiting intestinal absorption of potentially allergenic food antigens and infectious agents. A wide variety of bacterial and viral agents found in the respiratory and intestinal tract are recognized by sIgA antibodies, including *Escherichia coli*, *Streptococcus pneumoniae*, *Clostridium difficile*, *Salmonella*, *Rotavirus*, influenza virus, and the yeastlike *Candida albicans*.[17] The repertoire of sIgA antibodies specific for various antigens is derived from the microorganisms to which the mother is and has been exposed to. Specific antigen-triggered B cells from the mother's small intestine and respiratory tract migrate directly to the mammary glands of the breast where they differentiate into IgA-synthesizing plasma cells with sIgA secreted into the breast milk to be delivered to baby at feeding. Breast milk contains a multitude of components: oligosaccharides, lactoferrin, lysozyme, and nucleotides, which enhance the growth of beneficial microflora, and *Lactobacillus* and *Bifidobacterium*, which are known for their healthful immune-modulating effects. Because the sIgA immunity does not fully mature until the age of four, the initial inoculation of sIgA antibodies through breast milk is the first step toward decreasing the likelihood that a person will develop food allergies late in life. It is thought that during these four years, the immune system in the gastrointestinal tract is primed for later years. This way, all of the exposure within the first four years will form the necessary IgA antibodies in the gastrointestinal tract so that these antigens are always caught before they enter the bloodstream.[18]

Secretory IgA is what gives us the ability to eat a foreign substance without eliciting an immune response from the body. Because the gastrointestinal system is always directly exposed to the external environment—bacteria, food, and viruses—its function then revolves around forming a type of barrier on the mucosa so that these antigens, viruses, and bacteria basically slide through the gastrointestinal tract as inertly as possible. Intestinal permeability comes into play here as well, for the integrity of the gastrointestinal tract is first and foremost in providing a strong physical barrier against allergens and microorganisms. Second, the gastrointestinal tract is lined with organized and disorganized lymphoid tissue from which sIgA is secreted. Secretory IgA is different from other antibodies because it does not bind to a complement to begin an inflammatory process, but rather, it inhibits microorganisms from attaching to the intestinal mucosa. Secretory IgA also traps antigens in a mucus layer, which then makes it easier for the body to remove it.

Maintaining healthy bowel habits and ensuring a healthy flora in the gastrointestinal tract promotes sIgA. People's current exposure to antibiotics, synthetic foods, and food that isn't digest well disturbs the balance of the intestinal flora and sIgA levels drop. Finding those foods to which you are reactive and eliminating them from your diet is the first step to gastrointestinal and overall health. Eliminating these foods greatly decreases inflammation in the body and allows the gastrointestinal tract to heal and begin functioning optimally.

ALTERNATIVE TESTS

Following are several tests that are not part of the conventional group of tests run to determine reactions to food; however, many people—both patients and alternative practitioners—find that they offer additional insights into a person's dietary needs, especially when it comes to food combinations, and additional information to supplement standard and routine testing. These were also discussed in some detail in chapter 3.

EAV/VEGA—Skin resistivity is tested against a series of foods. When a food does not respond well, skin resistivity changes. This method identifies food the body is sensitive to—there is no allergic component or a genetic component. This method has had high correlation with IgG food-allergy tests.

Carroll Food Intolerance Test—This test looks at what types of foods (e.g., sugar, grain, fruit, dairy) a person genetically lacks the enzymes to digest well. It also gives food combinations (e.g., fruit with sugar) a person does not digest well. This method has been successful in helping people decrease their levels of inflammation. It is often used in conjunction with IgG Food Antibody Assessment Panels, and practitioners find that some food allergies resolve once these intolerances are removed from the diet.

Coca pulse test—The Coca pulse test measures the reaction of the autonomic nervous system to the stress of a food. It detects functional changes in the body after ingesting a particular food. After ingesting a small quantity of a particular food, if the pulse rises more than four beats per minute, it is considered to be a reaction to that particular food. A rise in pulse indicates that this food is a stressor to the nervous system.

IgG delayed test—In my clinical practice, many patients have already received the classical IgE skin test and some have also had a RAST test for IgE antibodies. Yet, occasionally, a progressive doctor, usually an allergist, has also done a few IgG tests for foods specifically. By the time patients have received their results, incorporated the knowledge gleaned from these tests, and put them into practice, they are feeling somewhat better. Yet they still have allergic burdens to be identified and explored. I attribute this in part to the narrow testing range of the items explored, so in our clinical practice, we will use IgG, IgE, and IgA testing that looks at approximately 100 foods, then we do additional testing for common herbals, spices, and environmental allergens. This type of testing is more complete, as it includes a more comprehensive testing of immunological responses to foods and environmental allergens commonly found in our environment. A patient can order an IgG delayed test at www.CPMedical.net and can gain access with the following pin No. 587556.

Many of my patients have benefitted from more comprehensive testing. Usually, they have already tried many therapies, some of which have brought relief but not resolution to their problem. For example, one patient came in with difficulty falling asleep. She had always considered herself to be a light sleeper; however, when an IgG Food Antibody Assessment Panel was done and she removed the offending foods, within a month's time she noticed an improvement in her sleep pattern. Before removing the offending foods, she had trouble falling asleep, would wake throughout the night, and would have trouble falling back asleep. After removing the offending foods, she had no difficulty falling asleep and was able to sleep through the night. She also lost weight that she had not been able to lose since the birth of her two-year-old child.

Another patient was a previously hyperactive child who had been diagnosed with attention-deficit hyperactivity disorder and was considered a problem at school. His family took him to a holistic physician where an IgG Food Antibody Assessment Panel was preformed. The child's IgG Food Antibody Assessment Panel report revealed significant elevated antibody levels to dairy, egg, gluten, wheat, and some fruits and vegetables. Within two weeks of following the customized elimination and rotation diet guideline, his behavior dramatically improved. He now engages in constructive and directed play and pays attention in school. His appearance has also changed in a positive way.

As evidenced by these patients, symptoms of food allergies, particularly delayed sensitivities, vary widely. Conventional medical doctors frequently treat the symptoms without considering the possible causes; patients are simply given medicine to keep the symptoms in check. However, I find that the symptoms become worse over time if the underlying cause is not addressed. This leads to more medications and stronger medications to control the symptoms, yet the symptoms are actually the body's attempts to communicate with you. Patients become more and more dependent on medications. I have found that removing the cause of the symptoms can make a world of difference. My patients have often been able to stop many symptom-targeted medications as well as supplements they used to manage food allergy symptoms. The patients gain more control over their health, which makes a lasting and profound change in their well-being.

Along with food allergy information, I find that patients also do well following a general guideline of foods that suit their genetic footprint better. Everyone is born with the inherent ability to produce certain enzymes to digest food. People of different genetic backgrounds digest foods differently. Just as some people have predisposing factors for certain diseases, some people do better with certain foods than others. This is why the more information we have about how our body responds to foods, the better we are able to provide our body with the optimal fuel for growth and regeneration.

One of the better known diets is the D'Adamo Eat Right for Your Type diet, which is also called the Blood Type Diet. This particular diet is based on how certain blood types react to particular types of foods. Diets such as these can be the foundation of our daily food choices, which are then further informed by such tests as the ELISA IgG food panel, EAV, and Carroll Food Testing. These tests further individualize the foods that work best for your particular genetic makeup. Additional information about this test is also discussed in chapter 3.

EAT RIGHT FOR YOUR TYPE DIET

D'Adamo has defined four types of basic dietary needs based on your ABO blood type, which include:

- Type O: high-protein foods, especially deep ocean fish and sea vegetables such as kelp; large amounts of fresh, organically raised vegetables and some fruits.
- Type A: vegetables and vegetable oils, deep ocean seafood, legumes (beans and peas), grains, and fruits (especially pineapple).
- Type B: high-protein foods, especially deep ocean fish, along with a moderate amount of dairy and eggs; most grains and legumes (beans and peas) and large amounts of fresh, organically raised green vegetables and fruits.
- Type AB: high-protein foods, especially deep ocean fish and vegetables (kelp); dairy, most grains, legumes (beans and peas), and large amounts of fresh, organically raised vegetables and fruits, and fermented soy products.

  - Within these groups there is also a subgroup of blood types according to the Lewis method of secretors and nonsecretors: Secretors make greater amounts of sIgA than nonsecretors. Secretory IgA is one of the first immune barriers in the gastrointestinal tract, respiratory tract, and genitourinary tract. Therefore, it is genetically more advantageous to have high levels of sIgA for greater protection against foreign matter trying to make its way into the bloodstream.

Another important concept within the D'Adamo diet is the lectin concept. Lectins are a type of protein molecules in foods, particularly grains, beans, and seeds, and they are able to bind with sugar molecules on the cells that make up the body.[19] The immune system is not involved in this particular reaction; thus, it cannot be measured by IgG Food Antibody Assessment Panels. Lectins are thought to influence inflammatory disorders such as weight gain and rheumatoid arthritis by causing the cells to—in effect—become sticky, or agglutinated. The agglutination process builds up in particular parts of the body, depending on the particular affinity of the lectin to a sugar portion of the cells.

Lectins are not broken down by stomach acid or protein-digesting enzymes. Many microorganisms make use of these lectins to attach themselves to their cell host. The human body also uses lectins to trap foreign matter and to expose them more efficiently so that the immune system may mount an inflammatory response against them. Each and every lectin is unique to a particular binding site. What they have in common is that they all bind to the sugar containing part of molecules that are on cell membranes.

Many of the lectins found in food bind to cell receptors that line the gastrointestinal tract. When these lectins bind with the cells, the end result is inflammation. For example, gliadin, a component of wheat gluten, activates acute inflammation, which can then result in inflammatory bowel disease as well as infectious or autoimmune diseases.[20] Dietary lectins also increase polyamine levels in the gastrointestinal tract, which can lead to bad breath damage to intestinal villi (which then leads to malabsorption) and may contribute to colon precancerous states.[21] Lectins do not affect everyone in the same manner. The action of lectins in the body largely depends on your genetic makeup. The concept is similar to why a person who smokes his or her entire life and never develops lung cancer while the smoker's partner develops the disease from the secondhand smoke. Everyone has antibodies to certain dietary lectins that are genetically determined, and each one of these types of antibodies will cause reactions in different places in the body.

Two good examples are rheumatoid arthritis and weight management. Lectins have a particularly high affinity for glycoprotein-rich connective tissue and proteoglycans in the skin. When lectins attach to these cells, the result is a stiffening and inflammation of joints. Studies have also shown that lectins can play a role in weight management. Certain receptors in fat cells see lectins as if they were insulin and react by forming more fat. Wheat germ agglutinin is known to cause fat cells to make more fat, and because it is not really a hormone, the body never tells the cell when to stop.[22] It makes sense then that carbohydrate-based diets do not work on a permanent basis. In the case of weight management, lectins play a double role—that of making more fat in fat cells and of increasing inflammation, which also increases weight by increasing water retention in the body.

Along with lectin awareness, testing for celiac disease is indicated even if other tests do not indicate a sensitivity or immune response to gluten/gliadin. In the United States, 1 in 133 people are thought to be affected with gluten-sensitive enteropathy[23] (celiac disease). Because of the varied nature of the symptoms, this disorder is frequently missed or is not diagnosed for many years. Celiac disease test panels test for anti-tTG (antitissue transglutaminase), IgA and IgG antibodies, total IgA, and antigliadin antibodies (IgG). The table shows the conditions that suggest a diagnosis of celiac disease:

Anti-tTG Antibodies, IgA	Total IgA	Anti-tTG Antibodies, IgG	Antigliadin Antibodies (AGA), IgG	Diagnosis
+	+			Presumptive celiac disease
–	+	–	–	Symptoms not likely due to celiac disease
–	–	+	+	Possible celiac disease, false-negative anti-tTG, IgA due to total IgA deficiency

Total IgA is important because it tells us the general state of intestinal immunity. When it is below normal levels, it is assumed that the body will not be able to mount a significant response to gliadin/gluten and a negative anti-tTG cannot be considered a true negative. An intestinal biopsy usually follows a positive or equivocal test result. The biopsy is used to make a definitive diagnosis of celiac disease.

It may seem like a great feat to avoid all of the foods that can potentially make you sick. With all this information, it is easy to feel as if there is nothing that can be eaten comfortably and without worry. Although it is true that eating in a way that is optimal for *your* body requires some discipline and creativity, it is not impossible. Remember that the body's reaction largely depends on the state of inflammation in the body. In other words, if you ingest foods that increase the inflammation in the body, such as refined sugars, refined grains, synthetic foods, fried foods, sodas—and you do not exercise and you live in a very toxic environment—your level of inflammation will be great. Likewise, your reactivity to the food you consume and the environment in which you live will be tremendous. The more you avoid foods that are toxic to you, the healthier you will feel and the more active you can be. Increased activity increases your sense of well-being and decreases inflammatory by-products in the body. So, once in a while, if you decide to eat a piece of pie, the repercussions will not be so great. The more you do to keep your body free of inflammation, the more you create a healthy cycle—in other words, the more you do to stay healthier, the better you feel, the better your body works, and the more you want to do better for your body. Although it does take time and dedication to be mindful of what you put into your body, the end result is a healthier, more vital you. In the end, it becomes a balancing game—what is more important, your health or the momentary pleasure of eating something that makes you sick? There is a flip side of a healthy cycle—one that leads to further inflammation and breakdown, lack of vitality, and chronic disease. The choice is always in your hands.

NOTES

1. Woof J, Kerr M. IgA function—variations on a theme. *Immunology.* 2004;113:175–177.

2. Wines BD, Hogarth PM. IgA receptors in health and disease. *Tissue Antigens.* 2006;68(2):103–114.

3. Johansson SG, Hourihane JO, Bousquet J, et al. A revised nomenclature for allergy. *Allergy.* 2001;56:813–824.

4. Lieberman P, Kemp SF, Oppenheimer J, Lang DM, Bernstein IL, Nicklas RA, et al. The diagnosis and management of anaphylaxis: an updated practice parameter. *Am Acad Allergy Asthma Immunol.* 2005;115(suppl):S483–S523.

5. Lieberman P, et al. (2005). The diagnosis and management of anaphylaxis: an updated practice parameter. *American Academy of Allergy, Asthma and Immunology,* S483–S523.

6. Amlot PL, Kemeny DM, Zachary C, Parkes P, Lessof MH. Oral allergy syndrome (OAS): symptoms of IgE-mediated hypersensitivity to foods. *Clin Allergy.* 1987;17:33–42.

7. Ortolani C, Ispano M, Pastorello E, Bigi A, Ansaloni R. The oral allergy syndrome. *Ann Allergy*. 1988;61(6 Pt 2):47–52; Eriksson NE, Formgren H, Svenonius E. Food hypersensitivity in patients with pollen allergy. *Allergy*. 1982;37:437–443.

8. Sloane D, Sheffer A. Oral allergy syndrome. *Allergy Asthma Proc*. 2001;22:321–325; Gershwin ME, German JB, Keen CL, Foschi FG. Adverse reactions to foods. *Nutrition and Immunology: Principles and Practice*. Totowa, NJ: Humana Press; 2000:238.

9. Asero R. How long does the effect of birch pollen injection SIT on applied allergy last? *Allergy*. 2003;58:435–438; Bucher X, Pichler WJ, Dahinden CA, Helbling A. Effect of tree pollen specific, subcutaneous immunotherapy on the oral allergy syndrome to apple and hazelnut. *Allergy*. 2004;59:1272–1276.

10. Yoshiike T, Aikawa Y, Sindhavananda J, et al. Skin barrier defect in atopic dermatitis: increased permeability of the stratum corneum using dimethyl sulfoxide and theophylline. *J Dermatol Sci*. 1993;5:92–96.

11. Eigenmann PA, Sicherer SH, Borkowski TA, Cohen BA, Sampson HA. Prevalence of IgE-mediated food allergy among children with atopic dermatitis. *Pediatrics*. 1998;101:E8.

12. Fadal RG. *Introduction to Food Allergy and Other Adverse Reactions to Foods*. LabCorp Clinical Monograph from Resident & Staff Physician. New York: Romaine Pierson Publishers; 1988:1–10.

13. Yusoff NA, Hampton SM, Dickerson JW, Morgan JB. The effects of exclusion of dietary egg and milk in the management of asthmatic children: a pilot study. *J Royal Soc Health*. 2004;124(2):74–80.

14. Mayer L. Mucosal immunity. *Pediatrics*. 2003;111(6 Pt 3):1595–1600.

15. Saarinen UM, Kajosaari M. Breastfeeding as prophylaxis against atopic disease: prospective follow-up study until 17 years old. *Lancet*. 1995;346:1065–1069.

16. Zeiger R. Food allergen avoidance in the prevention of food allergy in infants and children. *Pediatrics*. 2003;111:1662–1671.

17. Goldman AS. The immune system of human milk: antimicrobial, anti-inflammatory, and immunomodulating properties. *Pediatr Infect Dis J*. 1993;12:664–672.

18. Takasugi M, Sugano M, Yamada K. Measurement of total and food component-specific IgA in human saliva. *Food Sci Technol Res*. 2002;8:273–275.

19. Braun J, Sieper J. Rheumatologic manifestations of gastrointestinal disorders. *Curr Opin Rheumatol*. 1999;11:68–74.

20. Jones DS, ed. *Textbook of Functional Medicine*. Gig Harbor, WA: The Institute for Functional Medicine; 2005:30.

21. Luk GD, Desai TK, Conteas CN, Moshier JA, Silverman AL. Biochemical markers in colorectal cancer: diagnostic and therapeutic implications. *Gastroenterol Clin North Am*. 1988;17:931–940.

22. Ponzio G, Debant A, Contreras JO, Rossi B. Wheat germ agglutinin mimics metabolic effects of insulin without increasing receptor autophosphorylation. *Cell Signal*. 1990;2:377–386; Shechter Y. Bound lectins that mimic insulin produce persistent insulin-like activities. *Endocrinology*. 1983;113:1921–1926.

23. Celiac disease test. 2007. Lab Tests Online. Available at: http://www.labtestsonline.org/understanding/analytes/celiac_disease/test.html. Accessed March 21, 2009.

CHAPTER 6

Eat Well and Prosper

A great deal of dietary advice is available today. However, the one concept that is frequently overlooked is that each person is unique. A food that is a good choice for your neighbor may not be a good choice for you, and vice versa. Additionally, it is important for everyone to assess why they eat what they are currently eating. We must eat to live, not live to eat. The purpose of eating is health and wellness, and eating with intention is the only way to accomplish this goal.

Designing a healthful diet for patients can sometimes prove difficult. Testing is available to assess which foods may be an individual's unique allergen or sensitivity offenders to help with specific dietary plans. In clinical practice, I find the 96 IgG Food Antibody Assessment Panel the most important tool. It measures both IgG and IgE antibodies, unlike many of the traditional food allergy tests, which only measure IgE antibodies. IgE allergy reactions are fairly easy to recognize as they often have immediate and observable reactions. The IgG reactions, however, are generally more gradual reactions, thus making them more difficult to recognize without proper testing. IgG reactions can take up to 72 hours to develop. The 96-food sensitivity test uses enzyme-linked immunosorbent assay (ELISA) methodology. A patient's serum sample is added to a plate coated with purified food proteins and glycoproteins. If there are antibodies to any of the specific food or inhalant proteins in the patient's serum, a binding reaction will occur. The degree of antibody-antigen binding is dependent on the concentration of antibodies present in the patient's serum, so this is what is measured.

Food allergies can present with a wide variety of symptoms. Commonly attributed symptoms seen in type I hypersensitivity reactions include swelling of the mucous membranes and throat, constriction of smooth muscle in the lungs, hives and itching, redness, and rash. Delayed-type hypersensitivity reactions may manifest as diarrhea, constipation, spastic colon, itchy or red anus, gas, bloating, nausea, fatigue, and rash. Other symptoms attributed to food reactions are joint pain, headaches, and difficulty concentrating.

THE GASTROINTESTINAL SYSTEM AND ALLERGIES

The gastrointestinal system plays a critical role in the development of food allergies, as approximately 70 percent of the immune system is located in the digestive tract. In the stomach and small intestines, gastric acid and digestive enzymes, such as pepsin, amylase, lipase, and protease, break down food to absorbable molecules. Ideally, the stomach and intestines act as a semipermeable barrier, only allowing desirable molecules into the blood stream. However, when the intestines are affected by infection, inflammation, or malabsorption, the barrier function is compromised. This allows molecules usually too large to pass through the intestinal wall to pass into the bloodstream. This may lead to sensitization to food proteins as the immune system responds to these abnormally large molecules as antigens.

Other causes of increased intestinal permeability include inadequate levels of beneficial bacteria in the intestines and the presence of parasites, which lead to inflammation of the intestinal lining. Beneficial gut microflora, also known as probiotics, provide numerous functions in the intestines. Probiotics such as *Lactobacillus acidophilus* and *Bifidobacterium bifidum* assist in the absorption of nutrients, help maintain the intestinal barrier, compete with pathogenic bacteria and yeast, and can produce some vitamins. Adequate levels of microflora can be adversely affected by antibiotics, medications, diarrhea, constipation, chemotherapy, radiation, and poor diet. Additionally, hydrochloric acid is required in the stomach to maintain the gastric pH of 3. This extremely acidic environment is necessary to eliminate pathogenic bacteria and yeast. Gastric acid also activates the pancreatic digestive enzymes to continue with the proper breakdown of food. These enzymes are required for food to be broken down into smaller molecules. Inadequate levels of hydrochloric acid and active digestive enzymes can allow large molecules to be absorbed, which contributes to the sensitization seen in food allergies.

DIET AND ALLERGIES

The standard American diet is problematic. Various dietary regimens are recommended by practitioners, whether it is called the ancestral diet, the blood-type diet, or others. These diets have one thing in common: eating with intention and planning healthful, nutrition-rich meals. The standard American diet consists mainly of foods devoid of nutrients and endogenous enzymes. Americans also tend to eat the same few foods on a daily basis, increasing the likelihood of developing food allergies to those foods. A potato is a potato regardless of whether it is mashed, french fried, au gratin, scalloped, or hash browned. Likewise, whether dairy products are in the form of cheese, ice cream, whipping cream, or yogurt they are all typically derived from cow's milk. It is also imperative to drink adequate amounts of purified water, to flush out endogenous and exogenous toxins and undesirable chemicals from the body.

Additionally, most Americans do not eat enough fruits and vegetables. According to the National Health and Nutrition Examination Survey's (NHANES) 19th session in the second series of assessments of Healthy People 2010, most Americans do not eat the United States Department of Agriculture (USDA) recommended intake of at least two servings of fruit and at least three servings of vegtables per day. In 1988–1994, an estimated 27 percent of adults met the USDA guidelines for fruit and 35 percent met the guidelines for vegetables. In 1999–2002, 28 percent of adults met the guideline for fruit and 32 percent of adults met the vegetable guidelines, showing a significant decrease in vegetable consumption over time. In addition, only 11 percent of adults met the USDA guidelines for both fruits and vegetables in 1988–1994 and 1999–2002.[1] Methods of agriculture contribute to the problem: at least 60 percent of cultivated soils have growth-limiting problems with mineral-nutrient deficiencies and toxicities, and about 50 percent of the world population suffers from micronutrient deficiencies due to poor soil fertility, low levels of available mineral nutrients in soil, and improper nutrient management.[2]

A diversified diet is important to limit repeated exposure to the same potentially allergenic proteins and to ensure intake of the essential nutrients. I recommend the 3–2–1+1 diet to my patients, which promotes eating foods in a ratio of 3 vegetables + 2 fresh fruits + 1 multigrain + 1 protein as many times a day as needed. A diversified diet is also important to minimize cross-reactivity, which is when the immune system responds to proteins with similar structure or partial similarities rather than to specific antigens. Many pollens and foods will cause cross-reactions. Commonly reported cross-reactions include ragweed pollen allergies with melons and bananas; birch pollen with apples, carrots, hazelnuts, potato, pear, plum, nectarine, cherry, apricot, and almonds; mugwort pollen with celery, apple, and kiwi; latex with bananas, kiwi, avocado, chestnuts, and chickpeas[3]; Brassicaceae family with nuts, legumes, corn, and Rosaceae fruit[4]; and shellfish with other types of shellfish and dust mites.[5]

Organic Food

Eating organic foods, when possible, is important for overall health. Not only are organic foods free from pesticides and synthetic food additives, but they are also higher in nutritional value and are not genetically modified. Studies have shown that foods grown organically have higher levels of nutrients such as vitamins, minerals, and flavonoids. For example, one study showed that the levels of quercetin and kaempferol were 79 percent and 97 percent higher, respectively, in organic tomatoes compared with conventionally grown tomatoes.[6] Another study showed that organically grown blueberries were significantly higher in beneficial constituents compared with conventionally grown blueberries; they had higher levels of fructose and glucose sugars, malic acid, total phenolics, total anthocyanins, and higher antioxidant activity.[7]

Intake of food additives such as monosodium glutamate, sulfites, azo-dyes (tartrazine, sunset yellow, azorubin, amarant, cochineal red), benzoates, sorbates, butylated hydroxyanisole/butylated hydroxytoluene (BHA/BHT), and parabens may be a problem for persons with allergies. Studies have shown that sulfites, a common food preservative, can cause asthma and anaphylaxis.[8] Probably the most well-known allergy trigger is tartrazine (FD&C Yellow No. 5), an approved azo-dye present in many drugs and food products. Tartrazine sensitivity is most frequently manifested by hives and asthma. Also interesting to note, tartrazine reactions are more common in persons with sensitivities to aspirin or nonsteroidal anti-inflammatory drugs.[9] In another study, patients with clinical symptoms suggestive of allergy to food antigens were exhaustively evaluated for food allergies via history, skin-prick tests, blood tests, and elimination/challenge evaluation. Subjects in whom food allergies could not be identified underwent oral provocation with different food additives. The results showed that 57.89 percent of patients were positive for reactions to dyes, 34.21 percent for benzoates, and 7.81 percent for acetylsalicylic acid.[10]

Avoiding Genetically Modified Organisms

Genetically modified organisms are organisms such as plants in which the DNA has been modified. There is very little safety data on the long-term effects of eating genetically modified foods as the U.S. Food and Drug Administration has stated that these foods are no different than the nonmodified version. However, preliminary research using animals suggests that these foods have adverse health affects on numerous organ systems.[11] Researchers have also demonstrated a link between genetically modified potatoes and cancer,[12] as well as increased allergenicity of some genetically modified foods.

Acid–Base Balance

Researchers suggest that ancestral preagricultural diets were net base-producing, meaning they produced an overall endogenous alkaline environment in the body. Based on NHANES data, the average American diet currently is net acid-producing. A base-producing diet is enhanced by the consumption of fruits, stalks, tubers and vegetables, whereas the consumption of meat, refined grains, fats, and oils enhance acidity in the body.[13] According to the researchers, the historical shift from net base-producing to net acid-producing diet is attributed to the replacement of plant foods in the ancestral diet by cereal grains and energy-dense, nutrient-poor foods in the contemporary diet. Thus, eating a more contemporary diets leads to a mismatch between the nutrient composition of the diet and genetically determined nutritional requirements for optimal systemic acid-base balance.[14] This shift toward diet-induced metabolic acidosis can have numerous adverse health consequences and has been associated with many chronic diseases such as cancer.

Essential Fatty Acids

Diets high in essential fatty acids and low in saturated fats also help support the immune system and modulate the allergic response. Regularly consuming oily fish, such as salmon, herring, mackerel, and trout is a great way to ingest adequate levels of omega-3 long-chain polyunsaturated fatty acids, such as DHA (docosahexaenoic acid) and EPA (eicosapentaenoic acid), which play significant roles in inflammation and immune function. Numerous studies support the use of essential fatty acids to help modulate allergic reactions such as asthma and eczema.[15] Elevated level of EPA measured in cell membranes is associated with a decreased risk of allergic sensitization and allergic rhinitis (hay fever).[16] Flaxseed oils, borage oil, evening primrose oil, and black currant oils are also good dietary sources for essential fatty acids.

Breast-feeding

Early exposure to allergenic proteins increases the risk of allergies and auto-immune disease. One study showed that children exposed to gluten-containing foods such as wheat, barley, or rye in the first three months of life had a fivefold increased risk of celiac disease autoimmunity compared with children exposed to gluten-containing foods at age four to six months.[17] In another large study, mothers of 1,500 children were surveyed for the presence of allergic rhinitis, wheezing, and eczema in the children, as well as duration of breast-feeding, tobacco smoke exposure, number of siblings, family income, level of maternal education, and parental history of allergies. Asthma (15.6 percent), wheezing (12.7 percent), allergic rhinitis (22.6 percent), and eczema (19.4 percent) were less frequent in exclusive breast-fed children compared with infants who receive partial breast-feeding or milk-formula feeding. Additionally, the risk of allergic diseases, eczema, wheezing, and ear infections were decreased in children with prolonged breast-feeding (greater than 6 months) than in those with short-term breast-feeding duration (less than 6 months). Thus, the researchers concluded that exclusive breast-feeding prevents development of allergic diseases in children.[18] Another study showed that early weaning from maternal breast milk was strongly associated with childhood asthma, as was having a family history of asthma and allergic rhinitis, urban place of residence, and having smokers as parents.[19]

THE REALITY OF TODAY'S DIET

At no other time in human history have people consumed food out of tins, boxes, or vacuum-sealed containers, microwaved their meals, eaten frequently at fast-food establishments, or fueled their bodies by stopping at a local convenience store. As a modern society we are creating a new historical paradigm for eating fast and, unfortunately, living faster and dying faster. But just a moment—people live longer than ever, right? Well, there is something to be said for quantity, but without quality it is less than glamorous.

Thanks to medical science we can bring people back to life from heart attacks, replace organs, and medicate ourselves with

Food is your best medicine. —Hippocrates (circa 400 B.C.)

prescriptions to limp along. There will be a time in the near future, however, when the life expectancy will plateau for the masses. Living by the seat of one's pants, eating whatever, whenever, is not a sustainable model. We are now seeing a surge in diabetes; in 2005, 1.5 million cases were diagnosed. As you read this sentence, some 43 million Americans are approaching full-blown diabetes. I do not want you to be one of them. It takes a decade or two of modern diet and lifestyle for the statistics to start showing up because the human body can take a lot of punishment before it gives up. You continue to read on and learn about proactive ways to defend your health because you are obviously committed to your health and the health of your loved ones. People who play the role of the ostrich and bury their heads in the sand instead of being proactive will face a premature date with what we term "reactive healthcare," It's like the thumb in the dike to prevent the flood of consequences of years of bad habits and choices.

If we heeded this part of Hippocrates' wisdom, we would be a healthier and happier society. You were likely born weighing about six to nine pounds; you obviously weigh a fair amount more than this currently. Using the foods you have consumed over the years to make new cells, your body duplicated all of its original cells. If you are tired of walking around as the cellular equivalent of a hamburger, bag of chips, cola drink, or french fry, then the following information

> What a great day to become the master of your health and life. —Chris D. Meletis, N.D.

will help you start making healthy changes. Our goal is your success. Today is the beginning of the rest of your life.

Enzyme-Rich Foods

Join us for a moment for a daydream. Imagine you are enjoying a warm spring day. A gentle breeze is blowing as you walk through a long-since-abandoned apple orchard. You stand in the middle of acres of budding trees and chirping birds. You look around and soak in the moment, the calm peace, and the awe of the season. Why don't you see years and years of fallen apples on the ground? The answer is simple: "enzymes."

Fresh fruits and vegetables have enzymes in them, and just the right enzymes to digest themselves. *Great, so what does that have to do with me?* You eat a fresh, uncooked, unprocessed apple full of enzymes and guess what? The apple's enzymes helps you digest it. If you eat a cooked apple, applesauce, or dried apple, those enzymes have been destroyed. This means your salivary glands, stomach, and pancreas have to work harder to digest the food, because there is no help from Mother Nature.

By not cooking and not processing your produce, you are not destroying heat-sensitive phytonutrients that have been shown to fight chronic and progressive disease states. So whenever possible, go raw or, if necessary, lightly steamed to retain enzymes and nutrient content to fuel your body right.

By eating more fresh produce and fewer processed foods, you also decrease your intake of preservatives and chemicals. This protects your digestive tract, and as you age, it will continue to work better. Follow this concept for a moment: You spend 20 years eating out of boxes that are more colorful than the food inside (unless they added color back to the dead food in the box). If you destroy the enzymes that naturally occur in the foods you eat, then to break down the foods your digestive tract has to make more enzymes like amylase (carbohydrate digestive enzyme), protease (protein digestive enzyme), lipase (fat digestive enzyme), and others. This decreases your body's capacity for optimal digestion later in life. It has been proven that fresh vegetables and fruits are life preserving. Even the government tells us to eat five to seven servings of vegetables and fruits per day. So get going and give your body a helping hand. To increase your ability to digest and absorb the food you consume on the run, use a daily digestive enzyme; it's an excellent investment in your health.

Same Food, Different Day

A wheat is a wheat is a wheat. The point is that macaroni, bread, batter, cold cereal, or bagels are all wheat. If you keep eating the same foods day in and day out, you are limiting your nutritional diversity. You are limiting your access to new and different minerals, vitamins, and phytonutrients. The key in life is moderation, nothing more nor less. Yet the average American mostly eats the same 25 foods day in and day out. Go through the exercise of writing down a week's diet and see if you are in a rut. Do you see the same foods time and time again?

You are limiting your body's full potential if you are not rotating what you eat. If you have this habit, you might be deficient in numerous nutrients. The average American has suboptimal levels of one or more nutrients. This is another reason we all would be wise to supplement our diets. Remember, supplements are not called substitutes, and you can't just take pills to make up for a crummy diet.

A major problem with lack of food rotation is that you increase the chance of creating a food allergy. If your body is continuously bombarded with any one thing it can get easily annoyed. Think about how experiencing the same thing over and over may bother your sense of harmony, whether it be a noise, the same reruns on television, the same barking dog when you are trying to sleep, the same worries, or whatever. So give yourself a break. Having been in medicine for years and having helped thousands of patients, I have learned a lot about even my own diet by performing IgG Food Antibody Assessment Panels and reading the laboratory-generated four-day rotation diet recommendations that come with the test results. I saw a list of foods that I had never heard of. I realized a long time ago that I had to increase the menu of foods on my list. I learned that some great-tasting foods are out there, that I did not even know about, like amaranth, quinoa, teff, spelt, ugly fruit, miso, and nori. It is time to broaden your horizons and spice up your life when it comes to what you eat.

Clinical Cases

The effects of food allergies can present as various symptoms and medical conditions. As every person is unique, each person's reactions to foods are also unique. Several clinical cases have been included to demonstrate the various reactions to foods as well as the dramatic improvement with dietary changes.

1. Allergic Triad. The healthy journey of 10-year-old A.G. is a story that starts and ends simply enough but takes a few interesting turns along the way. A.G. first presented at the age of four. Her mother reported the all-too-often symptoms of recurrent otitis media, excessive earwax, and year-round sinus congestion with postnasal drip. As a nutritionally oriented physician the first step I pursued was food-sensitivity testing. A.G., though a mere four years old, was a surprisingly willing participant and had a standard venipuncture for a 96 general food IgE and IgG Panel. The results revealed a high reaction to dairy, eggs, almonds, and peanuts. She also had numerous moderate reactions to lobster, asparagus, broccoli, and clams. Eliminating these foods from her diet was a prudent first step in her treatment, and A.G.'s mother was counseled on this fact. The only supplements recommended at this time were a comprehensive children's multiple, a fish oil blend rich in EPA and DHA, and a child's probiotic formula. The latter two were to help reestablish gut tolerance. Implementing the elimination and rotation diet plan for a four-year-old was no small feat. A.G. and her mother went on a field trip to the neighborhood natural foods market and found healthful alternatives the mother could use in A.G.'s meals. Food, one assumes provides nourishment, but "what is food to one man may be fierce poison to others" (Lucretius c. 99 B.C.–c. 55 B.C.). A concept that is so fundamentally true yet it never ceases to amaze me how overlooked a simple food-sensitivity test is in general practice; it is an easy-to-do test that can steer treatment into the land of profound results. At A.G.'s follow-up six-week visit symptoms had resolved, A.G.'s diet plan was reassessed, and the mother was given additional food choices for A.G. At 12 weeks, A.G was in the peak of health. As a bonus, the mother reported that A.G. had stopped wetting the bed. Unfortunately, A.G.'s story doesn't end here at happily ever after. Three years later, now 7-year-old A.G. returned to my office. She was quite run down; her sinus congestion had returned with a vengeance and she had swollen cervical lymph nodes, otitis media with excessive ear wax, erythematous and scaly ear canals, typical allergic shiners, and eczema on her arms and abdomen. Apparently, A.G.'s rhinitis had returned when she was five and her pediatrician prescribed a nasal steroidal spray and oral antihistamine to control the hay fever symptoms. However, the antihistamine had upset her stomach so much so that she was prescribed the acid

blocker cimetidine. With this, she could tolerate the medication routine, which also included a steroidal ear drop for her itchy ears, a hydrocortisone cream for the eczema, and an antibiotic. My course of action at this time was to "test, not guess," so I ordered a follow-up 96 general food IgE and IgG panel, in addition to a full chemistry and complete blood count. A noteworthy finding was eosinophilia which, partly explained the aspects of the classic atopic triad in A.G.: eczema and hay fever—yes—but fortunately not yet asthma. Also, her food antibody panel showed elevations for the same foods as before in addition to a few others. This was not the news I was looking for. Apparently, A.G. had done so well on the elimination and rotation diet plan that the mother decided to reintroduce the offending foods into A.G.'s diet. This was an error in judgment that I must take some responsibility for, as patient education can always go further. The order of treatment was the same as before. She was doing well on this regimen and was headed in the right direction. Very often, I find that children require very little intervention. They are resilient little creatures that only require a commonsense approach to treatment with persistence being the key to success. Within six weeks, A.G. was doing much better and, under the supervision of her pediatrician, was gradually being weaned off the prescription medications. Today, A.G. is a vibrant, rambunctious, and happy go-getter, who at the age of ten has taken an active role in preparing healthful school lunches with the careful guidance of her mother. Note: Since treating A.G. the laboratory I routinely use in my clinical practice, US BioTek, now offers an IgG finger-stick test that does not require a venipuncture. This is a simple and effective way of getting the results of a 96 IgG food panel within 7 to 10 days.

2. Migraine Headaches. Malcolm is a 10-year-old boy who is active in school, hockey, and family life. He has experienced debilitating migraine headaches that occur weekly or more frequently for the past few years. Family life revolves around his episodes; planned events are tentative and must be called off at a moment's notice at first sign of a headache. Car travel frequently triggers a migraine and the family must sit by the roadside waiting for Malcolm to feel better. IgG food sensitivity testing is recommended. Malcolm has a sophisticated palate for cheeses, especially stinky ones, and for chocolate. His IgG results indicate a severe reaction to all dairy and a moderate response to eggs. The whole family decides to go cold turkey and give up dairy products. Malcolm's six-year-old sister leads the way with an enthusiastic "yes" to her first drink of soy milk. At his one-month follow up, Malcolm had only suffered from two headaches but hadn't needed any medications. Over the course of eliminating the problematic foods his face gains a healthy shine and his eyes an enhanced clarity. His family is able to take a road trip to California during school vacation; he doesn't have a single headache during that trip

and had even goes on the rides at Disneyland. The family is much more relaxed; there is a palpable change in his parents as their fear for him has begun to subside. At the seven-month mark of having been off dairy and eggs Malcolm has no headaches. It is convincing that the IgG test made the difference for this child's life and for the sanity of his home life.

3. Sleepless in a New Town. The parents of a one-year-old boy seek help for his problem of waking every two hours at night, which began when they moved to a new town. Physical examination reveals a normal, healthy little boy. An IgG Food Antibody Assessment Panel is ordered through a lab in Seattle to rule out food allergies as a possible etiology. The results show a strong delayed-type hypersensitivity to dairy products. Upon withdrawal of dairy products from his diet, the child is able to sleep throughout the night in less than a week's time, although the problem recurs from time to time after accidental ingestion of dairy products.

4. Chronic Middle Ear Infections and Hyperactivity. An eight-year-old girl with chronic middle ear infections, inflammation of the throat, insomnia, hyperactivity, and dermatitis, is found through IgG Food Antibody Assessment Panel to have elevated antibody levels specific to dairy, egg, cucumber, and watermelon. She is advised to avoid all allergenic foods. The dermatitis and ear infections decrease considerably after three months. After four months she is less hyperactive, and her quality of sleep has greatly improved.

5. Intestinal Distress. A 40-year-old woman presents with a nine-month history of intestinal distress involving diarrhea, nausea, gas, fatigue, backaches, insomnia, and periodic numbness of her fingers. A full gastrointestinal investigation proves negative. She states that her stools are like "mud." IgG Food Antibody Assessment Panel reveals a strong delayed hypersensitivity to almond—her favorite snack. Eliminating almonds from her diet results in a quick resolution of all symptoms.

6. Allergic Child. A child who has developed reasonably well for the first two years starts to experience a series of frequent illnesses, including gastroenteritis, conjunctivitis, rhinitis, recurrent attacks of bronchitis, urticaria, and constipation. IgG Food Antibody Assessment Panel reveals the presence of severe delayed and immediate allergies to dairy products and egg. After removing these offending foods from his diet, the child regains his health.

7. Years of Constipation. A 38-year-old woman has suffered from chronic constipation for several years. Food-specific antibodies to dairy, egg, and baker's yeast are quite elevated, as assessed through ELISA food-allergy testing. After one month on the customized elimination and rotation diet guideline her bowel functions completely normalize.

8. Hyperactive Behavior. A six-year-old boy has a history of serious hyper-active behavior and is more than a handful for his parents. He is often in trouble at school and has difficulty playing with other children without getting "too rambunctious." The allergy test ordered through US BioTek shows elevated immediate and delayed reactivity to dairy, chicken, egg, cucumber, gluten, and citrus fruits. The parents are advised to eliminate the allergenic foods from the child's diet, and supplement with EFAs and probiotics. After three months, the child's hyperactive tendencies greatly improve. His teachers and classmates also note that he is more sociable.

CONCLUSION

It is essential to understand that each person is unique; thus, it is reasonable to assume that each person's ideal diet will also be unique. A health-promoting diet may be different for each person. Antibody testing, such as the IgG Food Antibody Assessment Panel has made evaluating those variables much more straightforward and reliable. To minimize allergic reactions, it is imperative to eat with intention and focus on nutrient-dense foods such as fruits and vegetables. Many allergic symptoms, as well as various other medical complaints, can be eliminated or minimized with individualized dietary interventions.

NOTES

1. Casagrande SS, Wang Y, Anderson C, et al. Have Americans increased their fruit and vegetable intake? The Trend between 1988 and 2002. Am J Prev Med. 2007;32(4):257–263.

2. Cakmak I. Plant nutrition research: Priorities to meet human needs for food in sustainable ways. Plant Soil. 2002;247(1):3–24.

3. American Academy of Allergy, Asthma and Immunology (AAAAI). The Allergy Report: Allergic Disorders: Promoting Best Practice. 1996–2005. Available at: http://www.aaaai.org/ar/working_vol3/072.asp. Accessed October 25, 2008; Branco Ferreira M, Pedro E, Meneses Santos J, et al. Latex and chickpea (Cicer arietinum) allergy: first description of a new association. Eur Ann Allergy Clin Immunol. 2004;36(10):366–371.

4. Figueroa J, Blanco C, Dumpiérrez AG, et al. Mustard allergy confirmed by double-blind placebo-controlled food challenges: clinical features and cross-reactivity with mug-wort pollen and plant-derived foods. Allergy. 2005;60(1):48–55.

5. Wu AY, Williams GA. Clinical characteristics and pattern of skin test reactivities in shellfish allergy patients in Hong Kong. Allergy Asthma Proc. 2004;25(4):237–242.

6. Mitchell AE, Hong YJ, Koh E, et al. Ten-year comparison of the influence of organic and conventional crop management practices on the content of flavonoids in tomatoes. J Agric Food Chem. 2007;55:6154–6159.

7. Wang SY, Chen CT, Sciarappa W, et al. Fruit quality, antioxidant capacity, and flavonoid content of organically and conventionally grown blueberries. J Agric Food Chem. 2008;56:5788–5794.

8.   Reus KE, Houben GF, Stam M, et al. Food additives as a cause of medical symptoms: relationship shown between sulfites and asthma and anaphylaxis; results of a literature review. *Ned Tijdschr Geneeskd*. 2000;144:1836–1839.

9.   Dipalma JR. Tartrazine sensitivity. *Am Fam Physician*. 1990;42:1347–1350.

10.   Ibero M, Eseverri JL, Barroso C, et al. Dyes, preservatives and salicylates in the induction of food intolerance and/or hypersensitivity in children. *Allergol Immunopathol (Madr)*. 1982;10(4):263–268.

11.   Ewen SW, Pusztai A. Effect of diets containing genetically modified potatoes expressing Galanthus nivalis lectin on rat small intestine. *Lancet*. 1999;354:1353–1354.

12.   Ermakova IV. Commentary on the report about the feeding of rats by Monsanto's GM russet Burbank Bt potatoes. *Agrarian Russia*. 2005;4:62–64. Available at: http://www.gmfreecymru.org.uk/pivotal_papers/feedingrats.htm. Accessed March 21, 2009.

13.   Sebastian A. Dietary protein content and the diet's net acid load: Opposing effects on bone health. *Am J Clin Nutr*. Available at: http://www.ajcn.org/cgi/reprint/82/5/921.pdf. Accessed on April 13, 2009.

14.   Sebastian A, Frassetto LA, Sellmeyer DE, et al. Estimation of the net acid load of the diet of ancestral preagricultural Homo sapiens and their hominid ancestors. *Am J Clin Nutr*. 2002;76:1308–1316.

15.   Gorelova Zhlu, Ladodo KS, Levachev MM, et al. Role of polyunsaturated fatty acids in diet therapy of children with allergic diseases. *Vopr Pitan*. 1999;68(1):31–35; Schalin-Karrila M, Mattila L, Jansen CT, et al. Evening primrose oil in the treatment of atopic eczema: effect on clinical status, plasma phospholipid fatty acids and circulating blood prostaglandins. *Br J Dermatol*. 1987;117(1):11–19.

16.   Hoff S, Seiler H, Heinrich J, et al. Allergic sensitisation and allergic rhinitis are associated with n-3 polyunsaturated fatty acids in the diet and in red blood cell membranes. *Eur J Clin Nutr*. 2005;59:1071–1080.

17.   Norris JM, Barriga K, Hoffenberg EJ, et al. Risk of celiac disease autoimmunity and timing of gluten introduction in the diet of infants at increased risk of disease. *JAMA*. 2005;293:2343–2351.

18.   Bener A, Ehlayel MS, Alsowaidi S, et al. Role of breast feeding in primary prevention of asthma and allergic diseases in a traditional society. *Eur Ann Allergy Clin Immunol*. 2007;39(10):337–343.

19.   Majeed R, Rajar UD, Shaikh N, et al. Risk factors associated with childhood asthma. *J Coll Physicians Surg Pak*. 2008;18(5):299–302.

CHAPTER 7

Airborne Allergens and Other Burdens: Don't Hold Your Breath; Create a Healthful Environment

An estimated 40 million Americans suffer from upper respiratory symptoms due to allergic reactions to indoor and outdoor airborne allergens. According to the National Institute of Allergy and Infectious Diseases (NIAID), allergic diseases are now a major cause of illness and disability in the United States. The cause for this surge in allergies is multifactorial; however, two main components of seasonal allergies include family history (genetics) and the environment—both internal and external. In this chapter, we will examine the impact of the environment on our health and discuss simple steps that can be taken to minimize exposure to airborne allergens so as to liberate part of the burden our bodies must carry from day to day in its daily role of maintaining optimal health.

Seasonal and perennial hypersensitivity-related symptoms seem to be increasing as a major cause of illness and disability in the United States. Hay fever alone is the fifth leading chronic disease among adults and a major cause of work absenteeism. Hay fever accounts for more than *4 million* missed work days a year at a total cost of more than $700 million in lost productivity.[1] Chronic allergy sufferers incur even higher medical costs than those with seasonal allergies. Studies have also found that chronic allergy sufferers have higher comorbidities, or more concomitant diseases, as a result of the chronic allergies. Disorders like sinusitis, bronchial asthma, nasal polyps, sleep disturbances, depression, and migraines are more frequent in people with chronic allergies than in people with seasonal allergies. The increased number of repercussions also increases the individual's outpatient payments; results in a higher use of polypharmacy (the use of more than one drug), such as antihistamines, nasal steroids, asthma medications, and decongestants; and increases the amount of money spent on drugs.[2] Sinusitis also goes hand in hand with allergy. Approximately 70 percent of people with allergies suffer from sinus infections, which makes allergies a strong predisposing factor for sinusitis.[3] Sinusitis, accounts for 11.5 million office visits and more than $2 billion in direct medical costs in the United States.[4]

Surprisingly, the risk is much greater from sitting in one's house, office, or school. Studies estimate that people typically spend 90 percent of their time indoors, so the risk to human health may be greater from indoor air pollution than outdoor air pollution. Recently, there has been more awareness about the importance of having clean air indoors as well as outdoors. This is particularly true for the elderly, children, and the chronically ill, who run a greater risk of secondary infections or health consequences because of their lowered immunity and lowered resistance to illness. There is now even a term for indoor pollution, "sick building syndrome," which is described as a set of symptoms that are associated with being in a particular building or in part of a building. Poor indoor air quality can be the result of inadequate ventilation, chemical contaminants such as adhesives, carpeting, upholstery, cleaning agents, and combustion products; chemical contaminants from outdoor sources; and biological contaminants, such as molds, bacteria, pollen, and viruses that accumulate inside the building.[5] Although sick building syndrome encompasses more than environmental allergies, these factors must be taken into consideration if you suffer from environmental allergy symptoms.

Symptom	Airborne Allergy	Cold	Flu
Cough	Sometimes	Mild to moderate	Can be severe
Fatigue and weakness	Sometimes	Mild	Up to 2–3 weeks
Extreme exhaustion	No	No	Prominent
General aches and pains	No	Slight	Can be severe
Itching eyes	Common	No	No
Sneezing and runny/ stuffy nose	Common	Common	Sometimes
Sore throat	Sometimes	Common	Sometimes
Fever	No	No	Up to 3–4 days
Complications	Sinus infection, asthma	Sinus/ear infection, asthma	Bronchitis, pneumonia

Symptoms of airborne allergens are nothing to sneeze at and vary based on what caused the symptoms and a person's genetic susceptibilities. Typical airborne allergy symptoms include generalized itching, watery eyes, conjunctivitis, runny or stuffy and itching nose, coughing, and postnasal drip. Fatigue, sore throat, and weakness can also be symptoms of an environmental allergy. These symptoms can often be confused with those of the common cold or flu; however, the generalized joint aches and pains and the presence of a fever rules out an allergy. The comparison chart shown here presents allergy, cold and flu symptoms.[6]

A common sign among allergic sufferers is what is termed an "allergic salute." This sign is a horizontal crease mark on the nose and may be visible in people with allergies who persistently rubs their nose upward to alleviate the constant runny nose and stuffiness. "Allergic shiners" are another telltale sign of allergies. These are dark circles under the eyes, which are caused by nasal congestion. Nasal congestion can be caused by other reasons than allergies; however, the end result is the same. When the mucosa of the nose becomes inflamed, the pressure that is built up within the tissues prevents incoming blood from draining from the superficial parts of the face, such as the skin under the eyes. As the blood pools in the superficial vessels under the eyes, it has a bruising effect and results in puffiness, leaving the person looking tired and run down. Aside from the stuffiness, a person with allergies must also put up with other symptoms, such as conjunctivitis, postnasal drip, headaches, and even possible nausea from the postnasal drip. These symptoms stem from the inflammatory chemicals or mediators, including histamine, cytokines, and leukotrienes, that are released in the body tissues as a result of an immune reaction to a particular allergen or allergens. These mediators can affect almost any tissue in the body. In the nose, for example, it can result in the familiar allergic symptoms of nasal itch, sneezing, and runny nose. Histamine in particular induces nasal itching, sneezing, and running and blockage of the nasal passages, which are characteristic of allergic rhinitis.

The most common indoor/outdoor allergy triggers include tree, grass, and weed pollens; mold spores; dust mites and cockroaches and their waste products (feces, proteins from exoskeletons); and dog, rodent, and cat dander. In addition, approximately 10 million Americans are allergic to cats.[7]

Allergies can be seasonal or perennial allergies. Seasonal allergies are most common in spring, summer, and fall depending on what trees, weeds, and grasses are in season. The pollen of these plants triggers a seasonal allergic rhinitis called hay fever. Perennial allergens, on the other hand, such as pet dander and dust mites, can trigger allergic rhinitis any time of the year. Mold allergy may be a seasonal or perennial trigger depending on how the exposure is taking place.

THE BIOLOGY OF THE ENVIRONMENTAL ALLERGY

As discussed in Chapter 4, the mechanism of reactivity for environmental allergens shares common reactive processes. In the simplest of terms, when a person with allergies comes in contact with the allergen, his or her immune system reacts by generating IgE antibodies to the particular allergen proteins. The antibodies, which are produced by plasma cells in the blood, then bind to mast cells, some of which can found under the mucous membranes of the target tissue, such as the nose, eyes and lungs. On second contact, the antigen binds to these bound IgE antibodies causing active release of mediators within the cells—histamine, for one—resulting in allergic inflammation ranging from a runny nose to red and watery eyes. The immunological basis for allergic disease is currently visualized through the T helper cell (Th)1/Th2 paradigm. CD4$^+$ T cells differentiate into polarized Th1 and Th2 cells each with their own combination of cytokines (inflammatory substances) to either enhance cell-mediated or humoral-mediated immunity. The development of allergic disease is the result of an overproduction of Th2 cytokines by allergen-specific CD4$^+$ Th2 cells, which amplify and prolong allergic inflammation. Many factors influence this polarization, including type of antigen, dose, type of antigen presenting cell, and co-stimulatory signals received by the T cell in addition to genetic factors. Further, the amount and type of cytokines produced by Th2 cells, for example, may change the specific functions of the humoral immune response and the type of antibody that is made—so depending on the cytokines, the immune response could be an IgE response or an IgG4 or IgG2 or IgA response, for example.[8] Each antibody isotype differs in its biological properties, functional location, and ability to handle different antigens. Briefly, as mentioned previously, IgE binds to allergens and triggers histamine release from mast cells. The IgE antibody is elevated in atopic allergies and worm infections. IgG antibodies are also increased in inflammatory conditions and are involved in neutralizing the antigen by activating complement and phagocytes. IgA is found in mucosal areas, such as the gut and the respiratory and genitourinary tracts, and is found in mucous secretions, tears, saliva, breast milk, intestinal juice, and bronchoalveolar fluid. In the gut, IgA in the form of secretory IgA (sIgA) is produced from initial exposure to food peptides for example, in the gut lumen and is involved in immune exclusion. Secretory IgA is produced by plasma cells in the lamina propria at the rate of three grams per day and excreted into the mucosal lumen, transferred by the epithelial cells. Secretory IgA binds and excludes antigens present in the intestinal tract to prevent excessive systemic absorption of dietary and other antigens, such as milk, soy, peanut, wheat, ovalbumin, gliadin proteins; as well as bacteria, viruses, protozoa, fungi and other parasites. IgA, which represents primary immune reaction has a half-life of about five to six days. In contrast, IgG, which is indicative of an ongoing immune reaction, has a half-life of around 20 to 24 days. The immune response to most common inhalant allergens includes not only IgE but also IgG and IgA antibodies, which indicate exposure and immunological sensitization.[9] Although the presence of specific IgE antibodies against inhalants is a distinctive feature of atopic patients, specific IgG antibodies can be detected in parallel. Albeit IgG antibodies can be detected in sera of both atopic and nonatopic patients, there is a propensity for higher IgG levels in atopic patients. This is not surprising as there is the bias toward the production of Th2 cytokines in atopic persons via such co-regulatory mechanisms as the IgG isotype switching of IgG4. These antibodies develop in parallel and are selectively stimulated by Th2 cytokines; elevated levels of this antibody class in atopic persons is reasonably expected.[10] The associated immunopathological threshold for IgG responses and the preferential expression of the subclasses and correlating clinical manifestations are an area of active investigation.

A case in point is that of people with cystic fibrosis, an inherited chronic disease that affects the lungs and digestive system of about 30,000 children and adults in the United States.[11] Cystic fibrosis is characterized by unusually thick, sticky mucus secretions, which can affect the lungs, pancreas, liver, and intestines as well as the sinuses that block ducts and passageways. In the lungs these secretions may block the airways and lead to infections. Colonization of the lower respiratory tract with *Aspergillus fumigatus* and the complicating hypersensitivity reaction allergic bronchopulmonary aspergillosis, in addition to a high frequency of atopy, is well recognized in patients with cystic fibrosis. All four IgG subclasses are present in elevated in people with an *Aspergillus* infection compared to healthy counterparts.[12] The *Aspergillus* IgG antibodies indicate exposure and immunological sensitization. Measuring these antibodies may aid in diagnosis and treatment, preventing potentially irreversible lung damage. A close association has been found between deterioration of pulmonary function and colonization with the *Aspergillus* fungus and *Aspergillus*-specific–IgG antibodies. The deterioration of the lungs is thought to be directly attributable to local pathogenicity of the fungus or hypersensitivity mechanisms mediated by the specific IgG antibodies[13]; interaction of specific IgG antibodies with the fungal antigens in the bronchial tree may activate the complement pathway contributing to lung damage.

Allergic fungal sinusitis, another immunological fungal hypersensitivity, may present as a concomitant finding resulting from the same fungus, but it has been shown to involve other fungi, including *Bipolaris spp.*[14] Patients with allergic fungal sinusitis are also often found to have elevated total IgE levels. More than half of these patients have a history of seasonal or perennial allergic rhinitis, a history of asthma, and fungal antigen-specific IgE and IgG antibodies by enzyme-linked immunosorbent assay (ELISA).[15]

SEASONAL ALLERGIES

Seasonal pollen allergies are generally caused by tiny pollen grains carried by the wind. Although most flowering plants use pollinators to reproduce, some varieties of plants, such as grasses and some trees, depend on the wind to transfer pollen to the female flowers. These migratory pollen grains can cause a strong immune reaction in the human body. Pollen grains come in a wide variety of shapes and sizes, though most are spherical or oval and have characteristic pores, furrows, and textures in the outer wall. These textures determine how easily the immune system can mount an immune response against the particular pollen grain. The most allergenic types of pollen include grass pollen, which affects over 95 percent of hay fever sufferers. Pollen grains can be breathed in through the nose or can land in the eyes and set up an allergic reaction. The antibody produced, IgE, for example, is specific for the type of pollen the individual is exposed to (i.e., oak pollen or ragweed pollen).

Some trees are better producers of allergenic pollen than others. Small, light, dry pollen granules are best for wind transport. Ragweed, which has been reported to have been collected more than 400 miles out to sea and 2 miles high in the air, is a good example of a highly allergenic pollen. A single ragweed plant may generate a million pollen grains/day. Adding insult to injury, people with allergies are often sensitive to more than one type of pollen. This will usually lead to one allergy attack after the other, depending on when different pollen grains are let loose during the season. Many species of grasses and plants have a similar pollen structure, so if you are allergic to one, you are allergic to the other, because the immune system cannot distinguish between two types of pollen grains with key similarities. On the other hand, some pollen grains, such as pine pollen, are less allergenic. Pine pollen is rather heavy; it tends to fall straight down and is therefore not widely disseminated and rarely reaches the nose. Additionally, its thick outer coat, also called the exine, may render it an unlikely allergenic candidate. However, certain theoretical and limited studies have demonstrated allergenicity of the pine pollen in certain circumstances.[16]

Aside from grass pollen, tree pollen can also be problematic to allergy sufferers. The common trees offenders are oak, western red cedar, ash, elm, birch, and hickory, to name a few. Weeds are also notorious allergic triggers. In North America, common allergenic weeds aside from ragweed include sagebrush, redroot pigweed, lamb's quarters, and English plantain. Among grasses, some prolific producers of allergenic pollens are listed in the table with their potential cross-reactors.

Grass	Genus[1]	Cross-Reactors[2]
Bahia	*Paspalum*	Johnson, maize, meadow, rye grass, redtop, meadow fescue, sweet vernal. Trees: Bottlebrush, melaleuca
Bermuda	*Cynodon*	Johnson, bahia, buffalo, salt and grama grass, rye grass, timothy, meadow grass, olive, wall pellitory, sunflower
Smooth brome	*Bromus*	Wheat, timothy, meadow grass, rye grass, redtop, meadow fescue, sweet vernal, velvet grass, barley
Meadow fescue	*Festuca*	Timothy, cocksfoot, meadow grass, rye grass, velvet grass, canary grass, redtop, meadow Foxtail,
Johnson	*Sorghum*	Maize, bahia, rye grass, cocksfoot grass, timothy, meadow, redtop, meadow fescue, and sweet vernal
Perennial rye	*Lolium*	Velvet grass, timothy, meadow grass, cocksfoot, canary, meadow fescue, redtop, meadow foxtail
Sweet vernal	*Anthoxanthum*	Rye grass, canary grass, meadow grass, timothy, cocksfoot, meadow fescue, velvet grass, redtop, meadow foxtail, wild rye grass
Timothy	*Phleum*	Rye grass, canary grass, meadow grass, timothy, cocksfoot, meadow fescue, velvet grass, redtop, meadow Foxtail

[1]Cross-reactivity is shown to other species within the genus.
[2]*Sources*: www.labspec.co.za/online/l_grass.htm; www.immunocapinvitrosight.com.

Pollen is one of the most widespread triggers for environmental allergy and is not easily avoided, short of mostly staying indoors, using an effective air filtration unit, and keeping a judicious eye on pollen counts to plan your daily activities accordingly. Pollen counts depend a great deal on the weather. Because pollen is carried by the wind, logically more pollen will be around on dry breezy days. Also, pollen counts tend to be highest in the early morning and evening.

PERENNIAL ALLERGIES

As previously mentioned, the most common aeroallergens that account for perennial symptoms are house-dust mites (*Dermatophagoides pteronyssus, D. farinae*), animal dander (cat and dog dander in particular), and mold.[17] Dust mites are microscopic bugs that are related to spiders. These organisms thrive in warm and humid environments, eat dead skin cells, and nest in clothes, pillows and other bedding, carpets, and upholstery. Your bedding alone may contain as many as 10 million dust mites. When a dust mite dies, its body disintegrates into small fragments, which, in addition to their feces, mix with dust and become airborne. Once airborne, these particles can be inhaled through the mouth and nose. In a person with allergies, sneezing, wheezing, watering eyes, and a runny nose can result. Although you probably can't eliminate dust mites completely, precautions can be taken decrease exposure to them: use allergen-impermeable bedding and upholstery covers, decrease room humidity with a dehumidifier, and launder bedding frequently in hot (130–140°F) soapy water. More comprehensive changes include the following: change curtains for blinds; use tile, linoleum, or wood flooring instead of carpet; and use synthetic fibers instead of wool, cotton, and down. Mites live for approximately 30 days, during which time the female lays approximately one egg/day. Vacuuming, mopping, and keeping the house free of clutter will reduce places where the mites like to live. Also, avoid laying carpet over concrete floors, which creates a moist warm environment favorable to mite growth. The dust mite is only one inhabitant found in house dust. House dust

Allergen	Cross-Reactors[1]
Cat dander	Dog, horse,[2] porcine[3]
Cockroach	Mite, crab, shrimp[4]
Dog dander	Cat, horse, porcine[5]
Dust mite	Cockroach and other insects, snail,[6] shrimp[7]

[1] Cross-reactivity between allergenic epitopes in vivo may not have correlation to cross-reactivity in a clinical setting.

[2] Cabañas R, López-Serrano MC, Carreira J, et al., Importance of albumin in cross-reactivity among cat, dog and horse allergens. *J Investig Allergol Clin Immunol.* 2000;10(2):71–77.

[3] Hilger C, Kohnen M, Grigioni F, Lehners C, Hentges F., Allergic cross-reactions between cat and pig serum albumin. Study at the protein and DNA levels. *Allergy.* 1997;52:179–187.

[4] Chiou YH, You CY, Wang LY, Huang SP. Detection of cross-reactivity for atopic immunoglobulin E against multiple allergens. *Clin Diagn Lab Immunol.* 2003;10:229–232.

[5] Mamikoglu B. Beef, pork, and milk allergy (cross reactivity with each other and pet allergies). *Otolaryngol Head Neck Surg.* 2005;133:534–537.

[6] Pajno GB, Morabito L, Barberio G. Allergy to house dust mite and snails: a model of cross-reaction between food and inhalant allergens with a clinical impact. *Pediatr Pulmunol Suppl.* 1999;18:163–164.

[7] Witteman AL, Akkerdaas JK, van Leeuwen J, van der See JS, Aalberse RC. Identification of a cross-reactive allergen (presumably tropomyosin) in shrimp, mite and insects. *Int Arch Allergy Immunol.* 1994;105(1):56–61.

combines particulates of clothing, carpet, rugs, and upholstered furniture with a mix of human slough, animal dander, insect body parts, mites, saliva, pollens and molds, laundry detergent residuals, cosmetic powders, and tobacco smoke. All of these particles have the ability to trigger, aggravate, and perpetuate allergic reaction in such common sites as the eyes, nose, and throat. Common indoor allergens and their cross-reactions are listed in the table.

MOLDS

Outdoors, molds play a key role in nature's recycling system by breaking down organic matter such as dead plants, wood fiber, and fallen leaves. The resulting mulch returns beneficial nutrients back into the soil for the native organisms. As already mentioned, molds reproduce by means of microscopic spores that float in the air like pollen. Airborne molds are found throughout the year and are affected by wind, rain, and temperature. Wet or damp conditions are favorable for mold growth.

More than 300,000 species strong, molds are found in virtually every environment, both outdoors and indoors, all year around. Encouraged by damp or humid conditions, molds begin growing when the spores land on a wet surface. High humidity may occur in shady damp areas such as a pile of decomposing leaves in the backyard, in a poorly ventilated house, or in a very humid region, such as the northwestern United States. Molds are a part of a diverse group of organisms called fungi, which are part of the natural environment and range from teeny tiny molds and yeasts to giant mushrooms. The production of spores is characteristic of fungi in general. These spores are transported through air, water, and insects. Airborne, molds can spread from outdoor to indoor environments where they can create a potential health problem. Molds, which live on plant and animal matter may be familiar to most people as the agent responsible for spoiling foods.

Indoors, molds should be avoided. They may begin to grow in indoor areas when spores land on wet or damp surfaces that are left unattended for prolonged periods. Mold growth can be found in a variety of places in the home: carpets, upholstery, potting soil of indoor plants, attics, basements, bathrooms, refrigerators and other food storage areas, garbage containers, and windowsills to name a few. Mold spores waft through the air continually but can settle into cracks and crevices where they can take hold. Molds are persistent and thrive wherever dampness and moisture are a problem. Although mold and dust are common to the indoor environment and are mostly a natural occurrence, there is a potential for serious health effects, including, as mentioned previously, asthma, allergic reactions, sneezing, itching, coughing, wheezing, shortness of breath, and chest pain. In a person who is unaware of his or her sensitivities, this may cascade into a spectrum of chronic health problems from low-level, long-term exposure. When in doubt you should be tested to identify exposure and offending articles should be removed from the environment.

When mold becomes a problem, clean it up through moisture control. Wet materials that cannot be thoroughly cleaned and dried within 24–48 hours are best thrown out. When the leftover bologna starts to develop a beard, it is time to throw it out. The green fuzzy spots on old bread and velvet splotches on tomatoes and other fruit are signs of mold growth that has already penetrated deep into the food by its roots. *Alternaria* genus for example may be found on wheat, barley, oats, peanuts, and polished rice and has been identified in Japanese pear black spot and early blight of potatoes and tomatoes. Soft foods, like tomatoes, processed meats, and fruits; porous foods, such as breads and baked goods; and foods with high moisture content, such as cottage cheese, jams, and jellies can be contaminated below the surface and should be discarded at the first signs of mold growth. As a general rule of thumb perishables should *not* be out of the refrigerator longer than two hours, and leftovers should be used up within three to four days to prevent mold growth. If you find something moldy in the fridge, throw it out; don't sniff it first because that will allow the pesky spores access to your respiratory tract. Wipe the area of the fridge clean and dry and check nearby food items that may have touched the spoiled food for cross-contamination—mold spreads quickly and easily.

The health risk due to dampness and toxigenic molds in the home and workplace is a subject of considerable interest as mold exposure is thought to be a risk factor for the development of asthma, allergy, and neuropsychological illness[18] Common molds found in moisture-damaged buildings include *Penicillium, Cladosporium, Aspergillus,* and *Stachybotrys,* to name a few. Chronic respiratory infections, eye and skin irritation, and other negative health effects have been found to be dependent on the mycotoxins of the particular species involved.[19] Chronic exposure to *Alternaria tenuis,* for example has been suggested to play a role in symptoms of neuropsychological impairment, and its mycotoxins exhibit both mutagenic and carcinogenic properties. In a case described by Anyanwu et al, the affected patient was experiencing general arthralgia and joint pain, cough, headache, and fatigue, in addition to impairment in intellectual processing, language, speech, abstract reasoning, and higher-order thinking. Significantly elevated serum IgG antibodies to three toxigenic molds were found, suggesting chronic exposure to *Alternaria tenuis, Epicoccum nigrum,* and *Pullularia pullulans.* Interestingly, there were no correlations between the toxigenic molds identified in her indoor environment and those found in her serum. The authors theorize that the toxigenic mold antigens, particularly *Alternaria tenuis,* led to changes in the brain structure and resulted in consequent mind and behavioral effects.[20]

Generally, there are no widely accepted common names to the molds. Synonyms found are usually other Latin names to avoid misleading and inaccurate references. From a taxonomical point of view, there is cross-reaction between the molds because they, as a group, contain and produce galactomannans with similar immunogenic and galactofuranosyl side chains. For cross-reactions to other allergens, cross-reactivity has been shown to other species within the fungus family. There is one reported case of cross-reactivity between raw mushroom and molds in a patient with oral allergy syndrome reported in the literature.[21] The table lists some common molds and ways to control their growth.

Common Mold	Possible Sources of Exposure	Measures of Control
Alternaria tenuis	Water-damaged areas (basements, old buildings), poor housekeeping, poor ventilation and poor air filtration, carpets, textiles, horizontal surfaces (often on window frames) Common in outdoor samples of soil, seeds, and plants Stored wheat, barley, oats, corn, and peanuts. Black spot of Japanese pear blight of tomato and potato.	Adequate air filtration and filtration system Hygiene/cleaning Moisture control
Aspergillus fumigatus	*Aspergillus* spp. are ubiquitous in the outdoor environment; soil, seed, and plant debris/decaying vegetation, and indoor air. Insulations used in the duct work of heating, ventilation and air conditioning (HVAC) systems[1]	Adequate air filtration and filtration system Hygiene/cleaning Moisture control Proper storage of food items away from excess moisture
Cladosporium herbarum	Most commonly identified outdoor fungus found on dead plants, woody plants, straw, and soil Air-handling units, heating, ventilating, and air conditioning systems of building, with or without a history of water damage[2] Painted metal surfaces of covering panels and register vents of heating, air conditioning, and ventilation systems[3] Food, paint, and textiles	Adequate air filtration and filtration system Hygiene/cleaning Moisture control
Penicillium notatum	*Penicillium* spp. spoilage in a wide variety of foods, including meat, cereals, nuts, cheese, eggs, fruit, breads, grains, and processed and refrigerated foods *Penicillium* spp. have also been observed to grow in damaged canned goods[4] Air-handling units, heating, ventilating, and air conditioning systems of building, with or without a history of water damage[2]	Proper storage of food items away from excess moisture Avoid prolonged storage of food sources in refrigerators and storage bins Adequate air filtration and filtration system hygiene/cleaning Moisture control

[1] Ezeonu IM, Price DL, Crow SA, Ahearn DG. Effects of extracts of fiberglass insulations on the growth of *Aspergillus fumigatus and A. versicolor. Mycopathologia.* 1995;132(2);65–69.

[2] Ahearn DG, Crow SA, Simmons RB, et al. Fungal colonization of fiberglass insulation in the air distribution system of a multi-story office building: VOC production and possible relationship to a sick building syndrome. *J Ind Microbiol Biotechnol.* 1996;16(5):280–285.

[3] Ahearn DG, Simmons RB, Switzer KE, Ajello L, Pierson DL. Colonization by *Cladosporium* spp. of painted metal surfaces associated with heating and air conditioning systems. *J Ind Microbiol Biotechnol.* 1991;8(4);277–280.

[4] Lewis P, Donoghue MB, Hocking AD, Cook L, Granger LV. Tremor syndrome associated with a fungal toxin: sequelae of food contamination. *Med J Aust.* 2005;182:582–584.

In summary, molds need a source of moisture, a source of carbon, and a favorable temperature to thrive. Key preventive measures against molds in the home include the following:

- Dispose of visible dirt and debris.
- Clean and decontaminate all heating, ventilation, and air conditioning systems (HVAC).
- Inventory all water-damaged areas, building materials, furnishings, carpet, and cabinets and determine the extent of drywall damage. Remove and dispose.
- Inventory all stored food supplies. Remove and dispose of items that have been improperly stored or stored for a prolonged time.

GENETICS AND ALLERGIES

As mentioned in the beginning of the chapter, both environmental and genetic factors play a part in the development of immune reactions against the environment. The interplay between these two factors is multifaceted and the two can either help or compromise each other, depending on the circumstances.

Experts suggest that there is a familial tendency to develop allergies in general, though not to any specific allergen; the approximate risk of a child developing allergy is 50 to 70 percent if both parents are affected versus about 20 to 40 percent if only one parent or sibling is affected. Nonatopic individuals can still carry a risk especially during times when the body's natural defenses are compromised, such as during infection or illness or after intensive contact from work sources causing sensitization. Other studies have also shown that there may be a gene that promotes the production of interleukin-4, a key protein essential in allergic reactions. Studies have shown that people of African-American descent have higher rates of allergies and asthma because of their genetic predisposition to produce higher levels of interleukin-4. It is believed that this might have been a mechanism to protect against tropical parasites. Without parasite infections here in North America, the overactive immune system then turns to harmless allergens and induces immune reactions to the environment.[22]

ALLERGIES AND THE ENVIRONMENT

Aside from genetic factors that can influence the ease by which the body creates immune responses against a host of environmental allergens, the environment in which we live also plays an important role in the development of allergies. Although we cannot control our genetic expression, we can modify our environment in such a way that it encourages the immune system to quiet down or we can expose ourselves to the very environment that makes our bodies most reactive to allergens.

Over the past 50 to 100 years, the incidence of environmental sensitivity has increased monumentally, particularly in urban settings. Studies have shown that people living in urban areas are more likely to develop allergies than their rural counterparts. Several factors may account for these differences:

1. Pollution in urban areas increases the inflammation of the respiratory tract, thereby affecting the integrity of this barrier in such a way that allergenic substances can enter the bloodstream.
2. Studies have found a higher incidence of allergy in persons who live above the ground floor; because of the vertical distribution of pollen, they are more likely to develop allergies.[23]
3. Living in cities typically means more exposure to stress, which lowers immunity. Lower sIgA production makes it easier for allergens to penetrate the bloodstream to create an allergic response in the body.
4. Different lifestyle options are related to urban versus rural life. This will be discussed later in more detail.
5. Initial exposure to pollen in urban dwellers may be less than in a rural setting; therefore, children do not acquire the necessary immunity (particularly IgA) to fend off potential allergens as they grow up.
6. Socioeconomic status and family size have a strong association to allergies. The higher the socioeconomic status and the smaller the family size, the greater the likelihood of developing allergies. This may have to do with initial exposure to environmental allergies as a child. This is particularly true with first-born children because new parents tend to be more careful in preventing the child from exposing themselves to dirt and so on. However, more research in this field is still necessary.

Our environment informs our body about where we live, who we share our space with, who is foe, and who is friend. Therefore, it follows that whatever we surround ourselves with will inform our body what it needs to do to function as best as possible. When it comes to the environment and allergies, heavily polluted areas provide a worst-case scenario for the allergy sufferer. Traffic-related air pollutants, like nitric oxide, can react with pollen to make it more immunogenic, which means the immune system recognizes it and mounts an allergic reaction to the pollen more easily than if it were unaffected by air pollution. The reason behind this lies in the damage air pollution can cause in the mucous membranes. The more we expose ourselves to polluted air, the more irritated the lining of our respiratory passages becomes. As with the bowel, an irritated mucous membrane in the nose, throat, and lungs also compromises the integrity of the barrier this lining should have. Any irritation in the mucosa opens up the lining to easier accidental transport of a foreign particle; thus, it is easier to create an immune response against this particle. What this exposure adds up to is just more susceptibility to immune reactions in polluted areas—and more cautionary steps that need to be taken to avoid exposure.

LIFESTYLE AND ALLERGIES

Lifestyle is the factor we have the most control over when it comes to allergies. Genetic tendencies cannot be changed, and we cannot live in the perfect environment; however, by providing our body with essential nutrients and avoiding foods and other exposures to reduce general inflammation will allow us to better cope with allergies. One reason allergic reactions can be so severe is because of a generalized inflammatory state in the body. For example, if we eat foods we do not digest well, that creates inflammation in the bowel and possibly creates immune reactions. If we also live in the city and are exposed to pollutants, another source of irritation is added. There we may work in an office space that has no natural air flow, is wired for Wi-Fi, and emits electromagnetic radiation, which lowers our resistance to stress. Furthermore, we may subsist on frozen entrees and little or no fresh vegetables or whole grains—which also increases inflammatory markers in our body. When allergens are added to the mix, the result is a fantastic cascade reaction of immune intolerance and reaction to the environment. This is an example of all the different insults that our bodies might encounter; however, steps can also be taken to *minimize* the insults our bodies have to endure in the course of the day.

For example, the following steps may be taken to reduce direct exposure to allergens:

- Save outside activities for late afternoon or after a rainfall to minimize exposure to pollen.
- Keep windows closed in the home and the car.
- Keep pets and clothing out of the bedroom.
- Shower daily before bed to remove pollen and other allergens that have accumulated throughout the day on the hair and skin.
- Leave shoes outside.
- Vacuum the entire house regularly, including upholstery.
- Change pillow cases on a daily basis.
- Use an efficient HEPA (high-efficiency particulate air) filter in the house to reduce dust floating in the air.
- Perform regular maintenance on air vents and furnaces.
- Improve indoor air pollution by investing in plants that clean the air, such as peace lilies, bamboo palm, spider plant, flowering mums and mother-in-laws-tongue.[24]

A more conventional method of dealing with environmental allergies uses allergen immunotherapy. A physician may sometimes use allergen-specific IgG or IgG4 to monitor a patient undergoing this therapy. Although IgG4 has been suggested to play a role as a blocking antibody that interferes with the binding of IgE to allergen.[25] increases in allergen-specific IgG4 titers are not predictive of the efficacy of the immunotherapy.[26] Immunotherapy is often initiated once a correlation of elevated IgE antibody from skin testing, patient symptoms,

suspected triggers, and allergen exposure is definite. Indications for immunotherapy include allergic rhinitis, allergic asthma, or stinging insect hypersensitivity with symptoms that are perhaps not adequately controlled by avoidance
measures and medications. Immunotherapy involves the subcutaneous injection of gradually increasing doses of a specific allergen the patient is allergic
to for the goal of increasing the patient's tolerance over time and minimizing
symptomatic expression. Immunotherapy is often associated with a shift from
a Th2 to a Th1 immune response to allergen. Moreover, allergen-specific IgG
offers a simple indicator for allergen exposure that may be used to evaluate the
effectiveness of environmental control measures. IgG antibodies against molds
and fungi, as mentioned earlier, are used as biomarkers to indicate exposure.

As stated previously, however, getting to the underlying cause of the allergies
is of utmost importance. Ruling out food sensitivities/allergies and intolerances,
as well as following a diet rich in vegetables, fruit, unrefined grains, and healthy
oils; exercising; and drinking plenty of water can be very beneficial to this condition. Furthermore, specific nutritional therapies, which will be discussed in a
later chapter, optimize the mucosa in the respiratory and gastrointestinal tracts to
minimize the inflammation and damage caused by past lifestyle choices. This approach remains much less invasive and results in a healthier, more vibrant you.

That said, it is important to remember that our understanding of allergy
remains far from complete. New discoveries are made almost on a daily basis
in this field. We do know that chemical irritants, such as air pollution, insect
sprays, tobacco smoke, and paint, can worsen airborne allergy symptoms. Although several factors may provoke the allergic response, heredity also plays a
major influence. Inhalant allergic reactions are multifaceted in nature regarding
symptomology and underlying immunologic mechanisms. Immediate-type hypersensitivity reactions through IgE are the best understood, but they represent
only a fraction of responses, the rest of which may be non–IgE-mediated and/
or involve mixed reactions. Factors that regulate the immunological response,
specifically IgG, is currently an area of active research; the biological function of IgG antibodies have been described briefly as one that both enhances
and suppresses the immune response to aeroallergens. Whatever the cause of
the allergies, one of the best ways to enhance your health, regardless of your
genetic makeup, is to give your body the best attention and care possible to
give it the strength and flexibility to deal with the ever-increasing complexity
of modern life.

BEYOND ENVIRONMENTAL ALLERGENS

So, now that we have looked at some of the science behind environmental allergens, let's take a glance at some other practical factors you and your loved ones
need to know about. Remember the saying, "the straw that broke the camel's
back"? Obviously, it was the total of all the straws—first, middle, and last—that
injured the camel. Likewise, total toxic exposures can lead to sickness, disease,
fatigue, weight gain, and simply not feeling well. The key to enjoying life to

the fullest is to get to be so healthy that you are thriving, not merely surviving. To achieve excellent health it is critical to limit toxins in your environment, water, and the air. So, now that you have learned about environmental allergens, let's look at other environmental factors that will help complete your protection awareness.

We would like to help you become aware of the dangers of environmental toxins. However, instead of subjecting you to information overload, we will give you a brief summary. We hope to raise your awareness enough that you will take action. Please take this information and proposed solutions seriously. It may save your life.

> It is the heightened level of awareness and healthy intent that protects us the most.
> —Chris D. Meletis, N.D.

CONCLUSION

Identifying and lessening environmental burdens is very important and should be part of one's overall health and wellness program along with controlling exposure to food contaminants and allergens. The human body has sufficient daily challenges to maintain wellness and health without undue burdens either directly or indirectly entering our lives as obstacles to optimal existence and healthy aging.

NOTES

1. *Chronic Conditions: A Challenge for the 21st Century.* Washington, DC: National Academy on an Aging Society; 1999.

2. Crown WH, Olufade A, Smith MW, Nathan R. Seasonal versus perennial allergic rhinitis: drug and medical resource use patterns. *Value Health.* 2003;6:448–456.

3. Slavin R. Comorbidities of allergic rhinitis and its impact on treatment. American College of Allergy, Asthma & Immunology. *1999–2003 Medical Association Communications.* Available at: http://www.cmecorner.com/macmcm/PCP2003/pcp_sp_2003_05. htm. Accessed November 5, 2008.

4. Slavin R. Comorbidities of allergic rhinitis and its impact on treatment. American College of Allergy, Asthma & Immunology. *1999–2003 Medical Association Communications.* Available at: http://www.cmecorner.com/macmcm/PCP2003/pcp_sp_2003_05.htm. Accessed November 5, 2008.

5. United States Environmental Protection Agency. Indoor Air Facts No. 4 *(revised) Sick Building Syndrome.* February 1991. Air and Radiation (6609J). Available at: http:// www.epa.gov/iaq/pdfs/sick_building_factsheet.pdf. Accessed November 5, 2008.

6. National Institute of Allergy and Infectious Diseases. 2008. Available at: http:// www3.niaid.nih.gov/topics/allergicDiseases/PDF/ColdAllergy.pdf. Accessed November 5, 2008; WebMD Medical Reference. 2007.

7. Asthma and Allergy Foundation of America. *Allergy facts and figures.* Available at: http://www.aafa.org/display.cfm?id=9&sub=30. Accessed November 5, 2008.

8. Umetsu DT, DeKruyff RH. TH1 and TH2 CD4+ cells in human allergic diseases. *J Allergy Clin Immunol.* 1997;100(1):1–6.

9. Platt-Mills T, Vaughan J, Squillace S, Woodfolk J, Sporik R. Sensitization, asthma, and a modified TH2 response in children exposed to cat allergen: a population-based cross-sectional study. *Lancet.* 2001;357:752–756.

10. Ishizaka A, Sakiyama Y, Nakanishi M, et al. The inductive effect of inter-leukin 4 on IgG4 and IgE synthesis in human peripheral blood lymphocytes. *Clin Exp Immunol.* 1990;79:392–396.

11. Cystic Fibrosis Foundation. *About Cystic Fibrosis.* Available at: http://www.cff.org/AboutCF/. Accessed November 28, 2008.

12. Skov M, Pressler T, Jensen HE, Hoiby N, Koch C. Specific IgG subclass antibody pattern to *Aspergillus fumigatus* in patients with cystic fibrosis with allergic bronchopulmonary aspergillosis (ABPA). *Thorax.* 1999;54:44–50.

13. Forsyth KD, Hohmann AW, Martin AJ, Bradley J. IgG antibodies to *Aspergillus fumigatus* in cystic fibrosis: a laboratory correlate of disease activity. *Arch Dis Child.* 1989;63:953–957.

14. Manning SC, Holman M. Further evidence for allergic pathophysiology in allergic fungal sinusitis. *Laryngoscope.* 1998;108:1485–1496.

15. Manning, Scott C., Holman, Marie. Further evidence for allergic pathophysiology in allergic fungal sinusitis. *Laryngoscope,* 1998, 108(10):1485–1496.

16. Freeman GL. Pine pollen allergy in northern Arizona. *Ann Allergy.* 1993; 70: 491–494.

17. Mackay IS, Durham SR. ABC of allergies: perennial rhinitis. *BMJ.* 1998; 316:917–920.

18. Anyanwu EC, Kanu I, Nwachukwu NC, Saleh MA. Chronic environmental exposure to Alternaria tenuis may manifest symptoms of neuropsychological illness: a study of 12 cases. *J Appl Sci Environ Manage.* 2005;9(3):45–51.

19. Muller A, Lehmann I, Seiffart A, et al. Increased incidence of allergic sensitization and respiratory disease due to mould exposure: results of the Leipzig Allergy Risk Children Study (LARS). *Int J Hyg Environ Health.* 2002;204:363–365.

20. Anyanwu EC, Kanu I, Nwachukwu NC, Saleh MA. Chronic environmental exposure to Alternaria tenuis may manifest symptoms of neuropsychological illness: a study of 12 cases. *J. Appl. Sci. Environ. Mgt.* 2005;9(3):45–51.

21. Dauby P-AL.; Whisman BA, Hagan L. Cross-reactivity between raw mushroom and molds in a patient with oral allergy syndrome. *Ann Allergy Asthma Immunol.* 2002;89:319–321.

22. Ansorge R, Metcalf E. Allergy Risk Factors: Scientists have revised their theories about how and why allergies are on the rise. *Prevention.* Available at: http://www.prevention.com/cda/article/allergy-risk-factors/3dfd323b0b803110VgnVCM20000012281eac____/health/conditions.treatments/allergies/0/0/2. Accessed November 28, 2008.

23. Armentia A, Asensio T, Subiza J, et al. Living in towers as risk factor of pollen allergy. *Allergy.* 2004;59:302–305.

24. Ed Hume Seeds: Houseplants That Help Purify The Air. Available at: http://www.humeseeds.com/purify.htm. Accessed November 29, 2008.

25. Nakaqawa T, Takaishi T, Sakamoto Y, et al. IgG4 antibodies in patients with house-dust-mite-sensitive bronchial asthma: relationship with antigen-specific immunotherapy. *Int Arch Allergy Appl Immunol.* 1983;71:122–125.

26. Allergen immunotherapy: a practice parameter. American Academy of Allergy, Asthma and Immunology. *Ann Allergy Asthma Immunol.* 2003;90(1 Suppl 1):1–40.

HELPFUL WEB SITES

American Academy of Allergy, Asthma and Immunology: http://www.aaaai.org/

Asthma and Allergy Foundation of America: http://www.aafa.org/

Complementary Prescriptions (Articles and Products for Allergy Support): www.cpmedi cal.net access code: 587556

Environmental Protection Agency (for more information on air-cleaning devices): http://www.epa.gov/

U.S. Department of Health and Human Services, National Institute of Allergy and Infec-tious Diseases: www.niaid.nih.gov

CHAPTER 8

Supplements to Control the Allergic Cascade

Numerous nutritional supplements have shown efficacy in regards to treating allergies. Many of these treatments positively modulate specific physiological pathways in the body to reduce the overactive immune response or decrease cellular products and resulting symptoms once the immune system is activated. Additionally, several supplements improve the functioning of the digestive system to help combat the activation of the immune system via the gut. Many of these supplements work synergistically and can provide beneficial activity for the immune and digestive systems.

NUTRIENTS

Essential Fatty Acids

Essential fatty acids are fats that are required in the diet and are important for numerous physiological functions. Probably the most well-known essential fatty acid supplement is fish oil. Oily fish, such as salmon, herring, mackerel, and trout, contain significant levels of the omega-3 long-chain polyunsaturated fatty acids DHA (docosahexaenoic acid) and EPA (eicosapentaenoic acid), which have the ability to affect inflammation and immune function. EPA and DHA compete with arachidonic acid, an omega-6 fatty acid, in inflammatory pathways. Arachidonic acid, commonly ingested in the diet from animal products, is the precursor of proinflammatory mediators, while EPA and DHA compete with arachidonic acid and increase production of anti-inflammatory cellular mediators. The balance of these mediators, known as eicosanoids, play a critical role in inflammation and, therefore, allergies. Western diets are dramatically increasing in omega-6 fatty acids leading to an imbalance of omega-6 in relation to omega-3 polyunsaturated

fatty acids, which in turn leads to an overproduction of the pro-inflammatory eicosanoids. Gamma-linolenic acid (GLA) is an omega-6 fatty acid found in black
currant oil, borage seed oil, and evening primrose oil. GLA is metabolized in the
body to series 1 prostaglandins, which also decrease the inflammatory response and
inhibit arachidonic acid from forming inflammatory eicosanoids known as leukotrienes.[1] Linoleic acid is also a precursor to GLA and can be supplemented in the
diet to support the anti-inflammatory pathway. Linoleic acid is commonly found
in the oils of corn, safflower, sesame, soybean, sunflower, walnut, and grape seeds.

The average American diet is estimated to contain 10 times more omega-6
fatty acids compared with omega-3 fatty acids. This increases the production of
proinflammatory eicosanoids, which increases the likelihood of allergic (atopic)
conditions. This imbalance alters the balance of T helper cells type 1 and type 2,
thus favoring the production of allergy-inducing IgE antibodies.[2] Research indicates that an elevated level of EPA measured in cell membranes is associated with
a decreased risk of allergic sensitization and allergic rhinitis (hay fever). Similarly,
an increased intake of the omega-3 fatty acid alpha-linolenic acid is associated
with a decreased risk of allergic sensitization and allergic rhinitis.[3] A recent study
showed that supplementation with GLA and EPA in patients with asthma showed
a decrease in leukotriene levels, use of rescue bronchodilators, self-reported asthma
status, and use of a bronchodilator medication.[4] Researchers have demonstrated
that supplementation with omega-3 fatty acids in children with allergic diseases
resulted in an improvement in fatty acid levels in plasma and red cell membranes,
cellular and humoral immunity status, and eicosanoid synthesis, as well as positive clinical changes.[5] Another interesting study examined GLA levels in mothers
and infants to assess the role essential fatty acids play in the prevalence of atopic
disorders. The study found that the breast milk of allergic mothers contained less
GLA than that of healthy nonallergic mothers, and atopic (allergic) infants had
less GLA in phospholipids than healthy infants.[6] Studies have also found that
supplementation with oral evening primrose oil in patients with atopic dermatitis
(eczema) resulted in a statistically significant improvement in the overall severity
and grade of inflammation, the percentage of the body surface involved by eczema, and dryness and itching.[7]

Quercetin

Quercetin is a dietary flavonoid found in buckwheat tea, green tea, apples, ber-
ries, brassica vegetables, onions, and red wine. Quercetin exhibits antihistamine,
anti-inflammatory, and antioxidant activity. Histamine is a chemical mediator responsible for allergy symptoms such as hives, constriction in the lungs, itchy and
watery eyes, congestion, and sneezing. Numerous studies have demonstrated that
quercetin inhibits the release of histamine from particular white blood cells known
as mast cells and basophils.[8] In addition, quercetin has been shown to decrease
asthmatic reactions in animal models similar in effectiveness to the pharmaceuticals cromolyn sodium and dexamethasone.[9] Using similar animal models, quercetin has also been shown to inhibit anaphylactic smooth-muscle contraction.[10]

N-Acetylcysteine

N-acetylcysteine (NAC) is a derivative of the amino acid L-cysteine. NAC is used for antioxidant and anti-inflammatory activity and can be converted intracellularly to the potent antioxidant glutathione. Glutathione is a naturally occurring tripeptide that protects cells from toxic free radicals and is involved with immune system function. Glutathione is not absorbed when taken orally; thus, supplementing with NAC is an effective way to increase glutathione levels. NAC has been used in the treatment of bronchitis and other lung conditions as an expectorant or mucous thinner, as well as for its anti-inflammatory and antioxidant effects.[11] Selenium is also important to supplement with NAC, as it is required for the synthesis of the enzyme glutathione peroxidase. Glutathione peroxidase is the enzyme responsible for catalyzing the reaction in which reduced glutathione synthesizes water from hydrogen peroxide. Hydrogen peroxide and other highly reactive oxygen intermediates cause cellular damage. Increased free radicals such as nitric oxide are associated with allergies, asthma, and elevated IgE levels,[12] thus making antioxidant support crucial to allergy therapy.

Alpha-Lipoic Acid

Alpha-lipoic acid is a coenzyme that is used medicinally for its powerful antioxidant activity. It is metabolized to dihydrolipoic acid, and both molecules exhibit antioxidant free-radical scavenging activity. Alpha-lipoic acid has broad-spectrum effects in the body as it is both water and fat soluble and can regenerate endogenous antioxidants such as vitamins C and E, glutathione, and coenzyme Q10, helping to recycle these antioxidants in the body.[13]

Vitamin C

Vitamin C (ascorbic acid) is a water-soluble vitamin found in many fruits and vegetables and is required in the diet in humans. Vitamin C is used particularly for antioxidant and immune-modulating activity, and it has some antihistamine effects. As an antioxidant, vitamin C can protect cells from reactive oxygen species known to cause tissue damage. Research indicates that low vitamin C levels are associated with elevated plasma histamine levels.[14] Individuals with asthma have been shown to have significantly lower levels of plasma and leukocyte vitamin C compared with healthy control subjects, as well as an increase in overt vitamin C deficiency. In fact, one study showed that leukocyte vitamin C was deficient in 92.0 percent of subjects with asthma versus only 8.0 percent of control subjects.[15] Studies have shown that ascorbic acid supplementation of 1500 milligrams per day attenuated exercise-induced airway narrowing in subjects with asthma.[16] Another study showed that two grams of vitamin C significantly improved lung function after a histamine challenge in patients with allergic rhinitis one hour after taking it, compared with the placebo group.[17] Additional research found a fivefold increase in bronchial hyperreactivity among those patients with

the lowest intake of vitamin C.[18] Researchers have shown that vitamin C deficiency is not uncommon. One study found that 6 percent of subjects had plasma
vitamin C concentrations indicative of overt vitamin C deficiency and another
30.4 percent of the subjects showed subclinical vitamin C depletion.[19] In addition, estrogen and oral contraceptives, and smoking and other forms of nicotine have been shown to increase vitamin C excretion causing measurably lower
plasma levels.[20]

Vitamin E

Vitamin E is a fat-soluble vitamin that acts as an antioxidant and free-radical
scavenger of lipids and fats. Vitamin E exists in eight forms, including four
tocotrienols and alpha-, beta-, gamma-, and delta-tocopherols. The D-alpha-
tocopherol isomer is the natural form found in foods and has the most biological
activity. Vitamin E is used for antioxidant activity and protects cell membranes
from free-radical damage. Vitamin E modifies the leukotriene inflammatory
pathway, making it a potential therapy for allergies and asthma.[21] Leukotrienes
are derived from the 5-lipoxygenase pathway of arachidonic acid metabolism,
and production of leukotrienes is increased in patients with asthma. Vitamin E
has been shown to inhibit the activation of neutrophils, which, in persons with
asthma, results in the synthesis of leukotrienes in a dose-dependent fashion.[22]
Recent studies have shown that supplementation with gamma-tocopherol significantly decreased many of the reactions seen with allergic airway diseases in
animal models. In particular, there was a decrease in eosinophils (white blood
cells associated with allergies), inflammatory chemical mediators, cells that produce mucus, and mucus storage.[23] Although vitamin E deficiency is rare, one
study showed that decreased maternal vitamin E intake during pregnancy is associated with increased risk of childhood asthma at age 5.[24] Additionally, the
concentration of alpha-tocopherol in erythrocytes has been shown to be significantly lower in children with atopic dermatitis compared with healthy control
subjects.[25] Also, researchers have shown that a higher concentration of vitamin E
intake is associated with lower serum IgE antibody concentrations and a lower
frequency of allergen sensitization.[26]

Beta Carotene

Beta carotene is a carotenoid found readily in fruits, vegetables, grains, and
oils. It is converted to vitamin A in the body, and it is estimated that carotenoid intake provides approximately 50 percent of dietary vitamin A.[27] Beta
carotene has antioxidant activity, prevents lipid peroxidation, and may reduce
free-radical damage.[28] Patients with asthma have been shown to have decreased
levels of carotenoids in their blood compared with healthy control subjects,
despite similar intake levels.[29] One study showed that supplementation with
64 milligrams of beta carotene daily for one week decreased exercise-induced
asthma in 53 percent of subjects studied.[30] Animal models have shown that
supplementation with beta carotene decreased levels of the antibodies IgE and

IgG1 and decreased serum histamine levels during anaphylactic reactions.[31] Another study showed that supplementing beta carotene with vitamin E (alpha-tocopherol) in mice significantly suppressed both the antigen-specific and total IgE antibody levels. The authors suggested that this combination may be beneficial for preventing type I allergic reactions.[32]

Coenzyme Q10

Coenzyme Q10 (CoQ10) is a potent antioxidant that is an important cofactor for numerous cellular processes such as the production of cellular energy in the form of adenosine triphosphate (ATP). Studies have shown that serum and whole blood concentrations of CoQ10 are significantly decreased in patients with asthma.[33] In a randomized clinical trial, patients with asthma were supplemented with 120 milligrams of CoQ10, 400 milligrams vitamin E (alpha-tocopherol), and 250 milligrams of vitamin C daily. The results showed that antioxidant supplementation decreased the dosage of corticosteroids required by patients with asthma, indicating lower incidence of potential adverse effects of the drugs and decreased oxidative stress.[34] Another study showed that 40 percent of patients with various types of allergic conditions had dangerously low blood levels of CoQ10, similar to the levels seen in gravely ill cardiac patients.[35]

Magnesium

Magnesium is a critically important mineral, as it plays a role in more than 300 biochemical reactions in the body. Magnesium deficiency is not uncommon in the United States and is associated with numerous diseases. Patients with asthma have been shown to have decreased levels of red blood cell magnesium.[36] Numerous studies have investigated magnesium as a treatment for asthma. Research has shown that supplementation with oral, inhaled, and intravenous magnesium decreases bronchial reactivity and decreases allergen-induced skin responses in patients with asthma.[37] One study showed that as magnesium intake declines, the incidence of allergies and asthma increases.[38]

BOTANICAL MEDICINE

Green Tea (*Camellia sinensis*)

Green tea contains several active constituents, such as catechins, flavonoids, polyphenols, and caffeine, which are believed to provide many of the beneficial actions of this herb. Catechins such as epigallocatechin (EGC), epigallocatechin gallate (EGCG), and epicatechin gallate (ECG) are potent antioxidants and may also have anti-inflammatory activity. In animal models, oral supplementation with the catechins EGC, ECG, and EGCG, as well as caffeine, was shown to inhibit passive cutaneous anaphylaxis suggesting that these constituents may provide significant protection against the type I allergic reactions.[39] An interesting study showed that the constituent in green tea, EGCG, blocks the production of histamine and IgE, two compounds in the body that are involved in triggering and sustaining allergic reactions. The study showed that a methylated form of EGCG can block the IgE receptor, which is a key receptor involved in an allergic response. The effect was demonstrated using human basophils, which are blood cells that release histamine.[40] Also, as a potent antioxidant, green tea may reduce oxidative DNA damage, lipid peroxidation, and freeradical formation.

Stinging Nettles (*Urtica dioica*)

Stinging nettle leaf contains several active constituents, such as carotenoids, vitamin C, vitamin E, calcium, potassium, and flavonoids, including quercetin and rutin. In a double-blind randomized study, a freeze-dried preparation of *Urtica dioica* improved allergic rhinitis better than placebo.[41] This effect may be due to the quercetin content, as quercetin stabilizes mast cells and inhibits the release of histamine.

Perilla Frutescens

Perilla frutescens, also known as Beefsteak plant, belongs to the Mint family, which also includes basil, sage, mint, and rosemary. *Perilla* contains rosmarinic acid and luteolin, which are believed to be the active constituents. Several studies have shown that *Perilla* supplementation is effective in managing allergic symptoms. In a randomized, double-blind, age-matched, placebo-controlled parallel group study, patients with seasonal allergic rhinoconjunctivitis (nose and eye symptoms) were supplemented with an extract of *Perilla frutescens* enriched for rosmarinic acid for 21 days. The results showed a significant decrease in overall allergic symptoms, including itchy nose, watery eyes, itchy eyes. The study also found a significant decrease in the numbers of neutrophils and eosinophils in the nasal fluid of the *Perilla*-treated group.[42] In a study using animals, supplementation with an extract of *Perilla* was shown to decrease mast cell–mediated immediate-type allergic reactions measured by a reduction in plasma histamine levels.[43] *Perilla frutescens* leaf extract was also shown to significantly suppress IgE and IgG1 antibody levels in mice. This study also showed a decrease in the chemical mediators associated with the allergic response.[44] In another interesting study, rosemary extract was evaluated in a mouse model of allergic asthma. The study found that rosemary extract prevents allergic airway inflammation as shown by its inhibiting the typical increase in the number of eosinophils, neutrophils, and mononuclear cells around the airways and those in the bronchial lavage fluid upon exposure to dust mites.[45] Luteolin has also shown benefit in treating allergic symptoms. One study showed that luteolin suppressed proinflammatory mediators and decreased allergic swelling in mouse models.[46] Luteolin also significantly modulates airway bronchoconstriction and bronchial hyperreactivity in experimental mice models of allergic asthma. Additionally, the study showed that luteolin decreased the chemical mediators associated with allergies as well as decreased levels of IgE antibodies.[47] Other researchers have shown that luteolin suppresses histamine release from mast cells.[48]

Ginkgo Biloba

Historically, ginkgo leaf extracts were used to stimulate circulation and improve brain function in Chinese medicine. Ginkgo has also demonstrated efficacy in the treatment of allergic symptoms. Ginkgo leaf extract was shown to significantly reduced airway hyperreactivity and improved clinical symptoms and lung function in patients with asthma.[49] Another study found that *Ginkgo biloba* leaf extract significantly decreased the release of proinflammatory mediators after an antigen challenge in anaphylactic lungs using animal models.[50] Additional research has shown that topical treatment with ginkgo for allergic contact dermatitis has been shown to significantly decrease skin reactivity in 68.2 percent of the subjects studied.[51]

Butterbur (*Petasites hybridus, Petasites officinalis*)

Butterbur exhibits several properties that make it beneficial for the treatment of allergic rhinitis and asthma. It has been shown to relax smooth muscle and decrease levels of histamine and leukotrienes. One study showed that supplementation with butterbur in patients with allergic rhinitis significantly decreased nasal allergy symptoms, improved quality-of-life scores, and reduced histamine and leukotriene levels in nasal fluids.[52] In a randomized, double-blind, parallel-group study, butterbur was shown to be as effective as cetirizine (Zyrtec) in relieving symptoms of seasonal allergic rhinitis.[53] A similar study showed that butterbur extract was as effective as the pharmaceutical fexofenadine (Allegra) for the treatment of allergic rhinitis.[54]

FIGHT ALLERGIES WITH OPTIMAL INTESTINAL HEALTH

Intestinal health can play a significant role in the allergic response. Approximately 70 percent of the immune system is located in the digestive tract. Intestinal permeability contributes to the development of food allergies. In one study, patients with food allergies or food hypersensitivities who were on allergen-free diets were found to have statistically significant differences in intestinal permeability compared with control patients. In fact, the researchers showed that the worse the intestinal permeability, the more serious the clinical symptoms in patients with food allergy and hypersensitivity. They also found that impaired intestinal permeability was present in all subjects with adverse reactions to food.[55] Testing for intestinal permeability has been shown to be reliable for the diagnosing food allergies among children.[56] To further elucidate the connections between intestinal permeability, allergies, and immune dysfunction, consider the example of a newborn infant. Infants have increased intestinal permeability in order to absorb complete immune proteins from their mother's breast milk. Studies have shown that infants given gluten-containing foods such as wheat, barley, or rye during the first three months of life have had a fivefold increased risk of celiac disease autoimmunity (reaction to gluten) compared with children exposed to gluten-containing foods at four to six months.[57] Early introduction of food is also associated with increased risk of food allergy. According to the American College of Allergy, Asthma and Immunology, the optimal age for introducing selected supplemental foods should be 6 months; dairy products, 12 months; hen's eggs, 24 months; and peanut, tree nuts, fish, and seafood at least 36 months.[58] Animal models have also shown that intestinal permeability can be induced from conditions such as increased psychological stress.[59] Increased intestinal permeability is also associated with gastrointestinal diseases such as ulcerative colitis and Crohn's disease.

Strengthening the Colon

Short-chain fatty acids (SCFAs) play an important role in intestinal health. SCFAs, primarily acetate, propionate, and butyrate, are produced in the colon by fermentation of dietary carbohydrates. More specifically, degradation-resistant starches and dietary fiber are fermented by colonic microflora. SCFA production depends on several factors, such as the fermentation substrate, the species and quantity of microflora in the colon, and the transit time through the intestinal tract. SCFA concentrations in the intestines vary markedly with diet,[60] yet have several important functions in the intestines.[61] Butyrate affects a variety of colonic mucosal functions such as inhibiting inflammation and carcinogenesis, reinforcing the colonic defense barrier, and decreasing oxidative stress.[62] SCFAs are absorbed by the cells that line the intestines and promote intestinal mucosal growth, as butyrate is the major energy source for enterocytes, which are the cells lining the colon. In addition, butyrate induces specific enzymes that promote mucosal cell restoration. SCFAs also stimulate colonic blood flow and fluid and electrolyte uptake[63] and enhance the motility of the intestinal tract by stimulating contractions and shorten emptying time for the ileum.[64] SCFAs, particularly butyrate, have been shown to stimulate the secretion of mucus, an important part of the intestinal mucosal barrier in the colon.

According to researchers, SCFAs play a role in many disease conditions, including digestive disorders, cancer, and cardiovascular disease. The SCFAs butyrate, acetate, and propionate have been shown to be effective anti-inflammatory and immune-modulating agents in human colon cancer cell lines.[65] Butyrate has been shown to inhibit proinflammatory markers and is being investigated for the role this plays in the prevention of inflammatory bowel disease and cancer.[66] Butyrate is also being studied for its use in the prevention of colon cancer, as it has been shown to promote cell differentiation, cell-cycle arrest, and apoptosis (programmed cell death) of colon cancer cells. In addition, butyrate has been shown to decrease DNA damage in human colon cells and colon cancer cell lines by approximately 50 percent.[67] Researchers suggest that the high occurrence of colon disorders seen in Western civilizations may be the result of a diet low in resistant starch and fiber and the resulting low production of SCFAs in the colon.[68] Studies have shown that deficient production of SCFAs may be involved in antibiotic-associated diarrhea, food allergies,[69] ulcerative colitis, and other intestinal disorders.[70] Therefore, increasing levels of SCFAs may reduce the risk of developing immune system dysfunction, cancer, gastrointestinal disorders, and cardiovascular disease.[71]

Modulating ammonia levels in the colon is also important for optimizing colon health. Elevated levels of colonic ammonia can potentially adversely effect health. Ammonia is produced in the colon by bacterial fermentation of nitrogen-containing substances such as protein. Ammonia levels in the colon increase as protein intake increases. Research indicates that even low levels of ammonia can have detrimental effects on the cells that line the colon. Ammonia is toxic to the colonic epithelial cells, which can lead to cell destruction and increased cell turnover.[72] Animal models have also shown that increased production of ammonia from eating a high-protein diet increased the incidence of colon cancer.[73] In addition, ammonia levels found in the colon in people eating a typical Western diet has been associated with increased viral infections, growth of cancer cells, cell toxicity, and altered nucleic acid (DNA, RNA) synthesis.[74]

NUTRITIONAL SUPPORT FOR THE COLON

Probiotics

Probiotics are beneficial bacteria. More than 400 different strains of bacteria reside in the intestines, and particular strains of intestinal microflora are required for optimal health and normal immune system function. Various studies have shown that proper intestinal microflora, such as *Lactobacillus* and *Bifidobacterium*, provide health benefits. Most importantly, probiotics can improve the barrier function of the intestines. They can also compete with and suppress the growth of pathogenic bacteria, as well as modulate or stimulate the immune response.[75] Probiotics are also important for nutrient and enzyme synthesis and absorption. Any imbalance of the intestinal microflora can result in immune system dysfunctions, such as allergies or inflammation. Environmental and dietary factors can affect levels of probiotics. Factors such as drinking chlorinated water, eating a low-fiber diet, or using antibiotics or other medications can deplete the levels of beneficial bacteria, thus making it important to replenish them for optimal immune function. Common probiotic supplements include *Lactobacillus acidophilus*, *Lactobacillus sporogenes*, *Bifidobacterium bifidum*, *Bifidobacterium longum*, and *Bifidobacterium infantis*.

Lactobacillus is a genus of gram-positive colonic bacteria named for their ability to produce lactic acid. Common species include *Lactobacillus acidophilus*, *Lactobacillus rhamnosus*, *Lactobacillus reuteri*, *Lactobacillus sporogenes*, and *Lactobacillus fermentum*. *Lactobacillus reuteri* is the most common *Lactobacillus* species in the gastrointestinal tract. These bacteria bind to the mucosal lining in the intestines where they suppress pathogenic bacteria by producing lactic acid and hydrogen peroxide. They also prevent pathogenic bacteria from adhering to the mucosal lining by competing for mucosal binding sites.[76] *Lactobacillus* inhibits pathogenic bacteria by competing with pathogenic microbes in the colon for binding to the epithelial cells that line the intestines,[77] producing lactic acid, and increasing epithelial mucous production. *Lactobacillus* also supports the intestinal barrier and suppresses bacterial translocation through the intestinal lining and into the circulation.[78]

The genus *Bifidobacterium* is a gram-positive anaerobe that produces lactic acid, but resides lower in the intestinal tract than *Lactobacillus*. Common species include *Bifidobacterium bifidum, Bifidobacterium breve, Bifidobacterium longum,* and *Bifidobacterium infantis. Bifidobacterium* produces antimicrobial substances that suppress many pathogenic organisms. Some species of *Bifidobacterium* bind to the intestinal epithelial cells and prevent attachment of pathogenic bacteria. *Bifidobacterium longum* is particularly resistant to stomach acid, which improves the ability of the bacteria to reach the colon intact when ingested orally.

There is a great deal of research regarding the positive health effects of probiotics. Supplementation with probiotics has been shown to benefit numerous medical conditions, including allergies, infections, inflammatory conditions, and gastrointestinal disorders. Specifically, supplementation with probiotics has been shown to modulate the immune system and affect such conditions as food allergies and allergic rhinitis.[79] Research has also shown that both *Lactobacillus* and *Bifidobacterium* can affect the sensitization to dietary antigens in infants and was shown to significantly decrease the extent and severity of atopic eczema in these patients, demonstrating the ability to affect both allergy prevention and treatment.[80] According to researchers, decreased levels of lactic-acid producing intestinal microflora in children increases the incidence of allergies and atopy. Animal models have also shown that *Lactobacillus* can decrease levels of IgE and IgG1 antibodies, which are often elevated in persons with allergic conditions, as well as decrease systemic anaphylactic food allergy reactions.[81] Other research has shown that supplementation with *Lactobacillus* decreases the number and severity of respiratory infections and absenteeism in children that attend day care.[82] Animal models of autoimmune arthritis indicate that supplementation with *Lactobacillus* protects against rheumatoid arthritis progression and reduces swelling, cartilage destruction, and proinflammatory mediators.[83] Another recent study showed that supplementation with probiotics and prebiotics in patients with colon cancer decreased cell proliferation and other cancer markers while stimulating the immune response.[84] In addition, these bacteria support immune function and may promote synthesis of secretory IgA antibodies, the antibodies that protect the mucosal lining, in response to pathogenic organisms. In fact, *Lactobacillus* has been shown to stimulate the immune system in healthy persons while suppressing the immune response in hypersensitive persons with overactive immune responses.[85] Thus, these various studies demonstrate the immune system benefits of replacing beneficial bacteria in the gut.

Fructo-Oligosaccharides

Fructo-oligosaccharides (FOSs) are plant sugars that act as prebiotics. Prebiotics are substances that selectively promote the growth and activity of beneficial bacteria in the colon.[86] These bacteria, in turn, produce enzymes that ferment the

FOSs, as they are not metabolized by digestive enzymes and pass through the small intestine undigested. This provides beneficial effects such as increased fecal mass, decreased pH, and production of SCFAs. As mentioned previously, the SCFAs created by fermentation of FOSs have numerous beneficial functions in the intestines. In addition, FOSs increase intestinal absorption of magnesium, calcium, and iron.[87] FOSs exhibit anti-inflammatory activity on intestinal inflammation as well.[88] FOSs can be found naturally in some fruits and vegetables, such as Jerusalem artichoke, soybeans, and asparagus.

Digestive Enzymes

Digestive enzymes are required to properly break down food into macromolecules. These enzymes are secreted by the pancreas to adequately digest carbohydrates, proteins, and fats. Persons with food allergies are often missing or are inadequately secreting natural digestive enzymes[89]; thus, supplementation may be beneficial. Supplementing digestive enzymes, such as lipase, amylase, protease, maltase, lactase, sucrase, phytase, and cellulose, can decrease absorption of inappropriately large molecules in the intestines, which can lead to allergic sensitization. Hydrochloric acid supplementation may also be considered to optimize gastric pH, which is necessary to activate the pancreatic digestive enzymes.

Glutamine

Glutamine, which is produced primarily in skeletal muscle, is the most abundant amino acid in the body. Although the body can make glutamine, in times of severe stress it cannot meet the increased demand; thus, it is a conditionally essential amino acid. Glutamine provides metabolic fuel for several cell types in the immune system and for the enterocytes, the cells that line the intestines. Glutamine is critical for intestinal health. Research indicates that glutamine supplementation stimulates proliferation and differentiation of intestinal cells and maintains mucosal integrity, thereby preventing intestinal hyperpermeability and bacterial translocation.[90] Glutamine is also important in regulating intestinal IgA, an antibody that protects the mucosal lining.[91] Researchers have found that glutamine administration has a protective effect that prevents or reduces the intensity of the increase in intestinal permeability, particularly in critically ill patients. Glutamine supplementation also decreases the frequency of systemic infections in this population.[92] Researchers came to a similar conclusion examining patients with gastrointestinal cancer treated with chemotherapy in which oral glutamine decreased intestinal permeability and maintained the intestinal barrier.[93] Research also indicates that glutamine supplementation may decrease systemic inflammation and increase killing of bacteria by the immune system, in addition to improving intestinal permeability and decreasing bacterial translocation.[94]

Licorice (*Glycyrrhiza glabra*)

Licorice is used medicinally for its anti-inflammatory, soothing, laxative, and antispasmodic activity. Most research on deglycyrrhizinated licorice has focused on upper gastrointestinal health, such as ulcer healing and dyspepsia. However, deglycyrrhizinated licorice provides benefit for many other inflammatory intestinal disorders as well. Licorice may be useful to help decrease inflammation and heal or soothe an irritated intestinal lining.

Berberine

Berberine is a constituent found in various botanicals, such as goldenseal (*Hydrastis canadensis*) and Oregon grape (*Mahonia aquafolium*). Berberine may be beneficial in optimizing colon health by maintaining proper gastrointestinal flora and inhibiting pathogenic microbes in the colon. Berberine exhibits significant antimicrobial activity against bacterial, fungus, mycobacteria, and protozoa. In particular, research has shown that berberine has activity against many strains of pathogenic microbes, such as *Eschericha coli*, *Staphylococcus aureus*, *Streptococcus pyogenes*, *Shigella boydii*, *Vibrio cholerae*, *Mycobacterium tuberculosis*, *Candida albicans*, *Candida tropicalis*, *Trichophyton mentagrophytes*, *Microsporum gypseum*, *Cryptococcus neoformans*, *Sporotrichum schenckii*, *Entamoeba histolytica*, and *Giardia lamblia*.[95] Berberine also exhibits anti-inflammatory activity by decreasing proinflammatory chemical mediators.[96] Berberine may also reduce intestinal permeability.[97]

Cabbage (*Brassica oleracea*)

Cabbage is a cruciferous vegetable that contains several important nutrients, such as vitamin K1, vitamin C, vitamin A, vitamin E, B vitamins, calcium, and amino acids, including glutamine. Research has shown that cabbage exhibits significant antioxidant activity.[98] Evidence also suggests that individuals who consume large amounts of cabbage and other vegetables from the Brassicaceae family have a lower risk of developing colorectal and stomach cancer.[99] Cabbage juice has been shown to be highly effective for healing the stomach. One study of 100 patients with peptic ulcer demonstrated that drinking four glasses of fresh, raw cabbage juice daily dramatically reduced pain and healing time. According to the study, more than two-thirds of the subjects were better within four days and 81 percent were symptom-free within one week.[100]

Slippery Elm (*Ulmus fulva*)

The inner bark rind of the slippery elm contains mucilage constituents that are used medicinally for demulcent and emollient effects. Demulcents are agents that form a soothing film over a mucous membrane resulting in decreased pain and inflammation of the membrane. Slippery elm stimulates nerve endings in the gastrointestinal tract, which leads to increased secretion of mucus, which, in turn, coats and protects the lining of the intestines from excess acidity, ulcers, ingested irritants, and toxins.[101] Slippery elm has also shown antioxidant activity in colon as a free-radical scavenger.[102]

Marshmallow (*Althaea officinalis*)

Marshmallow leaf and root contain mucilage sugars, which create a protective layer on mucous membranes resulting in soothing and protective activity.[103] The mucilage also has antimicrobial, spasmolytic, and wound-healing properties.[104]

Aloe Vera

Medicinally, the gel from the aloe vera leaf is used for anti-inflammatory, antioxidant, antibacterial, and antifungal activity. Constituents of the aloe latex are believed to induce mucous secretion from mucous membranes and induce movement in the intestines. Aloe is used for a variety of digestive complaints, such as constipation, inflammatory bowel disease, and ulcers, as well as for wound healing and other inflammatory conditions. In addition to its anti-inflammatory activity, aloe has been shown to have antihistamine activity, and it inhibits bradykinin, a pain-producing chemical mediator.[105] Specific to colon health, research on inflammatory bowel disease has shown that aloe provides antioxidant activity and decreases inflammatory mediators.[106] In another study regarding aloe and colon health, aloe vera gel was supplemented at a dose of 100 milliliters twice daily for four weeks in patients with mild to moderate active ulcerative colitis. The results indicated that 37 percent of subjects showed improvement and 30 percent of patients had clinical remission with the aloe treatment.[107]

N-Acetylglucosamine

N-acetylglucosamine (NAG) is the acetylated form of glucosamine. Glucosamine is required for the synthesis of glycosaminoglycans and glycoproteins known as mucopolysaccharides, which is a component of mucous membranes, among other things. NAG is deficient in persons with inflammatory bowel disease (ulcerative colitis and Crohn's disease), which may cause a decrease in the intestinal mucosal glycoprotein cover that protects the intestinal mucosa from damage.[108] In one study, NAG was supplemented at a daily dose 3 to 6 grams orally as adjunct therapy to children with severe treatment-resistant inflammatory bowel disease. The results showed that two-thirds of the children showed clear improvement and all cases biopsied showed histological improvement with a significant increase in epithelial glycosaminoglycans and intracellular NAG levels.[109]

Phosphatidylcholine

Phosphatidylcholine is a lipid component of biological membranes, such as the protective intestinal mucosal layer. Phosphatidylcholine has been shown to exhibit significant anti-inflammatory activity in human intestinal cells.[110] Decreased mucosal surface hydrophobicity (lacking affinity for water) is associated with increased colonic permeability. Treatment with lipids, including phosphatidylcholine has been shown to increase surface hydrophobicity in the colon and to reduce colonic permeability in animal models.[111] Animal models have also shown that supplementation with phosphatidylcholine inhibits the translocation of bacteria across the intestinal lining into the bloodstream in susceptible animals and prevents a postoperative decrease in intestinal mucosal mass.[112] In human studies, phosphatidylcholine has been shown to significantly benefit patients with ulcerative colitis. In one study, six grams per day of phospholipids rich in phosphatidylcholine was supplemented in patients with ulcerative colitis for three months. The results indicated that 53 percent of patients had clinical remission, 90 percent showed improvement in clinical symptoms, and 55 percent reported an improvement in quality of life in the patients treated with phosphatidylcholine.[113] Research also indicates that phosphatidylcholine works synergistically with butyrate to inhibit colon cancer cells.[114]

Gamma Oryzanol

Gamma oryzanol is a mixture of ferulic acid esters of sterol and triterpene alcohols extracted from bran, such as rice bran oil, that possess antioxidant properties. Research has shown that gamma oryzanol exhibits antiulcer properties in mice.[115] Researchers suggest that gamma oryzanol may be a therapeutic agent for inflammatory intestinal disease as it has shown significant antioxidant activity in mice models of colitis.[116] Rice bran oil, which is high in gamma-oryzanol content, has also been shown to modulate the immune response. In particular, it was shown to decrease T helper cell type 2 (pro-allergy) chemical mediators and IgE antibodies, which suggests an antiallergy effect.[117]

Larch Arabinogalactan

Larch arabinogalactan is a polysaccharide derived from the bark of the larch tree, primarily *Larix occidentalis* (western larch). Arabinogalactan is a nondigestible soluble dietary fiber that enters the large bowel intact. In the colon, it is fermented by colonic bacteria. These polysaccharides give larch its medicinal properties—it affects both the immune and digestive systems. Arabinogalactan is also approved by the U.S. Food and Drug Administration as a source of dietary fiber. Supplementation with larch arabinogalactan has been shown to increase the production of the SCFAs butyrate and propionate and to decrease the generation and absorption of ammonia in the colon. Research also indicates that larch arabinogalactan ingestion significantly enhances beneficial gut microflora, specifically increasing anaerobes such as *Lactobacillus* and *Bifidobacterium*.[118] Larch arabinogalactan also has immune-modulating activity.[119]

Fiber

Fiber intake increases butyrate levels in the body. It is well established that fiber supports colon health as it has been shown to be protective against colon cancer and to raise butyrate levels. Dietary fiber has been shown to benefit intestinal conditions such as inflammatory bowel disease, which may be related to the production of butyrate that occurs when fiber is fermented in the colon resulting in a decreased inflammatory response.[120] Studies have shown that a high-fiber diet is associated with a decrease in plasma levels of proinflammatory chemical mediators.[121] Additional research has shown that the higher the dietary fiber intake, the lower the levels of C-reactive protein (CRP), a marker used to measure systemic inflammation.[122] Fiber supplementation at a dose of 30 grams per day has been shown to be effective at reducing CRP levels.[123]

Vitamin D

Vitamin D is a fat-soluble vitamin that plays an important role in gastrointestinal health. The body requires brief exposure of the skin to sunlight to effectively make vitamin D. Supplementation of vitamin D should be with cholecalciferol (vitamin D3), as it is significantly more potent that ergocalciferol (vitamin D2). Recent research indicated that vitamin D deficiency may compromise the intestinal mucosal barrier, leading to increased susceptibility to mucosal damage and increased risk of conditions such as inflammatory bowel disease.[124] Studies have shown that patients with inflammatory bowel disease have decreased levels of vitamin D. In fact, vitamin D deficiency (serum 25-OH-D concentration less than 15 nanograms per milliliter) is present in 22 to 70 percent of patients with Crohn's disease and 45 percent of patients with ulcerative colitis.[125] Vitamin D supplementation should be considered to optimize gastrointestinal health, particularly in persons with decreased sun exposure or living in northern latitudes.

A resource that many of my patients use to gain access to certified Good Manufacturing Practice (GMP)high-quality supplements is www.CPMedical.net a professional Web site that requires a pin number (use No. 587556) for full access to the articles, newsletters and supplements.

CONCLUSION

Numerous natural products are available to help support the immune system and manage the symptoms associated with allergic conditions. Some treatments help decrease symptoms and reactivity, while others directly affect the sensitization of the immune system to antigens. Supplementing with antioxidants, whether as a nutrient or botanical, is crucial for allergy treatment. In addition, treating the gastrointestinal tract is also important for modulating the overactive immune response seen with allergies.

NOTES

1. Leventhal LJ, Boyce EG, Zurier RB. Treatment of rheumatoid arthritis with gammalinolenic acid. *Ann Intern Med.* 1993;119:867–873.

2. Kankaanpaa P, Sutas Y, Salminen S, Lichtenstein A, Isolauri E. Dietary fatty acids and allergy. *Ann Med.* 1999;31:282–287.

3. Hoff S, Seiler H, Heinrich J, et al. Allergic sensitisation and allergic rhinitis are associated with n-3 polyunsaturated fatty acids in the diet and in red blood cell membranes. Eur J Clin Nutr. 2005;59:1071–1080.

4. Surette ME, Stull D, Lindemann J. The impact of a medical food containing gammalinolenic and eicosapentaenoic acids on asthma management and the quality of life of adult asthma patients. Curr Med Res Opin. 2008;24:559–567.

5. Gorelova Zhlu, Ladodo KS, Levachev MM, et al. Role of polyunsaturated fatty acids in diet therapy of children with allergic diseases. Vopr Pitan. 1999;68(1):31–35.

6. Kankaanpaa P, Nurmela K, Erkkila A, et al. Polyunsaturated fatty acids in maternal diet, breast milk, and serum lipid fatty acids of infants in relation to atopy. Allergy. 2001;56:633–638.

7. Schalin-Karrila M, Mattila L, Jansen CT, et al. Evening primrose oil in the treatment of atopic eczema: effect on clinical status, plasma phospholipid fatty acids and circulating blood prostaglandins. Br J Dermatol. 1987;117(1):11–19.

8. Shaik YB, Castellani ML, Perrella A, et al. Role of quercetin (a natural herbal compound) in allergy and inflammation. J Biol Regul Homeost Agents. 2006;20(3–4):47–52.

9. Moon H, Choi HH, Lee JY, et al. Quercetin inhalation inhibits the asthmatic responses by exposure to aerosolized-ovalbumin in conscious guinea-pigs. Arch Pharm Res. 2008;31(6):771–778.

10. Fanning MJ, Macander P, Drzewiecki G, et al. Quercetin inhibits anaphylactic contraction of guinea pig ileum smooth muscle. Int Arch Allergy Appl Immunol. 1983;71:371–373.

11. Reichenberger F, Tamm M. N-acetylcystein in the therapy of chronic bronchitis. Pneumologie. 2002;56:793–797.

12. Cardinale F, de Benedictis FM, Muggeo V, et al. Exhaled nitric oxide, total serum IgE and allergic sensitization in childhood asthma and allergic rhinitis. Pediatr Allergy Immunol. 2005;16:236–242.

13. Packer L, Witt EH, Tritschler HJ. Alpha-Lipoic acid as a biological antioxidant. Free Rad Biol Med. 1995;19:227–250.

14. Johnston CS, Solomon RE, Corte C. Vitamin C depletion is associated with alterations in blood histamine and plasma free carnitine in adults. J Am Coll Nutr. 1996;15:586–591.

15. Shidfar F, Baghai N, Keshavarz A, et al. Comparison of plasma and leukocyte vitamin C status between asthmatic and healthy subjects. East Mediterr Health J. 2005;11(1–2):87–95.

16. Tecklenburg SL, Mickleborough TD, Fly AD, et al. Ascorbic acid supplementation attenuates exercise-induced bronchoconstriction in patients with asthma. Respir Med. 2007;101:1770–2778.

17. Bucca C, Rolla G, Oliva A, et al. Effect of vitamin C on histamine bronchial responsiveness of patients with allergic rhinitis." Ann Allergy. 1990;65:311–314.

18. Soutar A, Seaton A, Brown K. Bronchial reactivity and dietary antioxidants. Thorax. 1997;52:166–170.

19. Johnston CS, Thompson LL. Vitamin C status of an outpatient population. J Am Coll Nutr. 1998;17:366–370.

20. Lykkesfeldt J, Christen S, Wallock LM, et al. Ascorbate is depleted by smoking and replaced by moderate supplementation: a study in male smokers and nonsmokers with matched dietary antioxidant intakes. Am J Clin Nutr. 2000;71:530–536; Thorp VJ. Effect of oral contraceptive agents on vitamin and mineral requirements. J Am Diet Assoc. 1980;76:581–584.

21. Food and Nutrition Board, Institute of Medicine. *Dietary Reference Intakes for Vitamin C, Vitamin E, Selenium, and Carotenoids*. Washington, D.C.: National Academy Press; 2000. Available at: http://www.nap.edu/books/0309069351/html/. Accessed March 23, 2009.

22. Centanni S, Santus P, Di Marco F, et al. The potential role of tocopherol in asthma and allergies: modification of the leukotriene pathway. *Biodrugs*. 2001;15(2):81–86.

23. Wagner JG, Jiang Q, Harkema JR, et al. Gamma-tocopherol prevents airway eosinophilia and mucous cell hyperplasia in experimentally induced allergic rhinitis and asthma. *Clin Exp Allergy*. 2008;38:501–511.

24. Devereux G, Turner SW, Craig LC, et al. Low maternal vitamin E intake during pregnancy is associated with asthma in 5-year-old children. *Am J Respir Crit Care Med*. 2006;174:499–507.

25. Hozyasz KK, Chełchowska M, Laskowska-Klita T, et al. Low concentration of alpha-tocopherol in erythrocytes of atopic dermatitis patients [in Polish]. *Med Wieku Rozwoj*. 2004;8(4 Pt 1):963–969.

26. Fogarty A, Lewis S, Weiss S, et al. Dietary vitamin E, IgE concentrations, and atopy. *Lancet*. 2000;356:1573–1574.

27. Hickenbottom SJ, Follett JR, Lin Y, et al. Variability in conversion of beta-carotene to vitamin A in men as measured by using a double-tracer study design. *Am J Clin Nutr*. 2002;75:900–907.

28. Manda K, Bhatia AL. Pre-administration of beta-carotene protects tissue glutathione and lipid peroxidation status following exposure to gamma radiation. *J Environ Biol*. 2003;24:369–372; Omenn GS. Chemoprevention of lung cancer: the rise and demise of beta-carotene. *Annu Rev Public Health*. 1998;19:73–99.

29. Wood LG, Garg ML, Blake RJ, et al. Airway and circulating levels of carotenoids in asthma and healthy controls. *J Am Coll Nutr*. 2005;24:448–455.

30. Neuman I, Nahum H, Ben-Amotz A. Prevention of exercise-induced asthma by a natural isomer mixture of beta-carotene. *Ann Allergy Asthma Immunol*. 1999;82:549–553.

31. Sato Y, Akiyama H, Suganuma H, et al. The feeding of beta-carotene downregulates serum IgE levels and inhibits the type I allergic response in mice. *Biol Pharm Bull*. 2004;27:978–984.

32. Bando N, Yamanishi R, Terao J. Inhibition of immunoglobulin E production in allergic model mice by supplementation with vitamin E and beta-carotene. *Biosci Biotechnol Biochem*. 2003;67:2176–2182.

33. Gazdik F, Gvozdjakova A, Horvathova M, et al. Levels of coenzyme Q10 in asthmatics. *Bratisl Lek Listy*. 2002;103(10):353–356.

34. Gvozdjáková A, Kucharská J, Bartkovjaková M, et al. Coenzyme Q10 supplementation reduces corticosteroids dosage in patients with bronchial asthma. *Biofactors*. 2005;25:235–240.

35. Ye CQ, Folkers K, Tamagawa H, et al. A modified determination of coenzyme Q10 in human blood and CoQ10 blood levels in diverse patients with allergies. *Biofactors*. 1988;1:303–306.

36. Zervas E, Papatheodorou G, Psathakis K, et al. Reduced intracellular Mg concentrations in patients with acute asthma. *Chest*. 2003;123:113–118.

37. Gontijo-Amaral C, Ribeiro MA, Gontijo LS, et al. Oral magnesium supplementation in asthmatic children: a double-blind randomized placebo-controlled trial. *Eur J Clin Nutr*. 2007;61:54–60; Beasley R, Aldington S. Magnesium in the treatment of asthma. *Curr Opin Allergy Clin Immunol*. 2007;7(1):107–110.

38. Hijazi N, Abalkhail B. Seaton A. Diet and childhood asthma in a society in transition: a study in urban and rural Saudi Arabis. *Thorax*. 2000;55:775–779.

39. Shiozaki T, Sugiyama K, Nakazato K, Takeo T. Effect of tea extracts, catechin and caffeine against type-I allergic reaction [in Japanese]. *Yakugaku Zasshi*. 1997; 117(7):448–454.

40. Fujimura Y, Tachibana H, Maeda-Yamamoto M, et al. Antiallergic tea catechin, (-)-Epigallocatechin-3-O-(3-O-methyl)-gallate, suppresses FcεRI expression in human basophilic KU812 cells. *J Agric Food Chem*. 2002;50:5729–5734.

41. Mittman P. Randomized, double-blind study of freeze-dried Urtica dioica in the treatment of allergic rhinitis. *Planta Med*. 1990;56(1):44–47.

42. Takano H, Osakabe N, Sanbongi C, et al. Extract of Perilla frutescens enriched for rosmarinic acid, a polyphenolic phytochemical, inhibits seasonal allergic rhinoconjunctivitis in humans. *Exp Biol Med (Maywood.)* 2004;229:247–254.

43. Shin TY, Kim SH, Kim SH, et al. Inhibitory effect of mast cell-mediated immediate-type allergic reactions in rats by Perilla frutescens. *Immunopharmacol Immunotoxicol*. 2000;22:489–500.

44. Ishihara T, Okamoto I, Masaki N, et al. Inhibition of antigen-specific T helper type 2 responses by Perilla frutescens extract [in Japanese]. *Arerugi*. 1999;48:443–450.

45. Inoue K, Takano H, Shiga A, et al. Effects of volatile constituents of a rosemary extract on allergic airway inflammation related to house dust mite allergen in mice. *Int J Mol Med*. 2005;16:315–319.

46. Ueda H, Yamazaki C, Yamazaki M. Luteolin as an anti-inflammatory and antiallergic constituent of Perilla frutescens. *Biol Pharm Bull*. 2002;25:1197–1202.

47. Das M, Ram A, Ghosh B. Luteolin alleviates bronchoconstriction and airway hyperreactivity in ovalbumin sensitized mice. *Inflamm Res*. 2003;52(3):101–116.

48. Kimata M, Inagaki N, Nagai H. Effects of luteolin and other flavonoids on IgE-mediated allergic reactions. *Planta Med*. 2000;66(1):25–29.

49. Li MH, Zhang HL, Yang BY. Effects of ginkgo leave concentrated oral liquor in treating asthma [in Chinese]. *Zhongguo Zhong Xi Yi Jie He Za Zhi*. 1997;17(4):216–218.

50. Harczy M, Maclouf J, Pradelles P, et al. Inhibitory effects of a novel platelet activating factor (PAF) antagonist (BN 52021) on antigen-induced prostaglandin and thromboxane formation by the guinea pig lung. *Pharmacol Res Commun*. 1986; 18(suppl):111–117.

51. Castelli D, Colin L, Camel E, et al. Pretreatment of skin with a ginkgo biloba extract/sodium carboxymethyl-beta-1,3-glucan formulation appears to inhibit the elicitation of allergic contact dermatitis in man. *Contact Dermatitis*. 1998;38(3):123–126.

52. Thomet OA, Schapowal A, Heinisch IV, et al. Anti-inflammatory activity of an extract of Petasites hybridus in allergic rhinitis. *Int Immunopharmacol*. 2002;2:997–1006.

53. Schapowal A, Petasites Study Group. Randomised controlled trial of butterbur and cetirizine for treating seasonal allergic rhinitis. *BMJ* 2002;324:144–146.

54. Schapowal A, Study Group. Treating intermittent allergic rhinitis: a prospective, randomized, placebo and antihistamine-controlled study of Butterbur extract Ze 339. *Phytother Res*. 2005;19:530–537.

55. Ventura MT, Polimeno L, Amoruso AC, et al. Intestinal permeability in patients with adverse reactions to food. *Dig Liver Dis*. 2006;38:732–736.

56. Laudat A, Arnaud P, Napoly A, et al. The intestinal permeability test applied to the diagnosis of food allergy in paediatrics. *West Indian Med J*. 1994;43(3):87–88.

57. Norris JM, Barriga K, Hoffenberg EJ, et al. Risk of celiac disease autoimmunity and timing of gluten introduction in the diet of infants at increased risk of disease. *JAMA*. 2005;293:2343–2351.

58. Fiocchi A, Assa'ad A, Bahna S; Adverse Reactions to Foods Committee; American College of Allergy, Asthma and Immunology. Food allergy and the introduction of

solid foods to infants: a consensus document. Adverse Reactions to Foods Committee, American College of Allergy, Asthma and Immunology. *Ann Allergy Asthma Immunol.* 2006;97(1):10–20.

59. Zareie M, Johnson-Henry K, Jury J, et al. Probiotics prevent bacterial translocation and improve intestinal barrier function in rats following chronic psychological stress. *Gut.* 2006;55:1553–1560.

60. Sanderson IR. Short chain fatty acid regulation of signaling genes expressed by the intestinal epithelium. *J Nutr.* 2004;134:2450S–2454S.

61. Shimotoyodome A, Meguro S, Hase T, et al. Short chain fatty acids but not lactate or succinate stimulate mucus release in the rat colon. *Comp Biochem Physiol A Mol Integr Physiol.* 2000;125:525–531.

62. Hamer HM, Jonkers D, Venema K, et al. Review article: the role of butyrate on colonic function. *Aliment Pharmacol Ther.* 2008;27(2):104–119.

63. Topping DL, Clifton PM. Short-chain fatty acids and human colonic function: roles of resistant starch and nonstarch polysaccharides. *Physiol Rev.* 2001;81:1031–1064.

64. Cherbut C, Aubé AC, Blottière HM, et al. Effects of short-chain fatty acids on gastrointestinal motility. *Scand J Gastroenterol Suppl.* 1997;222:58–61.

65. Tedelind S, Westberg F, Kjerrulf M, et al. Anti-inflammatory properties of the short-chain fatty acids acetate and propionate: a study with relevance to inflammatory bowel disease. *World J Gastroenterol.* 2007;13:2826–2832.

66. Andoh A, Tsujikawa T, Fujiyama Y. Role of dietary fiber and short-chain fatty acids in the colon. *Curr Pharm Design.* 2003;9:347–358.

67. Rosignoli P, Fabiani R, De Bartolomeo A, et al. Protective activity of butyrate on hydrogen peroxide-induced DNA damage in isolated human colonocytes and HT29 tumour cells. *Carcinogenesis.* 2001;22:1675–1680.

68. Scheppach W. Effects of short chain fatty acids on gut morphology and function. *Gut.* 1994;35:S35–S38.

69. Chen CC, Walker WA. Probiotics and prebiotics: role in clinical disease states. *Adv Pediatr.* 2005;52:77–113.

70. Rabassa AA, Rogers AI. The role of short-chain fatty acid metabolism in colonic disorders. *Am J Gastroenterol.* 1992;87:419–423.

71. Wong JM, de Souza R, Kendall CW, et al. Colonic health: fermentation and short chain fatty acids. *J Clin Gastroenterol.* 2006;40:235–243.

72. Robinson RR, Feirtag J, Slavin JL. Effects of dietary arabinogalactan on gastrointestinal and blood parameters in healthy human subjects. *J Am Coll Nutr.* 2001;20:279–285.

73. Bartram HP, Scheppach W, Schmid H, et al. Proliferation of human colonic mucosa as an intermediate biomarker of carcinogenesis: effects of butyrate, deoxycholate, calcium, ammonia, and pH. *Cancer Res.* 1993;53:3283–3288.

74. Visek WJ. Diet and cell growth modulation by ammonia. *Am J Clin Nutr.* 1978;31:S216–S220.

75. Fedorak RN, Madsen KL. Probiotics and the management of inflammatory bowel disease. *Inflamm Bowel Dis.* 2004;10:286–299.

76. deRoos NM, Katan MB. Effects of probiotic bacteria on diarrhea, lipid metabolism, and carcinogenesis: a review of papers published between 1988 and 1998. *Am J Clin Nutr.* 2000;71:405–411; Mack DR, Michail S, Wei S, et al. Probiotics inhibit enteropathogenic E. coli adherence in vitro by inducing intestinal mucin gene expression. *Am J Physiol.* 1999;276:G941–G950 McGroarty JA. Probiotic use of lactobacilli in the human female urogenital tract. *FEMS Immunol Med Microbiol.* 1993;6:251–264.

77. Lu L, Walker WA. Pathologic and physiologic interactions of bacteria with the gastrointestinal epithelium. *Am J Clin Nutr.* 2001;73;1124S-1130S.

78. Madsen KL, Doyle JS, Jewell LD, et al. Lactobacillus species prevents colitis in interleukin 10 gene-deficient mice. *Gastroenterology*. 1999;116:1107–1114.

79. Savilahti E, Kuitunen M, Vaarala O. Pre and probiotics in the prevention and treatment of food allergy. *Curr Opin Allergy Clin Immunol*. 2008;8(3):243–248; Giovannini M, Agostoni C, Riva E, et al. A randomized prospective double blind controlled trial on effects of long-term consumption of fermented milk containing Lactobacillus casei in pre-school children with allergic asthma and/or rhinitis. *Pediatr Res*. 2007;62:215–220.

80. Isolauri E, Arvola T, Sütas Y, et al. Probiotics in the management of atopic eczema. *Clin Exp Allergy*. 2000;30:1604–1610.

81. Shida K, Takahashi R, Iwadate E, et al. Lactobacillus casei strain Shirota suppresses serum immunoglobulin E and immunoglobulin G1 responses and systemic anaphylaxis in a food allergy model. *Clin Exp Allergy*. 2002;32:563–570.

82. Hatakka K, Savilahti E, Pönkä A, et al. Effect of long term consumption of probiotic milk on infections in children attending day care centres: double blind, randomised trial. *BMJ*. 2001;322:1327.

83. So JS, Kwon HK, Lee CG, et al. Lactobacillus casei suppresses experimental arthritis by down-regulating T helper 1 effector functions. *Mol Immunol*. 2008;45:2690–2699.

84. Rafter J, Bennett M, Caderni G, et al. Dietary synbiotics reduce cancer risk factors in polypectomized and colon cancer patients. *Am J Clin Nutr*. 2007;85:488–496.

85. Pelto L, Isolauri E, Lilius EM, et al. Probiotic bacteria down-regulate the milk-induced inflammatory response in milk-hypersensitive subjects but have an immunostimulatory effect in healthy subjects. *Clin Exp Allergy*. 1998;28:1474–1479.

86. Bouhnik Y, Vahedi K, Achour L, et al. Short-chain fructo-oligosaccharide administration dose-dependently increases fecal bifidobacteria in healthy humans. *J Nutr*. 1999;129:113–116.

87. Ohta A. Prevention of osteoporosis by foods and dietary supplements. The effect of fructooligosaccharides (FOS) on the calcium absorption and bone. *Clin Calcium*. 2006;16:1639–1645.

88. Lara-Villoslada F, de Haro O, Camuesco D, et al. Short-chain fructooligosaccharides, in spite of being fermented in the upper part of the large intestine, have anti-inflammatory activity in the TNBS model of colitis. *Eur J Nutr*. 2006;45:418–425.

89. Segala M, Ed. *The Life Extension Foundation's Disease Prevention and Treatment*. 4th ed. Ft. Lauderdale, FL: Life Extension Media; 2003:44.

90. Miller AL. Therapeutic considerations of L-glutamine: a review of the literature. *Altern Med Rev*. 1999;4:239–248.

91. Fukatsu K, Kudsk KA, et al. TPN decreases IL-4 and IL-10 mRNA expression in lipopolysaccharide stimulated intestinal lamina propria cells but glutamine supplementation preserves the expression. *Shock*. 2001;15:318–322.

92. De-Souza DA, Greene LJ. Intestinal permeability and systemic infections in critically ill patients: effect of glutamine. *Crit Care Med*. 2005;33:1175–1178.

93. Jiang HP, Liu CA. Protective effect of glutamine on intestinal barrier function in patients receiving chemotherapy [in Chinese]. *Zhonghua Wei Chang Wai Ke Za Zhi*. 2006;9:59–61.

94. White JS, Hoper M, Parks RW, et al. Glutamine improves intestinal barrier function in experimental biliary obstruction. *Eur Surg Res*. 2005;37:342–347.

95. Amin AH, Subbaiah TV, Abbasi KM. Berberine sulfate: antimicrobial activity, bioassay, and mode of action. *Can J Microbiol*. 1969;15:1067–1076; Scazzocchio F, Corneta MF, Tomassini L, et al. Antibacterial activity of Hydrastis canadensis extract and its major isolated alkaloids. *Planta Med*. 2001;67:561–564; Rehman J, Dillow JM, Carter SM,

et al. Increased production of antigen-specific immunoglobulins G and M following in vivo treatment with the medicinal plants Echinacea angustifolia and Hydrastis canadensis. *Immunol Lett*. 1999;68:391–395; Sun D, Courtney HS, Beachey EH. Berberine sulfate blocks adherence of Streptococcus pyogenes to epithelial cells, fibronectin, and hexadecane. *Antimicrob Agents Chemother*. 1988;32:1370–1374; Kaneda Y, Torii M, Tanaka T, et al. In vitro effects of berberine sulphate on the growth and structure of Entamoeba histolytica, Giardia lamblia and Trichomonas vaginalis. *Ann Trop Med Parasitol*. 1991;85:417–425.

96. Fukuda K, Hibiya Y, Mutoh M, et al. Inhibition by berberine of cyclooxygenase-2 transcriptional activity in human colon cancer cells. *J Ethnopharmacol*. 1999;66: 227–233.

97. Taylor CT, Winter DC, Skelly MM, et al. Berberine inhibits ion transport in human colonic epithelia. *Eur J Pharmacol*. 1999;368:111–118.

98. Isbir T, Yaylim I, Aydin M, et al. The effects of Brassica oleraceae var capitata on epidermal glutathione and lipid peroxides in DMBA-initiated-TPA-promoted mice. *Anticancer Res*. 2000;20:219–224.

99. van Poppel G, Verhoeven DT, Verhagen H, et al. Brassica vegetables and cancer prevention. Epidemiology and mechanisms. *Adv Exp Med Biol*. 1999;472:159–168.

100. Cheney G. Vitamin U Therapy of Peptic Ulcer. *Calif Med*. 1952;77:248–252.

101. *The Review of Natural Products by Facts and Comparisons*. St Louis, MO: Wolters Kluwer Co; 1999.

102. Langmead L, Dawson C, Hawkins C, et al. Antioxidant effects of herbal therapies used by patients with inflammatory bowel disease: an in vitro study. *Aliment Pharmacol Ther*. 2002;16:197–205.

103. Newall CA, Anderson LA, Philpson JD. *Herbal Medicine: A Guide for Healthcare Professionals*. London: Pharmaceutical Press; 1996; Martindale W. *Martindale the Extra Pharmacopoeia*. London: Pharmaceutical Press; 1999.

104. Gruenwald J, Brendler T, Jaenicke C. *PDR for Herbal Medicines*. Montvale, NJ: Medical Economics Company; 1998.

105. Klein AD, Penneys NS. Aloe vera. *J Am Acad Dermatol*. 1988;18:714–720.

106. Langmead L, Makins RJ, Rampton DS. Anti-inflammatory effects of aloe vera gel in human colorectal mucosa in vitro. *Aliment Pharmacol Ther*. 2004;19:521–527.

107. Langmead L, Feakins RM, Goldthorpe S, et al. Randomized, double-blind, placebo-controlled trial of oral aloe vera gel for active ulcerative colitis. *Aliment Pharmacol Ther*. 2004;19:739–747.

108. Burton AF, Anderson FH. Decreased incorporation of 14C-glucosamine relative to 3H-N-acetyl glucosamine in the intestinal mucosa of patients with inflammatory bowel disease. *Am J Gastroenterol*. 1983;78:19–22.

109. Salvatore S, Heuschkel R, Tomlin S, et al. A pilot study of N-acetyl glucosamine, a nutritional substrate for glycosaminoglycan synthesis, in paediatric chronic inflammatory bowel disease. *Aliment Pharmacol Ther*. 2000;14:1567–1579.

110. Treede I, Braun A, Sparla R, et al. Anti-inflammatory effects of phosphatidylcholine. *J Biol Chem*. 2007;282:27155–27164.

111. Lugea A, Salas A, Casalot J, et al. Surface hydrophobicity of the rat colonic mucosa is a defensive barrier against macromolecules and toxins. *Gut*. 2000;46:515–521.

112. Wang XD, Andersson R, Soltesz V, et al. Phospholipids prevent enteric bacterial translocation in the early stage of experimental acute liver failure in the rat. *Scand J Gastroenterol*. 1994;29:1117–1121.

113. Stremmel W, Merle U, Zahn A, et al. Retarded release phosphatidylcholine benefits patients with chronic active ulcerative colitis. *Gut*. 2005;54:966–971.

114. Hossain Z, Konishi M, Hosokawa M, et al. Effect of polyunsaturated fatty acid-enriched phosphatidylcholine and phosphatidylserine on butyrate-induced growth inhibition, differentiation and apoptosis in Caco-2 cells. *Cell Biochem Funct*. 2006;24:159–165.

115. Ichimaru Y, Moriyama M, Ichimaru M, et al. Effects of gamma-oryzanol on gastric lesions and small intestinal propulsive activity in mice [in Japanese]. *Nippon Yakurigaku Zasshi*. 1984;84:537–542.

116. Islam MS, Murata T, Fujisawa M, et al. Anti-inflammatory effects of phytosteryl ferulates in colitis induced by dextran sulphate sodium in mice. *Br J Pharmacol*. 2008;154:812–824.

117. Sierra S, Lara-Villoslada F, Olivares M, et al. Increased immune response in mice consuming rice bran oil. *Eur J Nutr*. 2005;44:509–516.

118. Robinson RR, Feirtag J, Slavin JL. Effects of dietary arabinogalactan on gastrointestinal and blood parameters in healthy human subjects. *J Am Coll Nutr*. 2001;20:279–285.

119. Kelly GS. Larch arabinogalactan: clinical relevance of a novel immune-enhancing polysaccharide." *Altern Med Rev*. 1999;4(2):96–103.

120. Rose DJ, DeMeo MT, Keshavarzian A, et al. Influence of dietary fiber on inflammatory bowel disease and colon cancer: importance of fermentation pattern. *Nutr Rev*. 2007;65:51–62.

121. Ma Y, Hébert JR, Li W, et al. Association between dietary fiber and markers of systemic inflammation in the Women's Health Initiative Observational Study. *Nutrition*. 2008;24:941–949.

122. Ma Y, Griffith JA, Chasan-Taber L, et al. Association between dietary fiber and serum C-reactive protein. *Am J Clin Nutr*. 2006;83:760–766.

123. King DE, Egan BM, Woolson RF, et al. Effect of a high-fiber diet vs a fiber-supplemented diet on C-reactive protein level. *Arch Intern Med*. 2007;167:502–506.

124. Kong J, Zhang Z, Musch MW, et al. Novel role of the vitamin D receptor in maintaining the integrity of the intestinal mucosal barrier. *Am J Physiol Gastrointest Liver Physiol*. 2008;294:G208–G216.

125. Pappa HM, Grand RJ, Gordon CM. Report on the vitamin D status of adult and pediatric patients with inflammatory bowel disease and its significance for bone health and disease. *Inflamm Bowel Dis*. 2006;12:1162–1174.

CHAPTER 9

Gastrointestinal Health: The Key to a Strong Health Foundation

The gastrointestinal system is complex. To understand how to optimize gastrointestinal health, it is imperative to have a basic knowledge of how the digestive system works, as well as a basic knowledge of commonly associated medical conditions. Diet and nutrition play a critical role in overall gastrointestinal health.

ANATOMY AND PHYSIOLOGY OF THE DIGESTIVE TRACT

The gastrointestinal tract consists of several organs. It is essentially a long hollow tube consisting of the mouth, esophagus, stomach, small intestine, large intestine (which includes colon), rectum, and anus. The solid organs that are part of the gastrointestinal system are the liver, pancreas, and gallbladder. These organs act together to break down food and absorb nutrients into the blood stream. The lining of the hollow organs is called the mucosa, and the mucosa is surrounded by two layers of smooth muscle that help move the food through the digestive tract. The movement of these hollow organs propels food and liquid through the tube and mixes the contents within each organ. Food moves from one organ to the next by wavelike muscle contractions called peristalsis. The liver and pancreas secrete digestive fluids and enzymes that help break down the food. The gallbladder stores bile, a digestive fluid, from the liver until it is needed. Digestion consists of four stages: ingestion of food, breakdown of that food, absorption of nutrients, and removal of undigested material. Food must be broken down into smaller molecules before it can be absorbed into the blood and carried to cells throughout the body to provide energy and build and nourish cells.

Digestion begins with the gastric cephalic phase, which occurs before food enters the stomach. The thought, smell, taste, and sight of food stimulate areas of the brain, such as the cerebral cortex, hypothalamus, and amygdala. Saliva production begins in the mouth and digestive enzyme production begins in the stomach. Digestion begins in the mouth where food is chewed and mixed with saliva. Saliva contains the enzyme amylase, which breaks down starches and moistens the food. The food then passes through the esophagus, which connects the back of the mouth at the pharynx to the stomach. The lower esophageal sphincter is a ringlike muscle that controls the passage of food into the stomach from the esophagus. No digestion takes place in the esophagus. The esophagus moves the bolus of food through by peristaltic contractions, whereby the two layers of muscles that surround the esophagus slowly contract to push the food through. Once a swallow begins, it becomes involuntary and proceeds under the control of the nervous system. The epiglottis is a flap at the top of the esophagus that closes during swallowing to prevent food from entering the trachea and the lungs.

The next phase, called the gastric phase, is stimulated by distention of the stomach from the food bolus and an increase in stomach pH. Several digestive products are secreted including gastrin, pepsin, intrinsic factor, hydrochloric acid, and small amounts of additional digestive enzymes. Intrinsic factor enables the absorption of vitamin B-12, and pepsin breaks down protein. The stomach is a hollow muscular organ that contracts to mix the food bolus with the digestive enzymes. Hydrochloric acid is a strong acid that generates a pH of 2–3 in the stomach. It functions by activating the enzymes, such as pepsin, which require a strongly acidic environment to become active and is inactivated over a pH of 5. Hydrochloric acid is also important to kill bacteria or other microorganisms in the food and protect the stomach and intestines from pathogens and bacterial overgrowth such as *Escherichia coli* and *Helicobacter pylori*.[1]

The stomach's inner lining, or mucosa, contains numerous glands to secrete digestive enzymes, as well as mucus to protect the stomach from the acidic pH. The stomach then slowly empties its contents into the small intestine, which can be modulated by the type of food in the bolus and the degree of muscle contraction by the stomach. Carbohydrates are the first to exit the stomach, followed by protein, and then by fats. Some smaller molecules can be absorbed directly from the stomach, such as alcohol. The liquefied food bolus, now called chyme, then passes into the duodenum, the first section of the small intestine, starting the intestinal phase. Here, the chyme is mixed with bile and pancreatic digestive enzymes. Bile is made in the liver, held in the gall bladder, and then released into the duodenum to emulsify fats for absorption. Also, some waste products are excreted from the liver in the bile for removal from the body. The pancreas secretes enzymes, including maltase, lactase, sucrase, amylase, lipase, trypsin, and chymotrypsin, that break down carbohydrates, protein, and fats. These enzymes are crucial for the proper and complete breakdown of the nutrients in the chyme. The pancreas also secretes sodium bicarbonate as a buffer to increase the pH of the acidic chyme entering from the stomach. The chyme is moved through the intestines by peristaltic waves of muscle contractions and passes through the duodenum to the jejunum and ileum, which are all parts of the small intestine.

The small intestine is lined with villi and microvilli, which are fingerlike projections that increase the surface area for absorption of nutrients. Most digested food and water molecules are absorbed through the small intestines. The absorbed nutrients are carried in the blood to the liver for filtering and removing toxins. Next, the chyme moves into the large intestine, which consists of the cecum, colon, and rectum. The large intestine absorbs water and electrolytes from the chyme and combines the undigested food, primarily insoluble fiber, with waste products to form feces. The colon and rectum then store the feces until it can be eliminated through the anus.[2] In addition, more than 400 different strains of bacteria reside in the colon. Particular strains of intestinal microflora are required for optimal health and for normal immune system function.

Another important function of the intestines is to act as a semipermeable barrier. This means that it actively selects which molecules or organisms can pass through into the bloodstream and which stay in the intestines. When intestinal permeability is increased, food and nutrient absorption is impaired. Dysfunction of the semipermeable barrier can allow larger molecules from the intestines to pass through into the blood, which can trigger immune system reactions because these large molecules are not recognized and are perceived as foreign. Progressive damage to the barrier may allow disease-causing bacteria, undigested food particles, and toxins to pass directly into the bloodstream. Dysfunctions in intestinal permeability are associated with numerous diseases, such as food allergies, irritable bowel syndrome (IBS), ulcerative colitis, Crohn's disease, chronic fatigue syndrome, psoriasis, autoimmune disease, arthritis, and heart disease. Dysfunction of the barrier can be caused by infection, trauma, medications; by consuming a less-than-optimal diet; or by other factors, such as psychological stress.[3]

Control Mechanisms

Food digestion is a complex process that is controlled both locally, with hormones, and via the nervous system. Several major hormones regulate the digestive system. The major hormones are produced and released by cells in the mucosa of the stomach and small intestine, released into the blood of the digestive tract, travel through the arteries, and return to the digestive system where they stimulate enzyme production and muscle contraction. Following is a list of these key hormones:

1. Gastrin, which is secreted from the stomach, is the major regulator of gastric acid secretion. Gastrin stimulates the gastric glands to secrete hydrochloric acid. The acid, in turn, stimulates the secretion of pepsinogen, the inactive form of the enzyme pepsin. Gastrin secretion is inhibited by a pH below 3.0. Gastrin is also important for normal cell growth in the lining of the stomach, small intestine, and colon.
2. Secretin is released from the upper small intestine in response to the presence of the acidic chyme entering the duodenum. Secretin causes

the pancreas to release high levels of bicarbonate to help neutralize the acidic chyme as it enters the small intestine.

3. Cholecystokinin (CCK) is released from the small intestines in response to the presence of food in the upper small intestine. CCK is the primary stimulus for release of digestive enzymes from the pancreas and release of bile from the gallbladder. This hormone is secreted in response to fats and peptones, partially digested protein, in the chyme. CCK also promotes normal cell growth of the pancreas.

4. Histamine is an amino acid derivative that is secreted in the stomach and increases gastric acid secretion.

5. Ghrelin is a polypeptide hormone primarily produced in the stomach. Ghrelin functions to stimulate appetite and gastric emptying. Levels of ghrelin rise before eating a meal and are lowest shortly after ingesting a meal.

6. Gastric inhibitory peptide is secreted from mucosal epithelial cells in the duodenum. It inhibits gastric motility, slows the secretion of acid, and induces insulin secretion.

7. Peptide YY is produced in the digestive tract in response to ingestion of food. Levels of peptide YY increase after a meal and inhibit stomach motility, slow gastric emptying, increases water and electrolyte absorption in the colon, and reduces appetite.

8. Motilin is secreted in the upper small intestine into the circulation during fasting at intervals of approximately 100 minutes, which triggers contractions that sweep the stomach and small intestine clear of undigested material.

9. Vasoactive intestinal peptide is a peptide related to secretin. It induces smooth muscle relaxation in such areas as the lower esophageal sphincter, stomach, and gallbladder; stimulates secretion of water into pancreatic secretions and bile; and inhibits gastric acid secretion.

10. Leptin is a hormone derived from adipose tissue. It functions by regulating energy intake and expenditure, including modulating appetite and metabolism. Leptin signals satiety, or fullness, to the brain. Interestingly, it circulates at levels proportional to body fat.

11. Other hormones may play a part in inhibiting appetite, such as glucagon-like peptide-1, oxyntomodulin (+), and pancreatic polypeptide.

The nervous system also regulates digestion. Nerves connect the digestive organs to the brain and spinal cord. The nerves that run from the brain stem release acetylcholine and adrenaline. Acetylcholine has several functions, including inducing the muscle layer of the digestive organs to squeeze with more force to push the food through the digestive tract. It also works synergistically with gastrin and histamine to stimulate gastric acid secretion of pepsin, hydrochloric acid, and mucus. Adrenaline has the opposite function. It relaxes the muscles of the stomach and intestine and decreases the flow of blood to these organs, slowing the digestive process. Local nervous reflexes are also found in the walls of the organs of the digestive tract, and they regulate digestion. These local nerves are stimulated by the presence of food or irritating stimuli. The vagus nerve, or cranial nerve 10, connects the brain stem to the organs in the abdomen. Vagus nerve activation generally reduces heart rate and blood pressure. Diseases of the organs of the digestive tract, such as infections can activate the vagus nerve as well as cause pain and emotional stress. Interestingly, researchers have shown that stimulation of the vagus nerve can improve symptoms of chronic major depression.[4] In addition, some intestinal hormones and peptides, including secretin and CCK, have also been shown to act as neurotransmitters and neuromodulators in the brain.

Further, pH balance also plays a role in controlling the process of digestion. The mouth, pharynx, and esophagus are generally weakly acidic, with a pH around 6.8. Salivary amylase functions at this pH. The pH of the stomach is very acidic, around 2–3. This inhibits salivary amylase and, thus, decreases the breakdown of carbohydrates in the stomach. Pepsin, on the other hand, is active at a pH of 1.8–3.5 but inactive at a pH over 5. The small intestine secretes bicarbonate to neutralize the acid chyme entering from the stomach. Secretion of secretin is activated by the presence of acidic chyme with a pH less than 4.5–5 in the duodenum. The pH in the duodenum is approximately 8, slightly basic, which is required for the pancreatic enzymes to function properly.

GASTROINTESTINAL DISEASES

Digestive disorders are quite common. According to the Centers for Disease Control and Prevention's most recent data, people made 41.3 million office visits to physicians and 15.1 visits to the emergency department for digestive system symptoms in 2004.[5] Frequently seen digestive disorders include IBS, gastroesophageal reflux disease (GERD), inflammatory bowel disease, including ulcerative colitis and Crohn's disease, celiac disease, diarrhea, constipation, indigestion, nausea, flatulence, and cancer. An estimated 60 to 70 million people are affected by overt diagnosable digestive diseases.[6] However, millions more suffer from subclinical gastrointestinal health issues that affect their ability to absorb nutrients from their diet, which has a dramatic impact on quality of life and predisposes them additional diseases. In fact, approximately 1.9 million people are disabled because of gastrointestinal diseases.[7]

Several basic gastrointestinal functional abnormalities can predispose patients to numerous diseases. For example, a condition known as hypochlorhydria, which is caused by low levels of hydrochloric acid, will cause a decrease in nutrient absorption, an increase in gastric inflammation, and is a risk factor for other diseases. It is also important to note that hydrochloric acid levels decrease with age. In fact, one study found that 80 percent of subjects, who had an average age of 84, were hypochlorhydric.[8] Also, increased production of ammonia in the colon can have adverse effects on the epithelial cells that line the colon. Ammonia is produced as a by-product of bacterial fermentation of protein and other nitrogen-containing substances in the colon. Increased production of ammonia from eating a high-protein diet was shown to increase the incidence of colon cancer in animal models[9] and increase the turnover of the colonic epithelial cells.[10] The typical Western diet is associated with increased levels of ammonia in the colon, which has also been linked to growth of cancer cells, cell toxicity, and altered nucleic acid synthesis, as well as increased viral infections.[11]

Intestinal permeability is also associated with numerous diseases. Many practitioners believe increased permeability leads to food allergies. Researchers have shown that patients with food allergy or food hypersensitivity have significantly increased intestinal permeability compared with the control groups. Additionally, the studies showed that the more severe the intestinal permeability, the more serious the clinical symptoms in these patients.[12] Intestinal permeability has also been associated with various other diseases, such as ulcerative colitis, Crohn's disease, and even chronic heart failure. In fact, one study showed that patients with chronic heart failure had a 35 percent increase in small intestine permeability and a 210 percent increase in large intestine permeability compared with control patients. The authors of the study suggest that chronic heart failure is a disorder in which intestinal permeability and absorption are altered, which may be a contributing factor to both the origin chronic inflammation and malnutrition seen with chronic heart failure.[13]

Although the numerous gastrointestinal diseases arise because of various causes, there is one commonality. Dietary choices affect symptoms. Different foods can trigger flares in different patients. Thus, it is imperative for patient with any of these conditions to identify and eliminate possible food triggers.

Crohn's Disease

Crohn's disease, also known as regional enteritis, is a chronic inflammatory condition of the digestive tract. It can affect any place in the gastrointestinal tract but usually involves the lower small intestine, called the ileum, and the colon. The exact cause of Crohn's disease is unknown; however, evidence suggests that a genetic predisposition causes an immune response to a dietary, infectious, or other environmental agent. The immune response causes swelling and edema of the intestinal walls, leading to pain, ulcerations, and complications. Crohn's disease symptoms encompass a large range of severity and include abdominal pain, often in the lower right area, diarrhea, weight loss, fever, rectal bleeding and fissures, arthritis, and skin problems. Stunted growth may occur in children with Crohn's disease. Intestinal blockage is a possible complication as well as inflammation in the eyes or mouth, kidney stones, gallstones, and other diseases of the liver and biliary system. In addition, deficiencies of proteins, calories, and vitamins may be caused by the inadequate dietary intake, intestinal loss of protein, or poor absorption related to celiac disease. During an acute flare, foods such as hot spices, alcohol, milk products, and bulky grains can increase diarrhea and pain and should be avoided. Crohn's disease slightly increases the risk of cancer in the gastrointestinal tract. Approximately

70 percent of patients with Crohn's disease will eventually require surgery for the condition.[14]

Ulcerative Colitis

Ulcerative colitis, another chronic inflammatory condition of the gastrointestinal tract, is characterized by inflammation and ulcerations in the colon and rectum. Most commonly, this condition presents with bouts of bloody diarrhea and mucous in the stool. Ulcerative colitis can also cause fatigue, fever, abdominal cramping, weight loss, loss of appetite, joint pain, skin lesions, liver disease, eye problems, and anemia. Onset of the disease is most common in patients aged 15 to 30 years, but the incidence also increases around age 50 to 70. Complications include bleeding, toxic colitis, toxic megacolon, and colon cancer. The exact cause of ulcerative colitis is unknown. However, similar to Crohn's disease, it is believed that a genetic predisposition leads to an immune response in the colon to a dietary, environmental, or infectious agent. The immune system is thought to react abnormally to the bacteria in the digestive tract. Emotional distress and food sensitivities may trigger symptoms in susceptible patients.[15]

Irritable Bowel Syndrome

IBS, also known as spastic colon, is a common functional bowel condition. Approximately 20 percent of U.S. adults have symptoms of IBS. It generally presents with abdominal pain, constipation and/or diarrhea, cramping, and bloating. IBS is more common in women than men, and onset of symptoms generally occurs before age 35. IBS can be either the constipation-predominate or the diarrhea-predominate type, or patients may alternate between the two types. Intestinal movement, or motility, can be abnormal with either less than normal motility or increased motility accompanied by muscle spasms in the muscles that surround the colon. The cause of IBS is unknown, but diet, emotional factors, drugs, hormones, and psychiatric disorders may precipitate or aggravate the condition. Interestingly, patients with IBS have increased sensitivity to distention of the intestines, which causes a heightened perception of pain. Additionally, it appears that patients with IBS have a colonic response to foods or stress that would not cause symptoms in a person without IBS. Some patients develop postinfectious IBS, which are IBS symptoms that begin after an infection in the gastrointestinal tract. Researchers have also found that patients with IBS have abnormal levels of serotonin in the digestive tract. Although most people are familiar with serotonin as a neurotransmitter in the brain, 95 percent of the body's serotonin is actually found in the digestive tract. This is believed to cause the increase in pain receptor sensitivity in the digestive tract of IBS patients. Other researchers have found that some patients with IBS actually have a mild form of celiac disease. Many patients with IBS can control their symptoms with diet, stress management, and if needed, medications.[16] Clinically, food allergies and sensitivities are frequently found in patients with IBS, and dietary changes significantly improve symptoms.

Celiac Disease

Celiac disease, also known as nontropical sprue or gluten-sensitive enteropathy, is a digestive condition caused by an immune reaction to the gliadin portion of the protein gluten. Gluten is a protein found in wheat, rye, barley, and oats, and it is also an additive in numerous other food products, cosmetics, supplements, and medicines. The immune reaction to gliadin causes white blood cells to accumulate in the lining of the intestines, thus leading to damage of the villi and microvilli in the intestines. This, in turn, leads to severe malabsorption of nutrients. Persons with celiac disease may present with gastrointestinal symptoms such as chronic diarrhea, constipation, bloating, abdominal pain, vomiting, or fatty stools. However, they may also present with weight loss, fatigue, arthritis, unexplained iron-deficiency anemia, osteoporosis or bone loss, infertility, irregular menstrual cycles, skin rash, mouth sores, depression, or anxiety. Patients with celiac disease are at increased risk for autoimmune conditions such as type 1 diabetes, rheumatoid arthritis, Sjögren's syndrome, and autoimmune thyroid or liver diseases. Many of the associated conditions are due to long-term malnutrition. Symptoms and associated conditions vary between patients, likely because of variations in the extent of intestinal damage, age of onset, and exposure to gluten before diagnosis. Celiac disease runs in families, thus showing a genetic component. An estimated 1 in 133 people in the U.S. general population have celiac disease, and the prevalence is as high as 1 in 22 people who have a first-degree relative with the condition, and 1 in 39 people who have a second-degree relative has the disease.[17] Patients with celiac disease need to follow a gluten-free diet, thus avoiding wheat, rye, barley, and oats. These grains can generally be replaced with rice, soy, potato, amaranth, quinoa, or buckwheat flour.[18]

Gastroesophageal Reflux Disease

Gastroesophageal reflux disease (GERD) is a chronic recurrent condition with frequent episodes of stomach contents backing up into the esophagus. This occurs because of dysfunction in the lower esophageal sphincter, which connects the esophagus to the stomach. Generally, this sphincter remains closed unless food is entering the stomach. However, in patients with GERD, the lower esophageal sphincter opens spontaneously or does not close properly after food passes into the stomach. The result is food and gastric acid entering the esophagus. GERD is the most common gastrointestinal-related diagnosis given by physicians n the United States.[19] A 2000 National Heartburn Alliance survey estimated that 60 million Americans have GERD symptoms at least once a month and 25 million adults have daily symptoms.[20] GERD commonly presents with heartburn and acid regurgitation. However, it may also present atypically with chronic cough, noncardiac chest pain, laryngitis, and poor sleep. Several other conditions have been associated with GERD, including Barrett's esophagus (precancerous changes in the esophagus), esophageal cancer, gastritis (inflammation of the stomach), esophagitis (inflammation of the esophagus), respiratory conditions, sleep disorders, and various ear-nose-throat conditions. The numerous risk factors for GERD include obesity, weight gain and increasing body mass index, hiatal hernia, smoking, excess alcohol intake, IBS, a family history of upper gastrointestinal disease, some pharmaceuticals, manual work,[21] and increased intake of table salt, sweets or white bread, caffeine,[22] and carbonated beverages.[23] Persistent wheezing, asthma, and airway hyperresponsiveness in childhood and the teenage years has also been shown to significantly increase the risk for GERD.[24] Moderate-intensity exercise and diets high in fruit and dietary fiber appear to be protective.[25] Lifestyle and dietary modifications benefit patients with GERD, but they should avoid foods that trigger symptoms, such as tomatoes and tomato products, coffee, tea, chocolate, caffeine, alcohol, citrus, mint, garlic, onions, spicy foods, fatty and fried foods, and any known food allergies. Also, very low carbohydrate diets improve GERD symptoms. In fact, one study showed that diets containing less than 20 grams of carbohydrates per day significantly improved GERD symptoms in less than six days.[26] Diets high in the antioxidant vitamin C are also associated with less risk of GERD symptoms and complications.[27] Other recommendations include elevating the head of the bed four to eight inches, sleeping on the left side,[28] avoiding lying down two to three hours after a meal, losing weight,[29] quitting smoking, avoiding eating large meals, and avoiding pharmaceuticals that aggravate GERD.[30]

Gastritis and Dyspepsia

Gastritis, an inflammation of the stomach lining, can be caused by several different conditions. Generally, gastritis develops when the protective layer of the stomach is damaged because of deficient barrier function by the mucous lining, which then allows the acid to irritate and inflame the lining. Gastritis can be caused by prolonged use of nonsteroidal anti-inflammatory drugs (NSAIDs), such as aspirin or ibuprofen, infection with bacteria such as *Helicobacter pylori*, or excessive alcohol intake. Gastritis may also occur after major surgery, traumatic injury, burns, or severe infections. Other causes include pernicious anemia, autoimmune disorders, and chronic bile reflux into the stomach. It is important to remember that inflammation is part of the immune response; thus, controlling the immune system is imperative to deal with chronic inflammation. Gastritis often presents as pain and dyspepsia (upset stomach), but it may also be characterized by bloating, nausea, vomiting, or a feeling of fullness or burning in the upper abdomen.

Infection with the bacteria *H. pylori* is known to cause gastritis and ulcers. More than 50 percent of the population worldwide is infected with *H. pylori*, and the prevalence of this infection increases with age. *H. pylori* can cause atrophic gastritis, dyspepsia, stomach and intestinal ulcers, iron-deficiency anemia, stomach cancer, and lymphoma. Researchers have shown that in patients with *H. pylori* infection, 15 to 25 percent have ulcers in the duodenum, 13 percent have gastric ulcers, and 1 percent develop gastric carcinoma.[31] Researchers have also shown that *H. pylori* is responsible for most cases of stomach disorders. For example,

67 percent of patients with dyspepsia, 70 percent of patients with gastritis, 86 percent of patients with duodenal ulcers, and 71 percent of patients with gastric ulcers are infected with H. pylori, according to one study.[32] Additionally, with chronic gastritis, the cells that secrete the stomach juices stop working, which may lead to vitamin B-12 deficiency anemia and absence of hydrochloric acid.

Dyspepsia, or indigestion, is a general term used to describe discomfort or a burning feeling in the upper abdomen, nausea, bloating, belching, or vomiting. Generally, it results from eating too much or too quickly, eating fatty foods, or eating during stressful situations. Also, smoking, excessive alcohol intake, using medications such as NSAIDS that irritate the stomach lining, fatigue, and chronic stress can also cause indigestion. Dyspepsia may also be attributable to abnormal stomach motility. For many patients, avoiding the foods and situations that trigger the indigestion is the most effective treatment.[33]

Diarrhea and Constipation

Diarrhea and constipation are symptoms of an underlying disease. Diarrhea is loose watery stools that typically occur more than three times per day when the condition is acute. Constipation is when a person has fewer than three bowel movement per week, and the stools are usually hard and dry and may be difficult or painful to eliminate.

Acute (short-term) diarrhea usually resolves on its own. Chronic diarrhea can be more serious as it increases the risk of dehydration and may be a symptom of a more severe condition. Acute diarrhea is generally caused by an infection or medication. Some common causes of infections include such bacteria as Campylobacter, Salmonella, Shigella, and Escherichia coli; viruses such as rotavirus, Norwalk virus, and cytomegalovirus; or parasites such as Giardia lamblia, Entamoeba histolytica, and Cryptosporidium. Chronic diarrhea may be caused by Crohn's disease, ulcerative colitis, IBS, celiac disease, or food intolerances or it may occur after the gallbladder has been removed. It is important to avoid any known food allergies or sensitivities while having a bout of diarrhea. If the diarrhea is chronic, investigating possible food reactions is indicated. Additionally, a bland diet is often recommended while avoiding milk products, fried and fatty foods, caffeine, and sugary foods. Bland foods such as bananas, plain rice, boiled potatoes, toast, and crackers generally do not aggravate diarrhea.[34]

Constipation is a common gastrointestinal complaint, and approximately 4 million Americans report frequent constipation. It occurs when the colon absorbs too much water from the feces, which can occur if the colon's muscle contractions are slow or sluggish, causing the stool to move through the colon slowly. Acute constipation usually resolves without treatment. However, chronic constipation should be thoroughly investigated. Constipation is commonly caused by poor diet and deficient water and fiber intake, and it is associated with diets high in fat and low in fiber-rich foods such as fruits, vegetables, and whole grains. Many Americans do not eat the recommended daily intake of fiber. Constipation is also common during pregnancy, after childbirth, after surgery, and with some medications. Additionally, it may be due to IBS, endo-crine disorders, neurological disorders, laxative abuse, lack of exercise, and fre-quently ignoring the urge to defecate. Other, less common causes of constipation include intestinal obstructions such as tumors, strictures, or scar tissue. Proper hydration is important to decrease the risk of becoming constipated, as well as exercising, avoiding food allergies and sensitivities, eating high-fiber foods, and limiting high-fat foods.[35]

NUTRITIONAL SUPPORT FOR GASTROINTESTINAL HEALTH

Numerous products are available to support the digestive tract. Some provide generalized support for optimal functioning, and others provide specific activity to combat a disease or condition. First and foremost, the diet must be addressed to identify possible food sensitivities. Then, supplements should be considered for healing the gut or to optimize function. (See Chapter 8 for more detailed informa-tion on supplements.)

- *Replace deficient digestive enzymes.* Digestive enzymes, such as lipase, amylase, protease, maltase, lactase, sucrase, phytase, and cellulose, are required to properly break down carbohydrates, proteins, and fats. Sup-plementation can decrease absorption of inappropriately large molecules in the intestines. Hydrochloric acid supplementation may also be con-sidered to optimize gastric pH.
- *Replace probiotics.* Probiotics are beneficial bacteria such as *Lactobacillus* and *Bifidobacterium.* In the intestines, probiotics can improve the bar-rier function of the intestines, compete with and suppress the growth of pathogenic bacteria, modulate or stimulate the immune response,[36] and enhance nutrient and enzyme synthesis and absorption. Probiot-ics may also promote synthesis of secretory IgA antibodies, the anti-bodies that protect the mucosal lining. Probiotics supplementation has been shown to benefit numerous medical conditions, including allergies, infections, inflammatory conditions, and gastrointestinal disorders.[37] Fructo-oligosaccharides (FOSs) are plant sugars that are used as prebiot-ics, which are substances that selectively support the growth and activity of beneficial bacteria in the colon.[38] FOSs also exhibit anti-inflammatory activity on intestinal inflammation[39] and increase intestinal absorption of magnesium, calcium, and iron.[40]
- *Improve the intestinal barrier.* Proper intestinal barrier function is im-perative for gastrointestinal health. The amino acid glutamine is used as a fuel source for the cells that line the intestines. Glutamine supple-mentation stimulates the growth and maturation of intestinal cells and helps maintain the integrity of the mucosal barrier, thus preventing intestinal hyperpermeability and bacteria from crossing into the blood-stream.[41] Glutamine also regulates intestinal IgA, an antibody that pro-tects the mucosal lining.[42] N-acetylglucosamine (NAG) is required for

the synthesis of mucopolysaccharides, a component of mucous membranes. NAG is deficient in persons with inflammatory bowel disease, which may lead to a decrease in the protective intestinal mucosal glycoprotein.[43] Phosphatidylcholine is a lipid component of the protective intestinal mucosal layer that has anti-inflammatory activity,[44] decreases bacterial translocation across the intestinal barrier,[45] and has shown benefit in patients with ulcerative colitis.[46]

- *Heal existing infections and inflammation.* Berberine is a constituent found in various botanicals such as goldenseal (*Hydrastis canadensis*) and Oregon grape (*Mahonia aquifolium*) and is used to maintain proper gastrointestinal flora and inhibit pathogens in the colon. Berberine exhibits significant antimicrobial activity against bacteria, fungus, mycobacteria, and protozoa.[47] Berberine also exhibits anti-inflammatory activity.[48] Cabbage (*Brassica oleracea*) exhibits significant antioxidant activity,[49] can help heal the stomach from ulcers,[50] and decreases the risk of colorectal and stomach cancer.[51] Aloe vera is used for anti-inflammatory, antioxidant, antibacterial, and antifungal activity; for a variety of digestive complaints, such as constipation, inflammatory bowel disease,[52] and ulcers; and for wound healing and other inflammatory conditions. Gamma oryzanol exhibits antioxidant activity and antiulcer properties[53] and may have antiallergy effects.[54]

- *Demulcent herbs.* Demulcent herbs are used to form a soothing film over the mucous membrane. These herbs decrease pain and inflammation of the intestinal lining and increase the mucous secretions that coat and protect the lining of the intestines from excess acidity, ulcers, ingested irritants, and toxins.[55] Commonly used demulcent herbs include licorice (*Glycyrrhiza glabra*), slippery elm (*Ulmus fulva*), and marshmallow (*Althaea officinalis*).

- *Get adequate fiber.* Fiber supports colon health: it helps regulate colonic motility, protects against colon cancer, and raises butyrate levels. High-fiber diets are associated with a decrease in plasma levels of proinflammatory chemical mediators.[56] Short-chain fatty acids (SCFAs), such as butyrate, decrease inflammation,[57] reinforce the colonic defense barrier, and decrease oxidative stress.[58] SCFAs also stimulate colonic blood flow, enhance fluid and electrolyte uptake[59] and increase the motility of the intestinal tract.[60] Deficient production of SCFAs may be involved in diarrhea, food allergies,[61] ulcerative colitis, and other intestinal disorders.[62] Larch arabinogalactan is a nondigestible soluble dietary fiber that has been shown to increase the production of the SCFAs, decrease the generation and absorption of ammonia in the colon, and enhance beneficial gut microflora such as *Lactobacillus* and *Bifidobacterium*.[63]

- *Get adequate vitamin D.* Vitamin D is important for gastrointestinal health. Research has shown that low levels of vitamin D can compromise the intestinal mucosal barrier, leading to increased susceptibility to mucosal damage and increased risk of conditions such as inflammatory bowel disease.[64] In addition, patients with inflammatory bowel disease have decreased levels of vitamin D.[65]

Clinical Cases

1. *Crohn's disease.* A 43-year-old woman presented to the office complaining of severe diarrhea. Her history revealed a family history of Crohn's disease (brother); off-and-on troubles with gastrointestinal system since childhood; diarrhea and upper left quadrant (of abdomen) pain beginning in 1997; severe diarrhea and vomiting with upper left quadrant pain by 2000; and radiographs showed strictures at terminal ileum. In October 2004, her severe diarrhea and pain intensified and her physician recommended a computed tomography scan and surgery to remove nine inches of bowel. The biopsy showed no detectable food allergy, and the pain and diarrhea were still present after surgery. Her medications included prednisone, doxycyline, essential fatty acid agonist, acid reflux antagonist, and Imodium. The symptoms she presented with included more than 25 bouts of watery, urgent, painful diarrhea daily. Symptoms were worse in morning and were aggravated by raw, cold foods, especially vegetables. She was unable to get through most meals without having significant abdominal pains and urgency. Frustration and anxiety were moderate to marked and seemed to aggravate her symptoms. She tried a course of acupuncture treatments one or two times weekly and was re-evaluated every 10 to 12 treatments. Medicinal herbs aggravated symptoms severely and were discontinued. Within two and a half months, she was having six to nine bowel movements daily (down from more than 25) with significant decreases in urgency and pain. She also felt less anxious and frustrated regarding her condition. Progress seemed slower than expected, however, and she would have random setbacks of urgent diarrhea with no known cause, which would clear within a few days with Imodium.

   Upon recommendation, she consented to the IgG Food Antibody Assessment Panel. The test results revealed reactivity for foods in the dairy group, mushroom, asparagus, cucumber, carrot, blueberry, cranberry, banana, pineapple, almond, sesame, wheat gluten and gliadin breads (including rye, spelt, whole wheat), sugar cane, and chicken egg. The patient was quite surprised to see that just about every elevated food item or group was a significant part of her diet. She had always avoided dairy products in general, but most of the other foods were consumed daily, if not multiple times per day.

   Within a couple of days her condition improved notably. Her bowel movements were nearly under control and had a solidity not experienced previously. Urgency and pain were all but eliminated. After a few weeks with minimal symptoms, the patient ate a regular bagel and experienced diarrhea very similar to what she had experienced before treatment, although it did resolve by the end of the day without medication, which was new. The patient is now on a maintenance course of acupuncture, is able to take herbs, and continues to comply with her dietary guidelines.

2. *IBS and celiac disease.* J.S. was a 46-year-old man with a history of irritable bowel syndrome, chronic lower back pain, and anxiety. He had been experiencing intestinal problems since high school. Evaluations by gastrointestinal specialists indicated celiac disease, although dietary changes were ineffective in relieving his complaints. An IgG Food Antibody Assessment Panel showed elevations for yogurt, milk, and peanuts, which he had been eating every day. On removal of the moderate and high reactive foods from his diet, the patient experienced about a 30 percent improvement in IBS symptoms in about a week's time. Upon evaluation at eight weeks, the patient said he had seen about an 85 percent improvement in his gastrointestinal symptoms and had no recurring bouts of intestinal distress. His back pain and soreness had also improved. He no longer plans his day around finding bathrooms and has felt the most improvement in his symptoms since high school. He was highly allergic to six different foods, which he has since eliminated from his diet. We continued to monitor his progress over the next couple of months.

3. *Vomiting, bloody stools, and GERD in a child.* N.D. had experienced coughing/vomiting, bloody stools, and poor weight gain since the age of six months and had shown no improvement with antiemetic drugs. By the time N.D. was 2 years old he had a skin rash, secondary GERD, poor appetite, and growth retardation in both height and weight. He had a history of positive egg allergy shown by IgE testing. In the fall of 2006, the boy was taken to Children's Hospital for pediatric specialty support. By this time he had developed allergy to Zyrtec, was experiencing abdominal pain, and was placed on acid-blocking drugs as well as montelukast and loratadine to control his allergies and trouble breathing. An allergist at the hospital performed IgE skin testing, which showed positive reaction to peach and egg. Follow-up IgE skin testing in November 2006, however, showed negative reaction to egg. With this, the allergist concluded that N.D. was no longer allergic to egg. N.D. was now on daily doses of montelukast, loratadine, and ranitidine, and he carried an EpiPen for severe allergic reactions. Despite the negative IgE results, the specialists concluded that a food was likely causing a non-IgE mediated eosinophilia, but there was no effective treatment offered and no definitive food was named.

His current symptoms were eczema, poor weight gain, weekly vomiting, and coughing. I recommended the IgG Food Antibody Assessment

Panel, and a blood collection was done at his second office visit. The report showed reaction to egg, chicken, cheese, milk, wheat, amaranth, soy, beef, rye, spelt, and pea. Within two months, the mother noted that N.D. had experienced no vomiting since starting the elimination diet in July. Follow-up appointments revealed no coughing and no recurrence of vomiting.

4. *Chronic diarrhea after gallbladder removal.* A woman came to the office for testing a few months after her gallbladder was removed. After the surgery she had horrible diarrhea no matter what she used as a supplement. After following the results of an IgG Food Antibody Assessment Panel she hasn't had a single problem with diarrhea and has lost weight. She was able to return to work as a FedEx driver.

5. *Chronic diarrhea.* A 32-year-old man with a long history of explosive diarrhea had sought help from many gastroenterologists to no avail. Apart from blood studies, he underwent multiple endoscopies and biopsies. The biopsy reports invariably came back as nonspecific findings consistent with irritable bowel disease. The last gastroenterologist he saw suggested that he be tested for food allergies to assess for immediate and delayed reactivity to foods with an IgG Food Antibody Assessment Panel. The results revealed that he was highly allergic to egg white and gluten. By following the customized elimination and rotation diet guideline, he reported much relief from his symptoms, which only recurred upon further exposure to the reactive foods.

6. *Diarrhea, nausea, and gas.* A 40-year-old woman presented with a nine-month history of intestinal distress involving diarrhea, nausea, gas, fatigue, backaches, insomnia, and periodic numbness of her fingers. A full gastrointestinal investigation did not identify any disease processes. She stated that her stools were like "mud." An IgG Food Antibody Assessment Panel revealed a strong delayed hypersensitivity to almond—her favorite snack. Eliminating almonds from her diet resulted in quick resolution of all symptoms.

7. *GERD and nausea.* A 40-year-old woman had with a lifetime history of esophageal reflux and nausea often to the point of vomiting. Her many visits to gastroenterologists proved futile, as they were unable to diagnose her condition. She also had a history of anxiety, alternating constipation and loose stools, rosacea, fatigue, low libido, multiple chemical sensitivities, and upper respiratory infections. An IgG Food Antibody Assessment Panel revealed elevated antibody levels specific to dairy and egg. Reflux and nausea fully resolved within two days of removing dairy and egg products from her diet. In addition, her anxiety lessened, her stools normalized, and her energy level and libido improved. Her multiple chemical sensitivities diminished in severity and the rosacea improved throughout the following year.

8. *Chronic constipation*. A 38-year-old woman had suffered from chronic constipation for several years. An IgG Food Antibody Assessment Panel showed that food-specific antibodies to dairy, egg, and baker's yeast were quite elevated. After one month on a customized elimination and rotation diet guideline, her bowel functions completely normalized.

CONCLUSION

To understand how to optimize the health and function of the gastrointestinal tract, one must first have a basic knowledge of the anatomy and physiology of the digestive system. Any specific digestive disorders must also be considered. Finally, diet and supplements can be manipulated to individualize a treatment plan for optimal gastrointestinal health.

NOTES

1. Husebye E. The pathogenesis of gastrointestinal bacterial overgrowth. *Chemotherapy*. 2005;51(suppl 1):1–22.

2. The National Digestive Diseases Information Clearinghouse. Your digestive system and how it works. 2008. Available at: http://digestive.niddk.nih.gov/ddiseases/pubs/yrdd/index.htm#top. Accessed November 22, 2008.

3. Zareie M, Johnson-Henry K, Jury J, et al. Probiotics prevent bacterial translocation and improve intestinal barrier function in rats following chronic psychological stress. *Gut*. 2006;55:1553–1560.

4. Park MC, Goldman MA, Carpenter LL, et al. Vagus nerve stimulation for depression: rationale, anatomical and physiological basis of efficacy and future prospects. *Acta Neurochir Suppl*. 2007;97(Pt 2):407–416.

5. Centers for Disease Control and Prevention. Fastats-digestive diseases. 2008. Available at: www.cdc.gov/nchs/fastats/digestiv.htm. Accessed November 8, 2007.

6. Adams PF, Hendershot GE, Marano MA. Current estimates from the National Health Interview Survey, 1996. National Center for Health Statistics. *Vital Health Stat*. 1999;10:1–148.

7. Sandler RS, Everhart JE, Donowitz M, et al. The burden of selected digestive diseases in the United States. *Gastroenterology*. 2002;122:1500–1511.

8. Husebye E, Skar V, Hoverstad T, et al. Fasting hypochlorhydria with gram positive gastric flora is highly prevalent in healthy old people. *Gut*. 1992;33:1331–1337.

9. Bartram HP, Scheppach W, Schmid H, et al. Proliferation of human colonic mucosa as an intermediate biomarker of carcinogenesis: effects of butyrate, deoxycholate, calcium, ammonia, and pH. *Cancer Res*. 1993;53:3283–3288.

10. Robinson RR, Feirtag J, Slavin JL. Effects of dietary arabinogalactan on gastrointestinal and blood parameters in healthy human subjects. *J Am Coll Nutr*.2001; 20:279–285.

11. Visek WJ. Diet and cell growth modulation by ammonia. *Am J Clin Nutr* 1978; 31:S216-S220.

12. Ventura MT, Polimeno L, Amoruso AC, et al. Intestinal permeability in patients with adverse reactions to food. *Dig Liver Dis*. 2006;38:732–736.

13. Sandek A, Bauditz J, Swidsinski A, et al. Altered intestinal function in patients with chronic heart failure. *J Am Coll Cardiol.* 2007;50:1561–1569.

14. The National Digestive Diseases Information Clearinghouse. Crohn's disease. 2006. Available at: http://digestive.niddk.nih.gov/ddiseases/pubs/crohns/index.htm. Accessed November 22, 2008.

15. The National Digestive Diseases Information Clearinghouse. Ulcerative colitis. 2006. Available at: http://digestive.niddk.nih.gov/ddiseases/pubs/colitis/index.htm. Accessed November 22, 2008.

16. The National Digestive Diseases Information Clearinghouse. Irritable bowel syndrome. 2007. Available at: http://digestive.niddk.nih.gov/ddiseases/pubs/ibs/index.htm. Accessed November 22, 2008.

17. Fasano A, Berti I, Gerarduzzi T, et al. Prevalence of celiac disease in at-risk and not-at-risk groups in the United States. *Arch Internal Med.* 2003;163:268–292.

18. National Digestive Diseases Information Clearinghouse. Celiac disease. 2008. Available at: http://digestive.niddk.nih.gov/ddiseases/pubs/celiac/index.htm. Accessed November 22, 2008.

19. Shaheen NJ, Hansen RA, Morgan DR, et al. The burden of gastrointestinal and liver diseases, 2006. *Am J Gastroenterol.* 2006;101:2128–2138.

20. National Heartburn Alliance. Survey 2000 Results: A Community Perspective, 2000. Available at: http://www.heartburnalliance.org/press_heartburn_survey.php. Accessed April 21, 2009.

21. Mohammed I, Nightingale P, Trudgill NJ. Risk factors for gastro-oesophageal reflux disease symptoms: a community study. *Aliment Pharmacol Ther.* 2005;21:821–827.

22. Lohsiriwat S, Puengna N, Leelakusolvong S. Effect of caffeine on lower esophageal sphincter pressure in Thai healthy volunteers. *Dis Esophagus* 2006;19(3):183–188.

23. Hamoui N, Lord RV, Hagen JA, et al. Response of the lower esophageal sphincter to gastric distention by carbonated beverages. *J Gastrointest Surg.* 2006;10:870–877.

24. Hancox RJ, Poulton R, Taylor DR, et al. Associations between respiratory symptoms, lung function and gastro-oesophageal reflux symptoms in a population-based birth cohort. *Respir Res.* 2006;7:142.

25. Nocon M, Labenz J, Willich SN. Lifestyle factors and symptoms of gastro-oesophageal reflux—a population-based study. *Aliment Pharmacol Ther.* 2006;23(1):169–174; Nilsson M, Johnsen R, Ye W, et al. Lifestyle related risk factors in the aetiology of gastro-oesophageal reflux. *Gut.* 2004;53:1730–1735.

26. Austin GL, Thiny MT, Westman EC, et al. A very low-carbohydrate diet improves gastroesophageal reflux and its symptoms. *Dig Dis Sci.* 2006;51:1307–1312.

27. Veugelers PJ, Porter GA, Guernsey DL, et al. Obesity and lifestyle risk factors for gastroesophageal reflux disease, Barrett esophagus and esophageal adenocarcinoma. *Dis Esophagus.* 2006;19:321–328.

28. Kaltenbach T, Crockett S, Gerson LB. Are lifestyle measures effective in patients with gastroesophageal reflux disease? An evidence-based approach. *Arch Intern Med.* 2006;166:965–971.

29. Mathus-Vliegen EM, Tygat GN. Gastro-oesophageal reflux in obese subjects: influence of overweight, weight loss and chronic gastric balloon distension. *Scand J Gastroenterol.* 2002;37:1246–1252.

30. The National Digestive Diseases Information Clearinghouse. Heartburn, gastroesophageal reflux (GRE), and gastroesophageal reflux disease (GERD). 2007. Available at: http://digestive.niddk.nih.gov/ddiseases/pubs/gerd/index.htm. Accessed November 30, 2008.

31. Sokic-Milutinovic A, Todorovic V, Milosavljevic T. Pathogenesis of Helicobacter pylori infection—bacterium and host relationship [in Serbian]. *Srp Arh Celok Lek.* 2004;132(9–10):340–344.

32. Hashemi MR, Rahnavardi M, Bikdeli B, et al. H pylori infection among 1000 southern Iranian dyspeptic patients. *World J Gastroenterol.* 2006;12:5479–5482.

33. The National Digestive Diseases Information Clearinghouse. Indigestion. 2008. Available at: http://digestive.niddk.nih.gov/ddiseases/pubs/indigestion/index.htm. Accessed November 22, 2008.

34. The National Digestive Diseases Information Clearinghouse. Diarrhea. 2007. Available at: http://digestive.niddk.nih.gov/ddiseases/pubs/diarrhea/index.htm. Accessed November 22, 2008.

35. The National Digestive Diseases Information Clearinghouse. Constipation. 2007. Available at:http://digestive.niddk.nih.gov/ddiseases/pubs/constipation/index.htm. Accessed November 22, 2008.

36. Fedorak RN, Madsen KL. Probiotics and the management of inflammatory bowel disease. *Inflamm Bowel Dis.* 2004;10:286–299.

37. Savilahti E, Kuitunen M, Vaarala O. Pre and probiotics in the prevention and treatment of food allergy. *Curr Opin Allergy Clin Immunol.* 2008;8(3):243–248; Giovannini M, Agostoni C, Riva E, et al. A randomized prospective double blind controlled trial on effects of long-term consumption of fermented milk containing Lactobacillus casei in pre-school children with allergic asthma and/or rhinitis. *Pediatr Res.* 2007;62:215–220.

38. Bouhnik Y, Vahedi K, et al. Short-chain fructo-oligosaccharide administration dose-dependently increases fecal bifidobacteria in healthy humans. *J Nutr.* 1999;129:113–116.

39. Lara-Villoslada F, de Haro O, Camuesco D, et al. Short-chain fructooligosaccharides, in spite of being fermented in the upper part of the large intestine, have anti-inflammatory activity in the TNBS model of colitis. *Eur J Nutr.* 2006;45:418–425.

40. Ohta A. Prevention of osteoporosis by foods and dietary supplements. The effect of fructooligosaccharides (FOS) on the calcium absorption and bone. *Clin Calcium.* 2006;16:1639–1645.

41. Miller AL. Therapeutic considerations of L-glutamine: a review of the literature. *Altern Med Rev.* 1999;4:239–248.

42. Fukatsu K, Kudsk KA, et al. TPN decreases IL-4 and IL-10 mRNA expression in lipopolysaccharide stimulated intestinal lamina propria cells but glutamine supplementation preserves the expression. *Shock.* 2001;15:318–322.

43. Burton AF, Anderson FH. Decreased incorporation of 14C-glucosamine relative to 3H-N-acetyl glucosamine in the intestinal mucosa of patients with inflammatory bowel disease. *Am J Gastroenterol.* 1983;78:19–22.

44. Treede I, Braun A, Sparla R, et al. Anti-inflammatory effects of phosphatidylcholine. *J Biol Chem.* 2007;282:27155–27164.

45. Lugea A, Salas A, Casalot J, et al. Surface hydrophobicity of the rat colonic mucosa is a defensive barrier against macromolecules and toxins. *Gut.* 2000;46:515–521.

46. Stremmel W, Merle U, Zahn A, et al. Retarded release phosphatidylcholine benefits patients with chronic active ulcerative colitis. *Gut.* 2005;54:966–971.

47. Amin AH, Subbaiah TV, Abbasi KM. Berberine sulfate: antimicrobial activity, bioassay, and mode of action. *Can J Microbiol* 1969;15:1067–1076; Scazzocchio F, Corneta MF, Tomassini L, et al. Antibacterial activity of Hydrastis canadensis extract and its major isolated alkaloids. *Planta Med.* 2001;67:561–564; Rehman J, Dillow JM, Carter SM, et al. Increased production of antigen-specific immunoglobulins G and M following in vivo treatment with the medicinal plants Echinacea angustifolia and Hydrastis canadensis. *Immunol*

Lett. 1999;68:391–395; Sun D, Courtney HS, Beachey EH. Berberine sulfate blocks adherence of Streptococcus pyogenes to epithelial cells, fibronectin, and hexadecane. *Antimicrob Agents Chemother.* 1988;32:1370–1374; Kaneda Y, Torii M, Tanaka T, et al. In vitro effects of berberine sulphate on the growth and structure of Entamoeba histolytica, Giardia lamblia and Trichomonas vaginalis. *Ann Trop Med Parasitol.* 1991;85:417–425.

48. Fukuda K, Hibiya Y, Mutoh M, et al. Inhibition by berberine of cyclooxygenase-2 transcriptional activity in human colon cancer cells. *J Ethnopharmacol.* 1999;66:227–233.

49. Isbir T, Yaylim I, Aydin M, et al. The effects of Brassica oleraceae var capitata on epidermal glutathione and lipid peroxides in DMBA-initiated-TPA-promoted mice. *Anticancer Res.* 2000;20:219–224.

50. Cheney G. Vitamin U Therapy of Peptic Ulcer. *Calif Med.* 1952;77:248–252.

51. van Poppel G, Verhoeven DT, Verhagen H, et al. Brassica vegetables and cancer prevention. Epidemiology and mechanisms. *Adv Exp Med Biol.* 1999;472:159–168.

52. Langmead L, Feakins RM, Goldthorpe S, et al. Randomized, double-blind, placebo-controlled trial of oral aloe vera gel for active ulcerative colitis. *Aliment Pharmacol Ther.* 2004;19:739–747; Langmead L, Makins RJ, Rampton DS. Anti-inflammatory effects of aloe vera gel in human colorectal mucosa in vitro. *Aliment Pharmacol Ther.* 2004;19:521–527.

53. Ichimaru Y, Moriyama M, Ichimaru M, et al. Effects of gamma-oryzanol on gastric lesions and small intestinal propulsive activity in mice [in Japanese]. *Nippon Yakurigaku Zasshi.* 1984;84:537–542.

54. Sierra S, Lara-Villoslada F, Olivares M, et al. Increased immune response in mice consuming rice bran oil. *Eur J Nutr.* 2005;44:509–516.

55. *The Review of Natural Products by Facts and Comparisons.* St Louis, MO: Wolters Kluwer Co.; 1999.

56. Ma Y, Hébert JR, Li W, et al. Association between dietary fiber and markers of systemic inflammation in the Women's Health Initiative Observational Study. *Nutrition.* 2008;24:941–949.

57. Tedelind S, Westberg F, Kjerrulf M, et al. Anti-inflammatory properties of the short-chain fatty acids acetate and propionate: a study with relevance to inflammatory bowel disease. *World J Gastroenterol.* 2007;13:2826–2832.

58. Hamer HM, Jonkers D, Venema K, et al. Review article: the role of butyrate on colonic function. *Aliment Pharmacol Ther.* 2008;27(2):104–119.

59. Topping DL, Clifton PM. Short-chain fatty acids and human colonic function: roles of resistant starch and nonstarch polysaccharides. *Physiol Rev.* 2001;81:1031–1064.

60. Cherbut C, Aubé AC, Blottière HM, et al. Effects of short-chain fatty acids on gastrointestinal motility. *Scand J Gastroenterol Suppl.* 1997;222:58–61.

61. Chen CC, Walker WA. Probiotics and prebiotics: role in clinical disease states. *Adv Pediatr.* 2005;52:77–113.

62. Rabassa AA, Rogers AI. The role of short-chain fatty acid metabolism in colonic disorders. *Am J Gastroenterol.* 1992;87:419–423.

63. Robinson RR, Feirtag J, Slavin JL. Effects of dietary arabinogalactan on gastrointestinal and blood parameters in healthy human subjects. *J Am Coll Nutr.* 2001;20:279–285.

64. Kong J, Zhang Z, Musch MW, et al. Novel role of the vitamin D receptor in maintaining the integrity of the intestinal mucosal barrier. *Am J Physiol Gastrointest Liver Physiol.* 2008;294:G208–G216.

65. Pappa HM, Grand RJ, Gordon CM. Report on the vitamin D status of adult and pediatric patients with inflammatory bowel disease and its significance for bone health and disease. *Inflamm Bowel Dis.* 2006;12:1162–1174.

CHAPTER 10

Water, Pets, Exercise, and Indoor Living: What Everyone Must Know

Numerous environmental modifications are suggested to combat allergies. Which recommendations are applicable to an individual will depend on the extent of the allergy symptoms and the type of allergies. In addition to minimizing common allergens, it is also imperative to limit environmental toxins, as toxin exposure has a strong correlation with exacerbating allergic reactions. Common indoor allergens include house-dust mite droppings, animal dander, cockroach droppings, and indoor molds, and indoor allergens are often responsible for perennial (all-year) allergies.[1] These allergens may only elicit minor symptoms in a person. However, the cumulative effect of these allergens plus food and chemical sensitivities may be enough to cause significant reactions. Avoiding these common allergens can decrease a person's total allergen exposure and may dramatically decrease overall reactivity.

BEDROOM

A person who sleeps eight hours per night spends roughly one-third of his or her time in the bedroom. Thus, controlling environmental allergens in the bedroom is critical and a priority for decreasing total allergenic exposure. Following are some suggested approaches.

1. Dust mites and their feces are common allergens. To decrease exposure to these allergens. cover the mattress, box spring, and pillows with zippered vinyl allergy covers to avoid breathing in these allergens at night.
2. Avoid using down-feather pillows and comforters as they tend to harbor dust and dust mites. If you do use them, cover them in zippered allergy covers.

3. Wash bedding weekly in hot water (130°F) and make sure it dries completely.
4. Limit decorations and window dressings in the bedroom as they collect dust.
5. Remove carpet from the bedroom if possible. Using washable rugs is better. Also, wash rugs frequently to remove allergens that may have been tracked in on footwear or dust that may have collected.
6. Use a high-quality HEPA (high-efficiency particulate air) filter in the bedroom to limit airborne allergen exposure at night.
7. Do not allow pets in the bedroom to decrease exposure to pet dander.
8. Wash one's hair before bed, particularly if one is allergic to pollens.
9. Do not keep coats, outdoor apparel, or items that are not laundered frequently in the bedroom.

IN THE HOME

We spend about 90 percent of our time indoors. Many of us do not realize that our indoor air is often more problematic than outdoor pollution. The following are tips to enhance our indoor air.

1. Keep air ducts for the home heating-cooling system clean, especially if the home is old or there are pets.
2. Keep windows and doors closed when the pollen count is high.
3. Avoid exposure to tobacco smoke. Airborne irritants can sensitize the respiratory tract and trigger or exacerbate asthma and respiratory allergies.
4. Carpet traps numerous allergens, such dust mites, mold, pet dander, and pollen and it may release toxic chemicals, such as formaldehyde. Limiting the amount of carpet throughout the house may be helpful. If you choose to have carpet, use short-fiber carpets so the allergens may be vacuumed up more easily.
5. Us a vacuum with a HEPA filtration system and clean it out regularly.
6. Mold, which grows in warm, moist areas, is another common allergen. Check all faucets and floors for possible leaks in pipes, and make sure bathrooms are well ventilated to decrease the growth of mold and mildew. Use a cleaning solution containing five percent bleach and a small amount of detergent to remove any visible mold.
7. Use a dehumidifier to reduce the humidity level to below 50 percent to decrease dust mites, mold, and cockroaches.
8. Conventional cleaning products contain numerous chemicals that may aggravate or trigger allergic reactions, particularly in persons with asthma. Using natural cleaning products, such as baking soda or vinegar in water, often works well.
9. To eliminate cockroaches, keep the home as clean as possible, take out trash frequently, and seal any cracks from outside the home. Also, clean

areas in the home where crumbs may accumulate, such as under the refrigerator and stove.

10. Avoid airborne irritants such as tobacco smoke, aerosols, paint, perfumes, and cleaning products as well as other strong odors because they may aggravate respiratory allergies.
11. Remove shoes outdoors to avoid tracking in potential allergens.
12. Formaldehyde is released from numerous household items, such as wood products and furniture, carpet, and textiles. Formaldehyde can aggravate the respiratory tract and trigger asthma and wheezing in some people.[2]

WATER

Water is a precious commodity nowadays. Most of our water sources are polluted and our tap water can be "enhanced" with fluoride, chloride and their permutated by-products. Water is the means by which we detoxify and move waste out of our body; therefore, it is extremely important to be aware of the quality of the water that we drink, cook with and bathe in.

1. Drink purified water. Heavy metals, such as lead and other chemical contaminants, may adversely affect immune function.
2. Check water quality regularly. In particular, check lead levels.

EXERCISE

Since we do live most of our lives indoors nowadays, it is important to make time to exercise our bodies on a regular basis. Historically, human beings walked at least 10 miles daily and were in constant movement throughout the day. Today, we are mostly sedentary and indoors. When we exercise it is important to take the following into consideration:

1. Do not exercise outdoors when the pollen count is high. Local and national pollen counts are available at several Web sites, such as the National Allergy Bureau at www.aaaai.org/nab.
2. Cold weather can aggravate asthma. Do not exercise outdoors in cold weather if you have cold-induced asthma.

OUTSIDE THE HOME

When we do wander outside, it is important to reduce our exposure to airborne allergens.

1. Check pollen counts regularly.
2. Lawns are often treated with pesticides. Avoid exposure to pesticides as much as possible as they have been shown to significantly modulate immune function.[3]

3. Limit exposure to freshly cut grass, mowing, and raking as these increase exposure to pollen and mold.
4. Drive with car windows closed when the pollen count is elevated.
5. Stay indoors when the pollen count or humidity is high.
6. Wear glasses or sunglasses to prevent pollen from coming in contact with the eyes.
7. Limit exposure to sensitizing and irritating agents.[4] Research has shown that outdoor air pollutants increase the risk of childhood asthma and allergic diseases.[5]

HELPING AVOID ENVIRONMENTAL ILLNESS

Millions of Americans suffer from some level of chemical sensitivity resulting from exposure to chemicals. Symptoms include dizziness, eye and throat irritation, chest tightness, and nasal congestion. Do you feel poorly after walking past a perfume counter? Does the smell of some things make you feel tired or dizzy or cause a headache? If so, you may be poisoned by it. Next time you or a loved one says, "This smell is making me sick," get away and stay away from it. Sometimes our bodies warn us when something is not right. Listen to the whispers.

Toxins are poisons from chemicals and pollutants. Another class of toxins, biotoxins, are produced by plants and insects. Some toxins are so deadly that they are used in chemical warfare. Other biotoxins will cause weight gain and may prevent you from losing weight. Toxins, like any poison, will make you sick or kill you depending on the toxic dosage, your general health, and your genetics. Toxins invade our bodies, drain our vitality, and cause free-radical damage, harming our DNA, brains, lungs, livers, and kidneys.

Environmental toxins are absorbed by the skin, eyes, and the respiratory and gastrointestinal tracts. Acute exposures and toxicity occur rapidly yet can have long-term or chronic consequences. Chronic exposures and toxicity occur over a long period of continuous or intermittent exposure. Toxicity can manifest with immediate or progressive symptoms. Unfortunately, the person suffering often mistakes this for part of the aging process or some unrelated series of symptoms.

What we cannot see or smell or feel can often be the most dangerous to our health. For example, radon gas is undetectable. This radioactive gas seeps from the ground into homes and workplaces. The Environmental Protection Agency (EPA) reports that there are about 14,000 deaths from lung cancer related to radon gas exposure in the United States each year. A simple radon home kit can help you detect if this is an issue for you. If you do not test your home, you will not know. A more familiar invisible gas, carbon monoxide, comes from gas or kerosene furnaces, appliances, fireplaces, wood stoves, and even autos in attached garages. Once again, a simple monitor can save your life.

Some common toxins are solvents, pesticides, herbicides, petroleum distillates, paints, pine oil, pest repellents, smoke (from burning oil, gas, kerosene, coal, wood, and tobacco products), aerosols, fumes (from new building materials like carpet, paint, furniture, pressed wood products, air fresheners), lead in paint and pipes, asbestos, chemicals in household cleaners, dusts, mold spores and toxins, airborne insulation, dust mites, pet dander, and more—in other words, things we are exposed to every day. Obviously we cannot entirely avoid all toxins, but we can take antioxidants and use proper ventilation, air filters, and common sense.

Commonsense ideas are to wear gloves and goggles when using any product that is supposed to be used only in a well-ventilated area. At the very least, a well-ventilated area means two windows are open and a fan is running. Leaving just an open window or door is woefully inadequate. If you are using an aerosol hair spray or cooking oil, hold your breath, close your eyes while spraying it, and leave the room long enough for the mist to settle. Keep children out of the area.

Some molds produce biotoxins that are so powerful that many of them are the basis for biological warfare. Mold spores like to grow on starch, and many modern construction materials provide that food—just add water. Today's buildings are sealed more tightly than ever before, which helps moisture build up inside. If you have had water come in contact with any sheetrock, wood, insulation, or carpet in your home, beware—especially if the mold is black. If your heating and air conditioning system is contaminated by mold, it has distributed airborne mold spores everywhere in your home.

Once the water source is removed, mold starts to die, and this is when it becomes dangerous. In an effort to survive, mold starts

> Just because you don't see it doesn't mean it can't kill you. —Chris D. Meletis, N.D.

producing powerful toxins (to kill other molds that might invade its endangered habitat). When you inhale these toxins, they invade every organ of your body. Your symptoms may include severe fatigue, headache, forgetfulness, disorientation, depression, weight gain, shortness of breath, asthma, and/or skin irritations. If you have any of these symptoms, take immediate action, have your home tested, and go see a reputable toxicologist.

If you go to any major city, you can literally see the air. Air pollution can come from factories, power plants, dry cleaners, vehicles, wildfires, home heating, and even dust. According to the EPA, "Air pollution can threaten the health of human beings, trees, lakes, crops, and animals, as well as damage the ozone layer and buildings."

To lessen your exposure to outdoor air pollution:

- Listen to weather advisories and air-quality alerts.
- Don't drive with your car windows down during rush hour.
- Try not to walk on busy streets.
- Avoid exposure to smoke, including barbecue grills (stay upwind).
- Stay well-hydrated so your mucous membranes are more resistant to damage.
- Don't do cardiovascular or aerobic exercise outdoors on high-pollution days.
- When air quality is poor, stay indoors and use an air filter.

HOLD YOUR BREATH INDOORS

EPA studies indicate that levels for many pollutants may be two to five times higher indoors than outdoors. Most people spend approximately 90 percent of their time indoors. Obviously, this is a serious health concern. Since tightly sealed homes began being built in the mid-1970s, asthma has increased in excess of 65 percent per year. We've locked all the indoor air pollutants in the home.

Young children inside homes and schools, the elderly, and those with debilitating health conditions are often indoors more often and thus suffer more from the harmful effects of indoor air pollutants. High-risk individuals are those that have allergies, asthma, and chronic obstructive pulmonary disease, or cardiovascular disease.

Dust can contain toxic substances, silica, dust mites, mold and mildew spores, cat dander, and viruses that can cause colds, flu, and more. Dust and many pollutants are readily inhaled into your lungs and are potentially absorbed throughout your body.

The consequences of exposure to indoor air pollutants can be immediate or cumulative. Symptoms can include but are not limited to the following:

- Irritation of eyes, nose, or throat
- Breathing/respiratory symptoms
- Increased number of illnesses
- Headaches
- Dizziness
- Fatigue
- Chronic and debilitating respiratory diseases
- Heart disease
- Cancer

TAKE A DEEP BREATH INDOORS

So what is a person to do? Use an air filtration unit that can filter around 250 cubic feet per minute and can remove 99 percent or more of airborne particles from the air that passes through it. Tabletop units usually filter fewer cubic feet per minute and remove a much lower percent of airborne particles. If you can find a unit that has a timer on it, that's ideal because you can set the unit to start running before you get home. Also, be certain the unit has an alarm or warning light that alerts you to change the filter, or you could be breathing polluted air and not know it. Get the best air cleaner you can find. It is a wonderful long-term investment for you and your family's health.

> Understanding the nature of the problem helps you make informed and effective decisions. —Chris D. Meletis, N.D.

RUSSIAN ROULETTE

Back away from the faucet slowly. If you have been drinking chlorinated and/ or fluorinated water, please stop. Why? Well, if chlorine is powerful enough to kill the things swimming around in a hot tub or public swimming pool, what else can it kill? One thing is for certain: It could very well disturb the balance of friendly bacteria in your colon, the same friendly bacteria that prevent invading microbes from proliferating. These bacteria also help produce vitamins like B-12 and K and help push toxic substances out of your body. Maintaining sufficient gastrointestinal bacteria helps minimize risk of food allergy burden and supports gut health.

For decades, unsuspecting people consumed trans fats, which led to premature deaths. Now unsuspecting people are drinking contaminated water, and this will produce the same results as trans fat consumption: early deaths.

We often take the purity of our tap water for granted—that's a big mistake. In a carefully researched, documented, and peer-reviewed study of the drinking water systems of 19 U.S. cities, the National Resources Defense Council (NRDC) found that pollution and deteriorating, out-of-date plumbing are sometimes delivering drinking water that can contribute to health risks. It is important to realize that many cities throughout North America depend on pre–World War II water-delivery systems and technology. Many city filtration systems are not properly designed to remove 21st-century contaminants like pesticides, industrial pollutants, arsenic, and other hazards.

Health experts acknowledge that there is no such thing as a safe level of arsenic (a carcinogen) for humans. Therefore, when the EPA set "safe" levels for arsenic, it created a controversy, which continues today. We will let you decide if you think any arsenic is safe. An NRDC study found 5 parts per billion in the drinking water of 22 million Americans. Regardless of what country you live in, you are probably drinking arsenic in your water if you do not have a filter to remove it. Another source of controversy is that there are other contaminants for which the EPA has not set mandatory compliance levels. In addition, many cities routinely fall into the EPA's level of concern for various contaminants. Some health experts think that when it comes to contaminants in drinking water, we are playing Russian roulette with our health. Results for specific cities are on the NRDC Web site at http://www.nrdc.org/water/drinking/uscities/contents.asp.

THE BIG THREE

To get anywhere close to providing quality water, each of the following three steps must be taken on a consistent basis by your regional and local water municipalities:

- The original water source (lake, stream, reservoir) must be protected from pollution.
- Pipes that convey the water must be well-maintained and not be a source of additional contamination.

- Modern treatment facilities must remove microbes such as parasites, viruses, organic and inorganic contaminants, pesticides, lead, arsenic, mercury, volatile organic chemicals, industrial pollutants, poisons, *Escherichia coli*, and other bacteria.

Is your water district removing 100 percent of these contaminants? Is your water life-sustaining or life-threatening?

SURVIVAL GEAR

If you think bottled water is the solution, think again. Not only is it expensive but the water industry is largely unregulated. Indeed, you can be ingesting a completely new set of contaminants. An NRDC study found that one-third of bottled water is contaminated by bacteria or other chemicals at levels exceeding the bottled water industry's own guidelines and/or state regulatory standards. In addition, the flexible plastic that most bottled water comes in can leech even more chemicals into the water.

If you do not own a quality water filter for cooking and drinking purposes, it is one of the best investments you can make. A good water filter removes viruses, bacteria, organic and inorganic contaminants, pesticides, lead, mercury, volatile organic chemicals, and other contaminants that pass through municipal or well-water systems. Some of the best filters available now incorporate an ultraviolet light to kill disease-causing bacteria or parasites. Water cleanses the 50–100 trillion cells of your body. The fluidity of your blood, the shock-absorbing capacity of your joints, and the cushioning of your brain are all water dependent. This is why it is vitally important to consume truly clean water.

> Give the gift of health to those that you care about. Educate them so they too can make informed decisions. —Chris D. Meletis, N.D.

NOTES

1. American Academy of Allergies, Asthma, and Immunology. Tips to Remember: Indoor Allergies. 2007. Available at: http://www.aaaai.org/patients/publicedmat/tips/indoor allergens.stm. Accessed October 1, 2008.

2. Krzyzanowski M, Quackenboss JJ, Lebowitz MD. Chronic respiratory effects of indoor formaldehyde exposure. *Environ Res.* 1990;52:117–125.

3. Li Q, Nagahara N, Takahashi H, et al. Organophosphorus pesticides markedly inhibit the activities of natural killer, cytotoxic T lymphocyte and lymphokine-activated killer: a proposed inhibiting mechanism via granzyme inhibition. *Toxicology.* 2002;172:181–190.

4. World Health Organization. *Prevention of Allergy and Allergic Asthma.* 2002. Available at: http://www.worldallergy.org/professional/who_paa2003.pdf. Accessed October 1, 2008.

5. Bener A, Ehlayel M, Sabbah A. The pattern and genetics of pediatric extrinsic asthma risk factors in polluted environment. *Eur Ann Allergy Clin Immunol.* 2007;39:58–63.

CHAPTER 11

Healthy Aging and Gaining Control over Your Wellness with a Sustainable Diet

Stress can hurt your health. No two people are alike and we react to the same stressful incidents differently. As the day unfolds, we are bombarded with stresses and adjust accordingly. The same holds true for our body. However, when our coping mechanisms are taxed the body's natural defenses collapse. This is the time when we start to feel sick.

As an analogy, imagine your body as a teacup. Everyone's teacup is different and made up of a special type of ceramic, molded into a unique shape and size. Throughout the day, months and growing years, we fill our cup with experiences, emotions and food. The tea that we fill our teacup with is our own brew that we make up as we go along. Ask yourself this: How much can your cup hold and is the tea good for you?

Let us look at this analogy in more detail for factors that influence our health:

1. The material the cup is made out of is your personal genetic profile. This comes from the genes you were born with that have been passed down through generations in your family. Genes determine your predisposition to disease, susceptibility to certain food allergies, and ability to metabolize different toxins.

2. The place where the cup sits—on a table in the dining room or in the kitchen cupboard—represents your surroundings, including the setting of your daily activities, home, and workplace. Are you next to an airport? Close to a farm? In an urban setting? In the country? What is your mode of transportation? Are the roads to work fraught with traffic or is it a leisurely drive? Where does your teacup live? This may reveal environmental stressors that you are unaware of. Environmental stress may have

a negative impact on your health and may influence the development of food allergies.

3. Fill your cup with the types of foods you eat and drink. What are your daily eating habits? Do you eat fast food, pack a healthy meal, or dine out lavishly? How much water do you drink in the course of a day? Are you consuming too much fat and sugar? How about caffeine? What do you think this tea looks and smells like? Simply put, your nutritional status affects your body's ability to manage stress. Poor nutrition in and of itself is a direct stress to the body and may predispose us to food allergies.

4. Evaluate your lifestyle. How much and how well do you sleep? Do you exercise? Do you experience loving, committed relationships in your life? Do you practice a spiritual belief? Are you satisfied with your personal interactions? What are your goals in life? How often do you get a chance to sit down and relax? Are you happy or sad? Complacent or mad? Do you see your cup as half empty or half full? These factors represent the temperature of your personal brew. Is it too hot to handle? Your perceptions and attitudes influence your coping mechanisms, digestion and health.

All of these factors determine how much your teacup can hold and how well. If your cup is too full it will overflow. This is the time when you begin to feel something is not right and symptoms emerge. In other words, you have exceeded your carrying capacity, or your ability to adapt efficiently. The symptoms you experience may range from a mild cold to a debilitating illness.

Now let's back up for one minute. Please understand the following concept, because it is very important. Everything we take into our body besides food, including the air we breathe, our life experiences, and our emotions, influence the nature of the many chemical messages we receive from the foods we eat. How we read this incoming news and information therefore depends on many factors, including genetics, immune status. and integrity of the gut wall. If the gut wall is healthy and our immune soldiers are competent, we are better able to read food messages as generally good. If on the other hand, the gut lining is weak and has a weak immune front our reading at this level may not be so good and we may mount a hostile reaction against our foods. Our immune cells fight back.

Think of the gut as your second brain. Just as the brain processes information into thoughts and actions, the gut processes information from our thoughts, actions, and the food we eat. Have you heard of the sayings "becoming sick with worry" or "that's absolutely nauseating"? These are examples of how our gut responds to our thoughts, and this can affect our digestion and immune front and can promote the development of food sensitivities.

What builds a strong and healthy gut wall? There are a number of factors to consider. Secretion of the right amount of digestive juices, availability of nutrients, beneficial bacteria (for example, *Lactobacillus acidophilus*), and a positive proactive attitude all play a part. Considerable research argues that a positive attitude influences the gastrointestinal tract in a beneficial way. Negative and worrisome thoughts, on the other hand, can literally eat away at the stomach making the gut lining thin and weak.

Equally important is the population of bacteria and other microorganisms present in the gut. Friendly bacteria such as *Lactobacillus acidophilus* and *Bifodobacterium* live within the gut in a mutualistic and loving relationship. Fiber derived from the foods we eat feeds these little critters. In turn, their growth helps to build a strong and healthy gut wall and a competent immune front. Nutrients such as vitamins, minerals, and essential fatty acids also help to nourish the gut wall and promote the growth and health of cells.

Digestive juices released by the stomach and pancreas help break down incoming foods and extract good messages for the body's growth and repair processes. If there is an insufficient amount of digestive juices made, the foods are not broken down sufficiently. The messages may then be misread and interpreted as hostile.

Compared with a healthy gut wall, consider what is called leaky gut syndrome or is clinically known as increased intestinal permeability. Literally, the junctions between the gut cells become leaky, which allows large food morsels that would otherwise be excluded to enter through the gut wall. These large morsels of food present too much information in an unreadable form, which we cannot use for our vital processes. It is hostile language and provokes our immune soldiers into action.

ORAL TOLERANCE

Oral tolerance simply means our immune soldiers do not react to the incoming food messages in a hostile way—they are tolerant. Under this state we are able to read the messages from our foods as beneficial for our body's growth and repair processes. An important antibody involved in this process is IgA. IgA antibodies are anti-inflammatory and protective in nature. A higher ratio of IgA to IgG has a special relation to tolerance induction. That's a good thing!

Oral tolerance is influenced by the population of friendly bacteria in the intestinal tract. Beneficial bacteria influence our immune soldiers in the gut wall and the type of chemical mediators they produce. With good mediators, IgA is produced in larger numbers than IgG, and oral tolerance is favored.

I HAVE MY FOOD ALLERGY TEST RESULTS, NOW WHAT?

In reviewing the results of your food allergy test, you may want to consider the following points:

- Not all bad reactions to food are caused by allergies. Other problems can be caused by food intolerances, food poisoning, and psychosomatic food aversions. Lactose intolerance is one popular example of a nonimmunological reaction to food, specifically food intolerance.

- You may show an elevated antibody level to a food you never eat. This may be due to a cross-reaction. Cross-reactions occur when an antibody to one food reacts to a similar protein structure found in another food item. The proteins may not be identical, but they are similar enough that the antibody reacts to both. In your gut, if you were to eat either food, the antibodies you have formed to one of the foods will cross-react to the other food item. Examples of foods that have cross-reactions include banana and pineapple or cow's milk and lamb. It is also important to note that you may be ingesting a source of your hidden food allergy that you are unaware of. Egg white, for example, is a common ingredient in baked goods and may be disguised with a fancy name under the ingredients list; albumin, globulin, livetin, ovalbumin, and ovovitellin are all egg-derived food components.
- The way food is prepared may affect how you react to it. Food preparation can alter proteins in such a way that a food may be more or less allergenic. For example, the whey portion of milk is altered by high heat. Therefore, people with a whey allergy may be able to tolerate heat-altered milk products such as evaporated, boiled, or sterilized milk. Butter is another example. Heating unsalted butter slowly over medium heat results in a special type of butter called ghee, or clarified butter. Clarified butter is 100 percent fat and devoid of milk solids, including proteins and lactose. Generally speaking, antibodies are formed to food proteins; therefore, clarified butter, which is devoid of proteins, may not cause an allergic reaction.
- Some medications can interact with the immune system. Corticosteroids, such as prednisone, suppress the immune system and hence antibody production. This may affect the results of the food allergy test. Generally, antihistamines will not interfere with the test results as they do not interfere with antibody production.

After you have received your food allergy test report and have identified your reactive foods, what next? You need to find ways to eliminate these allergenic foods from your diet.

ELIMINATION PHASE

This is a true test of your will power. You may have to give up some of your favorite foods. For many people the best way is to quit cold turkey. Face it, the more you put it off, the longer you will feel like a crummy little rowboat.

The amount of time you will need to give up your reactive food(s) varies from person to person and should be discussed with your doctor. Most people may start to reintroduce the foods into their diet three to six months after their complete elimination. Even so, reintroduction is best done on a rotation basis. After the elimination phase you may need to reassess your food allergies with a follow-up enzyme-linked immunosorbent assay before you start to munch again.

	Food	Bowel/Urine Habits	Mood	Activity/Exercise	Symptoms
Monday					
Breakfast					
Lunch					
Dinner					
Snacks					
Tuesday					
Breakfast					
Lunch					
Dinner					
Snacks					
Wednesday					
Breakfast					
Lunch					
Dinner					
Snacks					
Thursday					
Breakfast					
Lunch					
Dinner					
Snacks					
Friday					
Breakfast					
Lunch					
Dinner					
Snacks					
Saturday					
Breakfast					
Lunch					
Dinner					
Snacks					
Sunday					
Breakfast					
Lunch					
Dinner					
Snacks					

Keep a record of what you eat and how you seem to be affected by it. A diet diary can prove very helpful during the elimination phase. A diet diary is a daily recording of your food and supplement intake, bowel and urine habits, mood changes, symptoms, outside stressors, and exercise patterns. Besides identifying reactions to food, you can determine your level of stress and nutrient intake and look for possible patterns. A diet diary is easy to make. You may wish to use the diagram below as an example.

To design a diet diary of your own, place columns labeled with the days of the week on the left-hand side down the page, and columns for food intake, bowel habits, mood, activity, and symptoms across the top. With a conscientious effort, you can begin to determine your health patterns associated with foods. You may even discover patterns you never knew existed!

You must remember that you need to replenish any vitamin or other nutrients you may be losing during the elimination phase. For instance, if you relied on dairy for calcium, you will now need to seek other sources. You may want to add collard greens, figs, tofu, sardines, canned salmon with the bones, or broccoli as alternative calcium sources into your diet. When all else fails, there are also calcium supplements. The bottom line is to be certain you are getting enough minerals, vitamins, protein, carbohydrates, essential fats, fiber, and water in your daily fare.

ROTATION AND ELIMINATION DIET PLAN

It is often the case that eating too much of one food may cause you to be allergic to it. Rotation diets bring variety, decrease your exposure to allergenic foods, and may help prevent future allergies from developing. The purpose of the rotation diet is to minimize repetitive intake of the same foods day in day out. This may reduce the chance of developing future food allergies.

The lab I use in my clinical practice provides a booklet with allergy test results that includes an elimination and rotation diet guideline to follow with every food allergy assessment for increased compliance and convenience.

During the elimination and rotation diet, allergenic foods are avoided and nonallergenic foods are rotated by food families. This means no food is eaten more than once every four days and no foods of the same family are eaten more than once every two days. Some clinicians recommend that food families be rotated every four days. For example, day one may include the families saltwater fish, mustard, and morning glory; day two, bovine, goosefoot, and gourd; day three, crustaceans, fungus, and cereals, and day four, fowl, legumes, and composite. On day five, saltwater fish and members of the mustard and morning glory family are reintroduced as day one, and so on. This way you get nutrition through variety while not repeating the same food within any four-day period

Getting to know the food families is the first step to a successful rotation-style diet plan. Listed below are some examples of various food families and their members.

Family	Foods
Saltwater fish	Cod, flounder, herring
Mustard	Mustard greens, cabbage, broccoli
Morning glory	Sweet potato
Bovine	Beef, milk, cheese
Goosefoot	Beet, spinach
Gourd	Pumpkin, squash, melon
Crustaceans	Crab, lobster, shrimp
Fungus	Mushroom, yeast
Cereals	Corn, wheat, barley
Fowl	Chicken, eggs, turkey
Legumes	Navy bean, lima bean, kidney bean
Composite	Lettuce, endive, artichoke

Remember, the key to a successful elimination and rotation diet plan is variety. Variety is not only the spice of life, but it is also a good way to prevent food allergies.

Exercise your creativity and discover delicious choices. For instance, soymilk may be substituted on cereal for dairy milk, and grain or nut milks can be consumed on alternate days to soy. Also, flaxseed oil can be sprinkled on toast instead of butter, or scrambled tofu instead of scrambled eggs. The choices are endless and fun to explore!

Dining out can be especially difficult during the elimination phase. This is not a time to be passive about your order. Requesting specific food preparations in a restaurant is perfectly acceptable. You will be delighted at the willingness of the chef and your waitperson to fulfill your needs. Carrying snacks or nibbles with you just in case for those times when you simply cannot determine if a food item is okay, can also be helpful.

SIDE EFFECTS

One in four people who try to cut out a given food may experience withdrawal symptoms, such as fatigue, irritability, headaches, malaise, or increased hunger. These are all physical symptoms and are not psychological in nature.

Vitamin C and alkali salts (potassium bicarbonate and sodium bicarbonate) are helpful in alleviating the symptoms of withdrawal. Symptoms are self-limiting and should disappear within a few days.

It is important not to confuse withdrawal symptoms with other possible disorders. You should communicate any changes or new symptoms to your doctor. For example, if you are not getting enough calories, your symptoms may be due to low blood sugar, as opposed to withdrawal of a certain food from your diet.

IN A NUTSHELL

Be diligent. Allergenic foods are hidden everywhere! You must get accustomed to reading labels of packaged and prepared goods. Foods you want to avoid may be hidden in ingredient lists. To make this sleuthing easier for you, US BioTek provides a simple food family booklet with each elimination and rotation diet guideline to help you identify hidden and common food sources of your reactive foods.

Knowledge Is Powerful

Is food for pleasure, health, or sustenance? You are right if you answered, "All three." How do you find the balance where eating is still fun and rewarding, but also nourishing? After you find that balance, how do you maintain it? The answer is knowledge. Success in eating for wellness and health requires knowledge that leads to change.

Perhaps knowledge from a recent study will inspire you to change. For example, the Chicago Heart Association Detection Project in Industry has been studying risks of obesity for 32 years. Results published in January 2006 are startling. The two groups of people who were compared did not smoke and had normal blood pressure and cholesterol levels. One group was obese and one was normal weight. The obese group had a more than four times greater risk of hospitalization for heart disease and a 43 percent higher risk of death from heart disease. Stop and really think about that; it could save your life if it inspires you to change.

Perhaps knowing more about your heart's workload will inspire you to change. Every pound of weight gained adds 250 miles of blood vessels to the body. If you are 10 pounds overweight, then your heart is pumping an extra 2,500 miles. If you are 100 pounds overweight, your heart is pumping an extra 25,000 miles. Check your pulse and think about this; it could save your life if it inspires you to change.

Nutrition education has been uncommon, and our knowledge changes and grows with new scientific discoveries. Lacking this knowledge, most of us do not know how to make high-impact, health-promoting choices. Instead, we often make high-impact, health-depleting choices.

Has any of this knowledge inspired you to make some changes in your diet and lifestyle? To retain your new knowledge and inspiration you can write a note or draw a picture and then place it where you will see it every day. It could save your life.

Knowledge regarding how food affects your body can lead to positive changes. As you read the following sections on carbohydrates, protein, fat, and fiber, compare your diet with a healthy balanced diet and take notes. An honest comparison will make reaching your goal much easier.

> What you do not understand can kill you.
> —Chris D. Meletis, N.D.

Stop Eating Poison

Eating foods you are allergic to can make you sick. Some children, if they are allergic to a food, will develop vomiting, diarrhea, asthma, or a rash. If certain foods make you feel tired, achy, ill, or itchy, you may need testing for food sensitivity. You can perform the test at home with a simple finger stick, send it off to an international lab, and quickly get the results on how you react to the IgG Food Antibody Assessment Panel. Hundreds of our patients are now healthier because they know what foods they should avoid. A Web site where you can get this testing done without a doctor's prescription is the professional Web site: www. CPMedical.net, pin No. 587556. Sharing the results with your personal physician or health care provider is always important.

Carbohydrates

All we hear these days is carbs this and carbs that. Carbs stands for carbohydrates, one of the three major components of food. (The other two are the popular protein and the ominous fat.) There are two kinds of carbs, simple and complex. Simple carbs include table sugar, high fructose corn syrup, honey, maple syrup, juice, and soft drinks. Complex carbs include multigrain high-fiber bread, rolled oats, fruits, and vegetables.

What is the big deal about carbs and why are we so afraid of them? Perhaps because the standard American diet is very high in simple carbs and leads to altered body chemistry, obesity, and disease. Research has shown a connection between a diet high in simple carbs and elevated insulin and/or leptin (a protein believed to regulate fat storage), insulin and/or leptin resistance, elevated cholesterol, weight gain, diabetes, heart disease, strokes, and even Alzheimer's disease.

Medical science is just becoming aware of the glycemic index and the glycemic load of a food. The what? It may sound complicated at first, but understanding this is critical to your health, regardless of your age.

The glycemic index measures how high a food will cause blood sugar to rise after it is eaten. The food group that causes the greatest increase in blood sugar is carbohydrates. Both sugar and white bread have a glycemic index of 100. How a food compares to sugar or white bread determines that food's rating. The glycemic index ranks carbohydrates according to their effect on our blood glucose levels. Fortunately, we can refer to charts and not go through this process ourselves. Not all foods have been measured, but many have.

Just to make it a bit more complicated, some foods that have the same amount of total carbohydrate will have very different effects on blood sugar levels. Why? Because of how easily our bodies can digest the food. Foods that are digested quickly and easily make more carbohydrate available to the body. The glycemic load measures how available each food's carbohydrate is to the body. Thus, the glycemic load of a food is more informative than the glycemic index of that food. The following examples will make this clearer.

The glycemic index of an orange is rated 48 and a slightly underripe banana is rated 42. If that were the only rating considered, then you would conclude that the orange would increase your blood sugar more than the banana. But that would be wrong. An orange has more fiber and is digested more slowly than a banana. The glycemic load of the orange is 5 while the banana's is 11, more than twice that of the orange. Remember, that score is for a slightly underripe banana. (The riper the banana, the more the glycemic load rises.)

Processing a food removes fiber and the food is digested faster. For example, rolled oats have a glycemic load of 9 and Quaker Oats has a glycemic load of 24. The more-processed Quaker Oats raise the blood sugar more than two and a half times the level caused by the less-processed oats.

Using these examples, a breakfast of Quaker Oats with an underripe banana would result in a glycemic load of 35, but a breakfast of rolled oats with an orange would result in a glycemic load of 14. Can you see how the food you eat directly affects your blood sugar levels?

How do blood sugar levels affect your health and your waistline? If your blood sugar rapidly rises to a high level, this triggers an unhealthy chain of events. The higher it rises, the more triggers are pulled. One trigger results in stored fat and low energy. High blood sugar causes the body to store the food in fat cells where it is unavailable for use as energy for about three hours. Therefore, when you need energy during those three hours, it is pulled from your muscle cells, not your fat cells.

When a person eats too much sugar, a large amount of insulin is produced. Usually, the body will overcompensate, resulting in a low blood sugar level that tells the body to eat again in an effort to raise the blood sugar level. Welcome to a roller coaster ride no one wants. This is the get fat quick plan we all must avoid.

In contrast, if the blood sugar level gradually rises to a moderate level, the body is able to process and use the nutrients the food provides. A moderate blood sugar level causes the body to store the food in the form of energy that is available for use.

So, if you want to be fat and low on energy, eat foods with a high glycemic effect. If you want energy and less fat storage, eat foods with a low or moderate blood sugar effect. Of course, it is more complicated than that. Nutrients, toxins, satiety levels, hypoglycemia, insulin resistance, leptin resistance, and cholesterol levels will be discussed later.

The scientific and medical literature abounds with examples of how excess sugar intake causes accelerated damage to the body. Concern is growing because research is finding that simple carbs can cause your body to become more acidic and thus more prone to disease in general. Following is a list of some of sugar's metabolic consequences, drawn from a variety of medical journals and other scientific publications.

RESULTS OF EXCESS SUGAR INTAKE

Dramatic increase in triglyceride levels (fats in blood)
Accelerated onset and severity of diseases (e.g., kidney disease)
Lowered high-density lipoprotein (HDL) cholesterol (the good cholesterol) and increased low-density lipoprotein (LDL) cholesterol (bad cholesterol)
Chromium deficiencies
Decreased absorption and retention of minerals
Increased risk of cancers
Accelerated poor vision and blindness
Triggered hypoglycemia symptoms
Acid indigestion
Dramatic elevated risk for heart disease
Accelerated premature aging of the skin and body tissues
Tooth decay and gum disease
Increased probability of intestinal and colon disease
Increased inflammatory diseases
Increased risk of diabetes*

*Diabetes is an independent risk factor for a host of diseases. Truly understanding diabetes provides powerful motivation to make any necessary changes.

Carbs are not bad, but out-of-control carbs are killing all of us. And dessert is not bad—if you remember that the dessert plate is the *small* plate on the table. Fiber-rich food or carb-blockers slow or even eliminate the digestion of sugar. The key to regaining and maintaining a leaner, healthier you is moderation. Put the Carb Monster on a short leash and only let it out on rare occasions.

> When you indulge a sweet tooth or two, fiber is your friend. —Chris D. Meletis, N.D.

The Disappearing Act

Most simple carbs began life as more complex carbs. So what happened to change them? Before the industrial age, grains were processed by grinding them between stones, which removed the outer hull—rather like opening a package so that you can get to the contents. Modern processing uses machinery that grinds and grinds the grain until even the kernel is crushed—rather like opening the package and then stomping on the contents. Most of the nutrients and fiber are removed. To make up for the missing nutrients, some (not all) are added back in and then the package is labeled "enriched." Wait a moment, such items are sold as food! Webster's Dictionary defines food as: "something that nourishes, sustains." Is food with most of its natural nutrients removed still food? If you opened a package containing a computer and stomped on it, would it still be a computer?

During the enhancing process, a little extra sugar, salt, and flavor enhancer is often added. Thus, the technologically advanced, highly processed Western diet has added dessert sugar into our main-course foods. When eating these foods, the body becomes addicted to the unnaturally high levels of sugar and other substances. Processed foods whose ingredient list includes corn syrup or any other word ending in -ose (like sucrose, glucose, fructose, mannose) have had sugar added. (Note: The exception is sucralose, an artificial sweetener more commonly known as Splenda.) When we disturb the harmony found in nature, there is a price to pay. In this case, it is your health.

In many modern countries, complex, naturally nutritious food has been destroyed and limited human knowledge has tried to rebuild it. So much for common sense.

The excess sugar in the standard American diet was responsible for 1.5 million Americans being diagnosed with diabetes in 2005. An estimated 43 million are at risk of developing it soon. The standard American diet has killed millions in past decades. To stop this killer, we need to change our food choices.

If you do not make the decision to safeguard your health and the health of your loved ones, who will? By adopting a healthy diet and lifestyle, you will model that behavior for your family. Statistics show that if one or both parents are overweight, their children's risk of being overweight increases dramatically. Your personal decisions reach far beyond what you put in your mouth.

Eat Yourself Stupid?

If you eliminate all carbs from your diet (like some fad diets propose), tissues such as brain cells that are very glucose-dependent can become suboptimally nourished. So I guess you can eat yourself stupid or at least dull your mental performance. Carbs also give you energy for exercise. Healthy grains, fruits, vegetables, and some dairy foods are eventually converted to glucose that is used by the muscles and brain.

Fat and Lipids

Did you know that you need fat, even cholesterol, to live, and that your body produces cholesterol every day of your life? Without eating any meat or animal by-products, you will still produce cholesterol. Cholesterol is a lipid that is critical for the production of hormones and vitamin D, and it is incorporated into every cell of your body.

All fat has many calories compared with carbohydrates and proteins. Carbohydrates and proteins both provide four calories per gram of food; fat provides nine calories. Thus, fat needs to be used wisely.

Some fats (oils and lipids) are essential to your existence and are thus called "essential fatty acids." These include the omega-3, omega-6, and omega-9 oils. Omega-6 is readily available in a wide range of foods. Traditionally, fish has been a great source of omega-3 oil. Unfortunately, most of the fish in the world are now contaminated with toxins, PCBs (polychlorinated biphenyls), and mercury. Omega-3 oils are also found in flaxseeds, evening primrose oil, and perilla seeds. Omega-9 is in olive oil. We recommend that all our patients use only extra virgin olive oil for cooking. Olive oil is prominent in the Mediterranean diet, a diet that has been shown to increase longevity and decrease the onset of degenerative disease.

Now that we've talked about the good, let's discuss the bad and the ugly. Saturated fats are most commonly found in animal products. At room temperature, they are solid, stiff, or sticky. Are you surprised to learn they are likely to clog your arteries?

What once was tolerated in the food industry is no longer allowed. A recent U.S. government regulation requires that trans fat content be listed on processed foods. Why the change? One reason is that it is bankrupting our health care system. Trans fats (also called hydrogenated fats) are artificial. Take vegetable oil, add hydrogen gas and pressure until the oil becomes solid, and you have hydrogenated or trans fat.

Trans fat triggers excessive cholesterol production, increases the amount of LDL (bad cholesterol), and decreases the amount of HDL (good cholesterol). Need a way to remember which is good and which is bad? Think of the "L" in LDL as litter and the "H" in HDL as help. LDL litters your arteries and HDL helps control LDL litter.

Reading food labels is now a survival skill. Zero times three used to equal zero. However, as of January 2006 in the United States, zero times three on food labels just might equal 1.47. Foods containing less than 0.5 grams of trans fat per serving can now be labeled as containing 0 trans fat. The U.S. Food and

Drug Administration estimates that with the standard American diet, Americans consume an average of 5.8 grams of trans fats a day—a small but deadly number. If the food label includes words such as "partially hydrogenated oil," "hydrogenated oil," or "shortening," the product could have 4.9 grams of trans fat per serving. By law, the lists of ingredients are arranged so that the larger quantities are listed first. If the trans fats are among the first few ingredients, watch out. Because the grams are all listed per serving size, watch out for small serving sizes, too.

To load up on trans fats and speed your health's demise, eat processed foods, the No. 1 source for trans fats. The second source is any fried or heated oil products. Here is a short list of products high in trans fats:

- Chips (e.g., potato, corn)
- Cookies
- Crackers
- Doughnuts
- French fries
- Margarine
- Nondairy creamers, powdered or liquid
- Nondairy whipped toppings
- Shortening

> We have all been sold a bill of goods, not a sack full of real food. —Chris D. Meletis, N.D.

Notice that the top five on the list are also high in simple carbs, a double whammy to your health.

Protein

Protein provides the basic building blocks for the structure of your body. It is essential to sustain the muscles and overall integrity of your body. However, like King Midas with the golden touch, you can get too much of a good thing. Excess protein is hard on the kidneys and can contribute to numerous health issues, including osteoporosis. The key is to consume quality protein in proper proportion to other carbohydrates and fats.

Amino acids are the building blocks of protein. Most animal proteins are more complete than those found in grains such as corn, wheat, or lentils. Vegetarians must be careful to blend foods in their diet so as to obtain all the amino acids needed to form a complete protein.

For many people, consuming protein means eating animal products. However, animal fats have been linked to an increased risk of heart and other diseases. Did you know that toxins are stored in the fat cells? So when you eat animal fat you could be eating a very concentrated source of toxins—leftover hormones and antibiotics given to these animals. Toxins are poisons that can lead to cancers and other serious medical problems. Look for hormone-free, organic, or free-range lean meat. This way, you can have protein while limiting your ingestion of saturated fat and toxins. It makes sense to "go lean to be lean."

Which choice is healthier?

Choice No. 1: Grilled chicken breast on a leafy green salad
Choice No. 2: Lightly battered, deep-fried chicken on a leafy green salad.

If you guessed No. 1, you are right. Choice No. 2 introduces simple carbs in the batter and trans fats when it is fried.

Fiber (Dietary Sponge)

Fiber serves as the body's sponge. It absorbs toxins, sugar, calories, cholesterol, and hormones in the intestinal tract so they can be eliminated. Adequate fiber in the diet will result in two to three bowel movements per day. Yes, two to three per day is the health-oriented goal. Why so many? The longer the stool stays in your body, the drier and harder it becomes. That means your body is reabsorbing muddy toxic water, which increases the risk of disease. Consumption of sufficient fiber has been linked to lowered risk of heart disease, colon disease, and cancer. Can you see how drinking lots of water (80–90 ounces a day) and eating adequate fiber will help rid your body of germs and toxins?

The preceding dietary guidelines are important practical tips that can empower you as you seek to avoid food allergens and at the same time incorporate overall healthier eating habits. Following are 10 health tips from everyday healthy people who have dialed into their health potential.

10 ANTIAGING TIPS FROM MY PATIENTS

As a physician I have had the rare privilege of personally observing, hearing, and documenting the secret healthy aging tips from some of the healthiest young-old people around. Wise physicians learn much about themselves and life from their patients. Documented here are healthy aging tips from people who have captured the ability to truly optimize their health—those rare individuals who early on in their lives just got it, lived it, and now, well into their later decades, run circles around those half their age. Here are the secrets you and your loved ones need to know to enjoy a younger you through great health.

Tip No. 1: Enjoy Life

The difference between feeling like you are just surviving versus really and truly thriving is engaging life to its fullest. Certainly, not every day is a bed of roses, yet some that have gone through thick and thin over the decades report that successfully enjoying life depends on one's perspective.
Patient quote:

I've been through a lot over the years, but I've lived life to the fullest, even during tough times. I stay optimistic and realize that there is a season for all things, and just like the turtle and rabbit, it's perseverance and attitude that wins the race.

Tip No. 2: Maintain Good Hydration

Water and the accompanying essential electrolytes are literally the currency of life. Water bathes the 50–100 trillion cells in your body, keeping your blood thin, your brain cushioned, and your joints mobile. Minerals like magnesium, potassium, sodium, calcium, and chloride are electrically charged, and this electricity gives your cells the energy to live. Good hydration helps an electrical current flow between the inside and outside of your cells and sustains your vitality. All of my patients who are feeling younger longer with vibrant health are those who have prioritized hydration as a life decision. They tell me that their friends and family members who are underhydrated have gone from "grapes to raisins" or "plums to prunes" right in front of their eyes.

Patient quote:

> I'm not a scientist but I know that the earth's surface is covered with 70 percent water and the human body is supposed to be 70 percent water. This has to be more than a coincidence; who am I to argue with that design? So, I don't leave home without my water bottle.

Tip No. 3: Eat Lots of Fiber

The research is clear: We must consume more fiber to lessen our chances of dying prematurely from chronic degenerative diseases. These disease processes are the diametric opposite of where most of us want to go. So, if you want to stay younger longer, it is time to chew your food. If you can eat a meal with only a few chews per bite, you have a low-fiber meal. Fiber is chewy; it is what makes vegetables (like broccoli and cauliflower), fruits (like apples and pears), and true multigrain breads so healthy for us. Fiber not only helps scour and cleanse your intestinal tract, but it also helps mop up and absorb toxins in your body. Indeed, fiber is literally like a sponge, cleaning up and alleviating health-challenging burdens on a daily basis.

Patient quote:

> When I was growing up soda pop, candy, and sweets were not as common as today, I have concluded that more people die due to the advertising and promotion of these foods than anything else. We were given teeth to chew our foods, not to rot them out with sugar. It also causes diabetes and hurts our hearts.

Tip No. 4: Avoid Sugar

We are a society that is inundated with sugary food products. Sadly, 1.5 million Americans are diagnosed with diabetes each year. In addition, sugar has been shown to harden the 60,000 miles of blood vessels that nourish the very cells that make up your magnificent and dynamically created body. Clinically, I believe the reason so many people have lost weight, lowered their cholesterol, and felt better overall on the high-protein diets that became a fad over the past few years is not the high-protein but the low-sugar aspects of these diets. By definition, "refined sugar" (also known as the key component of junk food) is not natural; it goes against all common sense and has merely emphasized that the further from the natural source we go, the more we will find ourselves out of sync with the health, wellness, and vitality we all seek.

Patient quote:

I think junk food will bankrupt America. It is the plague of the modern world. It points out that just because we can do it, doesn't mean we should do it. Over the years, I have seen bad habits come and go. Someday, just like tobacco and bad fats, sugars will be regulated and foods will warn of the health hazards of consuming them. Mark my words, this will come to pass.

Tip No. 5: Have Faith

Invariably, patients who enjoy a happier existence have reported to me through the years that faith sustains them during difficult seasons in their lives and enhances and amplifies the exhilarating times as well. Faith represents a dynamic quality to our existence. Focusing on developing faith in yourself and focusing on the reality that there is a greater force at play in the universe helps keep things in perspective. Time and again, patients have related how they survived what seemed like virtually impossible hiccups in their lives. As they describe these journeys, they reveal that what sustained them was their faith in themselves and God, and having faith that things were going to get better. Indeed, those who stay younger longer are survivors of life and have learned to thrive and grow from adversity. They hold that life is not a destination but a journey.

Patient quote:

The best things that I have done for myself over the years are to eat well, get my sleep, pray daily, and have faith. It has been faith in myself and God that has allowed me to sustain hope, claim victory, and seek to move on to each and every day with positive anticipation that I will find good in the people that I meet and purpose in each and every day, even the harder ones.

Tip No. 6: Exercise

A governing law of physics aptly captures the essence and importance of exercise. A body in motion is likely to stay in motion; a body at rest is more likely to stay at rest. Over the years, the patients demonstrating the highest quality of life, without question, have stayed active or have gotten active. The concepts of inertia and momentum come into play here. If you sit around, not only will you collect dust, but you will also lose muscle mass, slow your metabolism, and prematurely age. If you keep the body limber, encourage your blood to flow and nourish the cells throughout your body, and stay lean, then you will have a stronger immune system and more energy and be more alert.

Patient quote:

> I have never been a runner; I like walking. I have done it from 11 months of age and now 80 years later, I still enjoy doing it. I attribute my energy and sense of just plain ol' feeling good to walking, drinking lots of good-quality water, working in the garden whenever possible, and eating my fresh vegetables that I grow myself.

Tip No. 7: Sleep

If you haven't been sleeping 120 days a year, you are falling short of your quota. We are each designed to sleep approximately eight hours a night—that is, one-third of each day. Many people in today's world claim they are too busy to sleep. Taking a deep breath and realizing the importance of sleep helps us appreciate that we should never skimp in the sleep department. During our sleeping hours our body restores itself, repairs the wear and tear of daily living, and processes the day's events. If you were to take a 40-year-old car and bring it back to its original condition, the process would be referred to as a restoration project. Well, regardless of how old your body is, it is the vehicle that transports you throughout life. If you want to enjoy being younger longer through radiant health, you need to schedule restoration time. Remember, the first four letters of restoration are r-e-s-t.

Patient quote:

> I have friends and family that just buzz around like bees; they seem to always be stressed and never seem to catch up. I have been a professional all my life and one of the things that has allowed me to accomplish some of my greatest personal and work goals has been sleep. I know that appears counterintuitive, but when I get a good night's sleep I wake with a clear mind, renewed energy. Often during sleep, and the moments of reawakening, many of the day's problems are answered with my rested and renewed mind.

Tip No. 8: Limit Fried Foods

The french frying of America has accelerated heart disease and cancer and put unnecessary wear and tear on our bodies. Whether it is the "super-size me" phenomenon or just the fact that we are eating too many processed foods, the consumption of adulterated oils is literally destroying our bodies. For decades, people have consumed pounds of trans fats and partially hydrogenated oil, totally unaware that it was raising their cholesterol, increasing free-radical damage within their bodies, and accelerating premature aging. Companies are finally starting to put information about trans fats on packaged foods. For those old enough to remember Saturday morning cartoons, the educational commercials between the cartoons proclaimed commonsense facts that escaped many (but not all) people, with such jingles as, "You are what you eat from your head to your feet." Indeed, if you eat junk food, fried foods, and unnatural oils (such as trans fats and partially hydrogenated oils), those will become your body's building blocks.

Patient quote:

> Ever since my kids were young during the 1970s, I have kept a watchful eye on what our family has allowed on the dinner table. I learned a lot about my eating habits and raising healthier kids thanks to the concept, 'You are what you eat.' I think if we all used a little more common sense, serious health problems would become more rare.

Tip No. 9: Minimize Chemical Exposures

The concept of better living through chemistry just doesn't have the same magical appeal that it did in the 1950s. Long gone are the days when getting the job done meant "the stronger it is, the better it is." Thanks to dedicated researchers and those who are not afraid to look at long-term consequences of chemical exposures, we now know that the fewer chemicals to which you and your loved ones are exposed, the better. *It is critical to remember that everything your body is exposed to must either be defended against or processed.* Thanks to official disclaimers in advertisements on television, on the radio, and in print materials, the public has become sensitized to the fact that prescription medications, while offering solutions to symptoms, are sometimes accompanied by serious side effects. Prescription drugs are chemicals that have medicinal purposes. Yet products to which we are exposed daily, like household cleaners, air fresheners, and detergents, require careful examination if you are serious about having great health. Will you include them in—or exclude them from—your body's daily battle?

Patient quote:

> I remember as a kid those hot summer days when we would stand in the fields, waiting for the crop dusters to fly over. The cool mist of the spray was our preferred place to play. Who would have ever thought that the same chemicals put upon our food were health hazards? Thanks to eating well in my later years, some grace from God, and now actively avoiding chemicals in my life whenever possible, I have found a balance and live life with a positive direction and clear intent when it comes to exposing myself and loved ones to potential hazards to our health.

Tip No. 10: Don't Stress

Stress happens. It is a fact of life. It is how we handle stress that determines if this silent killer is allowed to wreak havoc in our lives. More than ever patients are coming in with the signs and symptoms of stress. Yes, stress leads to all kinds of health problems ranging from, but not limited to, insomnia, irritability, weight gain, fatigue, increased infections, headaches, backaches, irritable bowel syndrome, and more. My single most important piece of advice is simple to conceive and essential to achieve:

Make time and focus your intent on "*destressing*" to avoid becoming "*distressed*" because once you are *distressed* you no longer enjoy a healthy state of being at ease. Thus, you have entered the realm of "*dis-ease*" that begets "*disease.*"

Patient quote:

I have survived two world wars and the impending woes of a chaotic and complex world. I haven't always had a healthy perspective, but now that I am blessed with the ability to yield to fate and God those things that are not within my immediate control, I realize that what I can do is be true to myself, do my best at any given moment, do better next time, and focus on the good in my life. I find the more I focus on the good, the more positive I allow myself to be, the happier I am, the healthier I am, and the more excited I am to have another day to truly live life. All worry does is steal the enjoyment of life. Trust me, it ain't worth it and doesn't solve any problems; it just makes them worse.

PARTING THOUGHT

I am privileged to be a physician; it is indeed a divine blessing that I am grateful for each and every day. It is an honor to assist, learn with, and work with patients committed to a healthier life for themselves, those they love, and all of humanity. May the tips in this chapter bless you abundantly with the peace and prosperity that come from embracing great health.

CHAPTER 12

Commonly Asked Questions about Allergies and Allergy Testing

WHAT IS AN ADVERSE REACTION TO A FOOD?

An adverse food reaction is any symptom that follows intake of a food. The symptom may be any perceptible change in how you feel and/or function.

A symptom may present, for example, as a rash, achy joints, or fatigue. Adverse food reactions are classified into three subgroups: toxic, psychological, and nontoxic food reactions. A toxic food reaction is commonly known as food poisoning, and it results from contaminants contained in the food. A psychological food reaction, or food aversion, is usually the result of a prior ill experience with the food and is largely psychosomatic in nature. A nontoxic food reaction is further divided into immune-mediated and non–immune-mediated groups. Non–immune-mediated food reactions include adverse reactions to food additives or pharmacological compounds, which can mimic allergy inflammation, and food intolerance due to an inherent enzymatic defect, such as lactose intolerance.

What is important to remember is why we have the desire and capacity to eat at the most fundamental level: to fuel our bodies and to build and repair the 50–100 trillion cells that make up the human body. Indeed, we ought to consume foods that sustain us most optimally and avoid foods that are detrimental. Identifying the foods that are individually best for one's unique biochemistry is of paramount important as we seek to eat to live and not live to eat. In other words, we seek food as nourishment, not poison unto the body.

WHAT ARE FOOD ALLERGIES?

A food allergy or hypersensitivity is an adverse food reaction for which an immunological basis is clearly defined. Immune-mediated adverse food reactions involve the production of antibodies to certain food antigens. These reactions depend on a person's sensitivity to some foods over others, which may occur for many reasons, including a genetic predisposition and current health status. Food allergies are classified as IgE-mediated and non–IgE-mediated reactions. In short, a food allergy or sensitivity can simply be looked at as a food that does not support one's individual biochemistry in a health-promoting manner. Symptoms vary— diarrhea, cramping, constipation, inflammation, bloating, and rash are just a few manifestations of a hypersensitivity reaction. A more complete list can be found in chapter 4.

IS LACTOSE INTOLERANCE A TYPE OF FOOD ALLERGY?

No. Unlike a food allergy, lactose intolerance is not mediated by the immune system. Instead, it is attributable to an enzymatic defect in the body, which does not allow for proper digestion of lactose (milk sugar). Food intolerance, in general, is one in which the sufferer has a "gut reactions"; however, the mechanism is not immunologic and in some cases is unknown.

WHAT MAY PROMOTE A FOOD ALLERGY?

The underlying cause of food allergies varies from person to person. Possible causes may include improper oral tolerance, stress, antigenic overload, compromised digestion, imbalance in gut microflora, and poor immune function. Over the past dozen-plus years I have discovered that food allergies appear to be exacerbated in persons who have used antibiotics.

HOW FREQUENT ARE FOOD ALLERGIES?

Food allergies may be very common and underrepresented as a major causative factor in a number of illnesses. As you read in the first couple of chapters, the medical literature shows that reactions vary. Some scientific reports suggest that the populace in general suffers from allergies at a rate in excess of 25 percent, that is, one in four people. Yet from my clinical experience I see a number closer to 50 percent of the general populace with some level of either overt allergy or health-altering food sensitivity. In my practice I find it is best to "test not guess."

WHAT ARE SYMPTOMS OF FOOD ALLERGIES?

Symptoms of food allergies are highly variable, ranging from constipation and skin rash to anxiety and depression.

HOW DO I GET TESTED FOR FOOD ALLERGIES?

In my clinical practice, I primarily use the enzyme-linked immunosorbent assay (ELISA) methodology for food antibody assessment because it offers a highly accurate and reliable means to determine immediate and delayed food reactions. A blood draw to obtain two milliliters of serum is all that is required for a complete 96 IgE/IgG Food Antibody Assay. A finger stick may also be used for IgG results only. A lancet is used to collect two or three drops of whole blood from the finger. The blood is absorbed onto microcollection strips, air dried, and mailed to the lab for assessment.

With this said, consulting your personal physician is always important, and if you know or believe you have had an anaphylactic (life-threatening) reaction, continue to avoid those foods or environment factors for a lifetime regardless of what any allergy test reports. It is always best to play it safe.

DO I NEED TO EAT OR AVOID CERTAIN FOODS BEFORE TESTING?

For most testing it is not necessary to eat any specific foods before testing. It is best to maintain your usual dietary habits and consume a variety of foods when possible. However, any food that has caused you to have an adverse reaction in the past should not be consumed before the allergy test. Certain adverse food reactions, namely anaphylaxis, can be fatal on secondary exposure to the offending food.

WHAT IS AN ANAPHYLACTIC FOOD REACTION?

An anaphylactic reaction to an ingested food is a life-threatening condition that causes swelling and constriction of the airways. It is an IgE-mediated hypersensitivity reaction that occurs immediately after a culpable food is ingested. This condition requires immediate medical attention. Do not eat foods that prompt an anaphylactic reaction under any circumstance.

DO I NEED TO DISCONTINUE MY MEDICATIONS BEFORE TESTING?

Anti-inflammatory and immunosuppressive medications, such as oral or intranasal corticosteroids (prednisone, beclomethasone, fluticasone, triamcinolone) and topical cortisone suspensions and creams, may affect systemic antibody production and hence test results. However, the dosage, route, half-life of medication, and duration of administration on systemic immune response are arguable. It is strongly advised that you discuss these variables with your health care practitioner who can consider these factors in more detail. The suggested period to abstain from these types of medications before testing ranges from two to eight weeks or until symptoms reemerge. Consult your practitioner before making any changes to your current medication regimen.

WHAT DO I DO WITH THE RESULTS OF MY TEST?

Different laboratories report results in different fashions. I use US BioTek food allergy testing with most of my patients. I have used this laboratory for well over a decade and I find their reports accurate, reproducible, user friendly, and self-explanatory. Each report comes complete with a four-day elimination and rotation diet guideline and a food family booklet for easy referral.

HOW LONG DO I NEED TO BE ON A SPECIAL DIET BEFORE I START SEEING RESULTS?

Food allergy–related symptom improvement may vary for each person. With proper treatment and dietary modifications retesting is recommended in three to six months. I routinely recommend retesting 3 to 6 months after the initial testing and avoiding reactive foods. Retesting will help distinguish permanent or semipermanent food reactions from those that arose from poor gastrointestinal health

CAN I HAVE WITHDRAWAL SYMPTOMS FROM ELIMINATING AN ALLERGENIC FOOD?

Yes. Believe it or not, you can easily become addicted to the foods we are allergic to! As with any addiction when you avoid the trigger you may develop withdrawal symptoms. Withdrawal symptoms are those that make you feel lousy and may include throat congestion, stuffy nose, diarrhea, fatigue, irritability, headaches, malaise, and increased appetite. Withdrawal symptoms should not be confused with other possible disorders, and you are advised to consult your practitioner about your specific symptoms. Keep in mind that withdrawal symptoms attributed to a food allergy are transient in nature. Some holistic practitioners attribute this short-term occasional symptom picture as a purging or detoxification process as the body transitions to a healthier state and the body's biochemistry finds a homeostatic wellness.

WHAT DO ELEVATED IgE ANTIBODIES TO CERTAIN FOODS MEAN?

Elevated IgE antibodies indicate an immediate immune-mediated allergic reaction to certain foods tested. This may manifest as a variety of symptoms that may last for a few hours to a few days after the culpable food is eliminated from the diet. Even if a suspected IgE or anaphylactic food does not appear on one's allergy list, one should continue to avoid known IgE reactions for a lifetime.

WHAT DO ELEVATED IgG ANTIBODIES TO CERTAIN FOODS MEAN?

Elevated IgG antibodies indicate a delayed immune-mediated reaction to certain foods tested. This may manifest as a variety of symptoms. Because ill effects are not felt immediately after intake of the suspect food, pinpointing symptoms to specific foods may prove challenging. Generally speaking, symptoms may manifest anywhere from a couple of hours to a few days after the culpable food is consumed. IgG antibodies live actively in circulation for about three weeks with a residual activity on immune cells lasting for at least a few months. Symptoms may therefore persist for weeks to months after omitting the culpable food from the diet.

WHAT IS THE DIFFERENCE BETWEEN IgE-MEDIATED AND NON–IgE-MEDIATED FOOD ALLERGIES?

IgE-mediated food allergies involve the production of IgE antibodies to certain foods, and it usually occurs immediately after the suspect food is ingested. These are defined as immediate food allergies because symptoms generally manifest within minutes to hours after the culpable food is consumed. A late-phase response peaks in about a day after contact and may last up to two days.

This classical food reaction occurs when IgE antibodies, bound to specific immune cells (mast cells), recognize and bind to the allergic food. This interaction triggers the release of chemical compounds, histamine and others, from the IgE-bound cell. These compounds cause much of the discomfort associated with allergy, including stomach cramping, diarrhea, skin rash, swelling, and anaphylaxis. The culpable food and resulting symptoms are unique to the individual affected.

Non–IgE-mediated food allergies involve antibodies other than IgE, namely IgG. Symptoms of an IgG-dependent food reaction may occur hours to days after ingestion of the suspect food and are therefore defined as delayed food reactions. In particular, IgG antibodies may bind to food antigens and form complexes in the circulation. These complexes may deposit in various tissues and trigger inflammatory reactions.

WHY DO MY RESULTS SHOW THAT I DO NOT HAVE A FOOD ALLERGY WHEN I KNOW I HAVE A REACTION TO THAT PARTICULAR FOOD?

Many different types of reactions to foods can occur besides an immune-mediated food allergy, including food intolerance, food poisoning, and a psychosomatic food aversion.

WHAT ARE CROSS-REACTIONS?

A cross-reaction is an important consideration in allergy assessment. When the immune system mounts a response to a protein of similar moiety to a known allergen, adverse reactions occur. This is especially evident between pollen, fruits and vegetables. Sensitization to latex, for example, has extensive cross-reactivity with certain foods, including avocado, potato, banana, tomato, kiwi, and pineapple. Natural rubber latex is a common ingredient in many products, including balloons, appliance cords, hearing aids, swimwear, condoms, rubber bands, and medical and dental supplies (e.g., masks, gloves, syringes, catheters, bandages).

DOES AN ALLERGIC RESPONSE TO GLUTEN MEAN
I HAVE CELIAC DISEASE?

A definitive diagnosis of celiac disease is obtained through a tissue sample taken from the small intestine where pathological damage is observed. An antibody response to gluten does not diagnose celiac disease, but it may warrant further investigation by your doctor.

AM I DOOMED TO HAVE THE SAME FOOD ALLERGIES
AS MY PARENTS?

Although there is a genetic component to the competency of the immune system, there are many lifestyle and environmental factors to consider that may influence the onset and progression of a food allergy. After you finish reading this book, you will know how to test for allergies and sensitivities, supplement with nutrients, and eat more healthfully so as to help minimize the likelihood of exacerbating your genetic predispositions.

CHAPTER 13

Examples of Allergy Liberation from around the World

The following cases have been compiled over the course of time and reflect the power of fueling the body properly. Indeed, it is not just the act of providing the right food, it is also the active process of avoiding the wrong food. A special thanks to US BioTek laboratory for sharing some of these stories from their international database of clients and physicians.

Regardless of the allergy or food intolerance testing that you choose to follow and implement, when the foods are properly identified, the body indeed can achieve a much higher level of wellness than often previously conceived.

DEBILITATING MIGRAINES

A young schoolteacher presented to the clinic as a first-time patient. She related her journey of having suffered from migraines since the age of 12; she was now experiencing upwards of two per week, that left her in bed, in a dark room, not able to move, talk, or function until the migraine passes. Her allergy results showed one very glaring IgG delayed reaction to peanuts. She was fairly nonreactive when it came to IgE reactions.

I instructed her to rigorously avoid peanuts, peanut butter, and all other sources of peanuts, including peanut oil. She reported back in two weeks that she was totally amazed that she had suffered from no migraines during that time. She was speechless. I had a couple of follow-up appointments with her to fine-tune other aspects of her health, and then she fell off the radar. Around the six-month mark she called to say her migraines had returned. I immediately inquired if she had resumed consumption of peanuts, and she stated that because she was well and symptom free she had indeed begun to eat peanuts again. I asked her to stop, and within a couple of days she regained her migraine-free status.

UNCONTROLLABLE IRRITABLE BOWEL SYNDROME

A young mother presented to my clinic with uncontrollable explosive diarrhea. Indeed, she related that often she could not make it to the bathroom quickly enough and would have an accident. I tested her for food allergies and found out that dairy foods were a problem. She went dairy free, avoided her IgG food intolerances, and is now doing 90 percent better. Now she need not worry about where the nearest restrooms are located when she goes out.

ASPERGER'S SYNDROME

In November 2004 I had an inquiry from the parents of a five-year-old boy who was diagnosed with Asperger's syndrome, nonverbal learning disorder, and sensory integration dysfunction. His school had also identified him as having autism spectrum disorder. The boy showed much impairment in communication and participating in social relationships, and he had restricted patterns of behavior. The parents were seeking advice on dietary intake, lifestyle, and supplementation that might improve his ability to function, and they had been pursuing alternative treatments in addition to the skills-based therapies that had already been in place for years.

Alternative biomedical testing and treatments to date had been largely unsuccessful and included the following:

- Testing for yeast/fungal overgrowth (negative)
- Testing for heavy metals, including mercury (negative)
- Attempts at elimination diets (unsuccessful and inconclusive)
- Vitamin supplementation (to date unsuccessful and inconclusive)

The one set of tests that had not been done was the assessment of underlying delayed food reactions. From a simple finger stick, a few drops of blood were all that was needed for a full 96 Food-Specific IgG enzyme-linked immunosorbent assay (ELISA) (US BioTek Laboratories). This is a quick, easy, and cost-effective procedure for the doctor to perform and is painless for the patient. Test results showed significantly elevated IgG antibodies to the foods shown in the table:

Casein	Yogurt
Cheddar cheese	Asparagus
Mozzarella cheese	Soy bean
Cottage cheese	Peanut
Whey	Banana
Milk	Pineapple
Goat milk	Egg white

Recommendations and dietary guidelines were given for diligent removal of all reactive products for six months, at which time we would rechallenge with dietary intake, if necessary. At the 60-day follow-up assessment, the child's mother and teachers had the following comments:

- He is happy and markedly calmer. He plays and shares with other children and is adapting well socially.
- He is reading near the average level for his age and is asking for books to read (which had not occurred previously).
- He bounds out of school happy and excited each day, whereas previously he was not happy and complained about the day.
- He has asked to have his siblings stay overnight in his room (which was previously unheard of).
- He is not only asking for homework but for extra homework, which was never the case previously.

Certainly, this case does not indicate that a cure for autism spectrum disorder has been discovered, but case management can focus on improved functional possibilities with favorable results. Immune-mediated reactions to foods activate pathways of inflammation that may affect downstream function. In this case, his food allergies may have been associated with cell injury and neurological impairment with the symptoms described.

The mother commented, "I have a hard time remembering how challenging it was six months ago. There are still challenges, but my son's behavior, social ability and learning ability are wonderfully different."

SICK AND TIRED

I suspected for many years that I had food allergies. In 2003, I was busy with personal activities and running my practice, so sitting down and eating whole foods was a tremendous challenge. Consequently, I relied on many protein (whey) shakes a day for my protein source in addition to lean protein sources, fruits, vegetables, and complex carbohydrates. Only on rare occasions did I eat any junk food. Still, I started noticing that I was losing a moderate amount of hair on my head and my resistance training workouts were regressing. In addition, I had dark circles under my eyes even though I was getting seven to eight hours of sleep a night.

In 2004, I decided to order numerous food panels. After getting my results back, I discovered that most of the food I was consuming tested positive, revealing significantly elevated antibody levels. Now it was time to make some radical changes in my diet. Initially, I completely eliminated any foods that were in the moderate and high categories. Results were positive (hair loss slowed, and dark circles [often called allergic shiners] began to fade). I took it a step further and completely eliminated foods that tested in the low category as well as ingredients (i.e., gluten) that were likely causing some negative results. Results were even better.

VOMITING

A two-year-old boy presented with a history of chronic vomiting that had occurred nearly on a daily basis his whole life. He also had chronic rhinorrhea, dysphagia, cough, and a tendency to aspirate thin fluids (i.e., water). He had seen a number of doctors and specialists, had undergone a swallow study and an adenoidectomy, and was recommended for an endoscopy, none of which provided an answer to his symptoms. An IgG antibody, however, revealed high reactions to dairy and egg, which were subsequently removed from his diet. In the eight weeks after he eliminated dairy and eggs from his diet, he only vomited four times: twice the first week and twice after accidental ingestion of dairy. His cough went away, the dysphagia resolved, and the rhinorrhea greatly improved.

FULL BODY ECZEMA

When S. was just a few hours old in the hospital, she had red spots on her face. The doctors told my husband and I that this was normal, and it would disappear after a few days. This was the start of a difficult and often painful journey away from sickness to health. S. was about one and a half months old when the rash worsened considerably, and her face was covered in a mass of severe sores. Smaller sores were on the rest of her body. Her clothes would become literally glued to her body and opened the sores when taken off. We went to every known specialist in our area to get help. As a mother, educated in natural medicine, I had always been against the use of steroid creams, at least when nothing was done to find the underlying cause. A potent steroid cream and Phenamin (an antihistamine) were the only treatments the doctors had to offer. I managed to resist for five months, but by then her skin was so bad that something had to be done. Of course I had also tried a lot of natural remedies in the meantime. I got a tip at the health center that S. might be allergic to something in my breast milk. To cleanse and eliminate I was advised to eat oat porridge cooked with water three times a day. I did, but unfortunately this did not work.

S. and I were then sent to a children's hospital for a week of treatment involving a course of steroid cream and allergy remedies. Skin scratch and serum IgE testing were performed. IgE antibodies to eight foods were tested (wheat, milk, egg, soy and cod, plus a few more). S. reacted to milk and egg but nothing else. After a few days of treatment S. was able to smile at us for the first time. The problem was that her eczema came back immediately when we stopped using the steroid cream, and we would have to stop some time.

We were desperate! A month after the visit to the children's hospital, I was told of a doctor practicing nearby who was getting good results treating atopic eczema. He had a drew a blood sample from me (since I was breast-feeding) and ordered 96 General Food Panel, for food-antigen-specific IgG and IgE antibodies. We kept S. away from all the foods to which I had elevated antibodies: milk, egg, corn, pineapple, apple, banana, cranberry, cucumber, broccoli, asparagus, and almond. In the beginning S. was much better, but she was not completely well. It seemed like we had not found everything. Yet because she was so much better we stopped using the steroid cream and allergy medicines. At the same time, we started a building-up treatment of her intestine and immune system. She was now a happy little girl at almost one year, even though she still often kept her parents awake at night with her itching, scratching, and occasional stomach pain.

One year went by where the status quo was maintained. She was doing okay but was not completely well.

Further treatment came in early 2005, when S. was two and a half years old. The doctors suggested we do a simple finger stick on S. for 96 General Food Panel IgG only test. The specimen collection went very well, as only a few drops of blood were required. The results were a shock, and we realized a lot had to be changed. I now had to bake bread without grains, and we already knew her type IV allergies (IgE reaction) against milk and egg. Good progress and a period free of symptoms followed the elimination of IgG- and IgE-reactive foods from her diet.

Late in the summer of 2005, some of her earlier symptoms began to reappear. Itching, sleepless nights, and small spots on her skin caused us all to worry. New action had to be taken, and this time the doctor suggested that we do the full IgG and IgE analysis to foods. S. is, after all, a very allergic little girl. Upon retesting, the results showed great improvement from the first test. We were definitely on the right track and making good progress with diet compliance. We have also found out that S. reacts to foods that are naturally high in histamine, such as tomato (e.g., ketchup). This is not an allergic reaction, but it gives her symptoms, so when we keep her away from these types of foods in addition to her IgG- and IgE-reactive foods, she is completely free of any symptoms. The other doctors tell me S. has grown out of her allergies. I know, however, that when she is given any of the foods she is allergic to (IgE and IgG reactions), her symptoms come back. With the help of the tests from US BioTek, we have now identified many of her damaging allergenic foods, and that has given us the grace period to allow her to heal.

RESPIRATORY INFECTIONS

A chiropractor shared the following interesting case. He has encountered several cases of young children with chronic respiratory infections and headaches who have been benefited from the testing. Located in a heavy dairy farming community, and the number of patients with high reactivity to dairy products is relatively amazing. The case of a five-year-old daughter of dairy farmers is a great example of the power of this testing. Simply put, without the testing this family would never have eliminated the dairy and she would undoubtedly still be suffering the consequences.

CYSTIC ACNE

For some time I've been sure of the connection between nonresponsive acne in adults and teens (that is, acne that does not clear up with antibiotics, prescription topicals such as Retin-A, and conventional over-the-counter acne skin care programs such as ProActiv) and until I began testing for food sensitivities, I was left only with dietary elimination as a means to try to pinpoint a person's allergen. Many of the patients we see at our facility have tried everything conventionally available with little or no result and are desperate for a fresh approach to solving their problem.

Our first test patient was Kim, an 18-year-old woman suffering from severe cystic acne. Her mother had spent hundreds of dollars on dermatologist appointments and prescriptions that worked only temporarily, if at all. When they visited our office for the first time, we did a thorough medical history and asked about prior failed attempts at managing Kim's acne. When I assured them that we were going to try an entirely new approach, I expected to meet with some resistance, but to my surprise they were eager to try an IgG finger-stick test. When Kim tested positive for dairy, banana, and wheat allergies I could see the relief in their faces. Kim had been eating all of those foods almost daily, which explained why her acne never seemed to improve. When these items were removed from her diet, Kim noticed a remarkable improvement in her acne within days and is now being treated to reduce the scars left from the years of battling cystic acne.

ACNE AND WELLNESS

At the age of 30, Tara was still suffering from acne that did not respond to oral or topical medications. She had spent countless amounts of money on dermatologist visits and could not understand why she still had acne as an adult, when her doctors had told her she would likely grow out of it. After submitting her blood for a standard food panel IgG test, she was found to be severely allergic to dairy, eggs, mushrooms, and yeast (both baker's and brewer's) all of which were regular staples in her diet. Upon eliminating those foods, Tara noted a dramatic improvement in her acne. She says she knows when she has accidentally had one of those foods because her acne flares up within 24 hours.

MIGRAINES

H.B. had a history of debilitating migraines, typically occurring three or more days per week, over the past 25 to 30 years. She had been to numerous doctors, including neurologists and psychiatrists, and she had been tested for allergies (IgE via radioallergosorbent test and skin testing) all to no avail. She was otherwise in great health and was totally skeptical about undergoing a finger-stick IgG Antibody Assay. The first month after the testing was done and the patient had followed an appropriate elimination diet, she had no migraines and has remained migraine free to date.

FIDGETY CHILD

A six-year-old girl underwent food antibody test and implemented the recommended dietary changes: removing wheat, dairy and eggs. After 24 hours, the parents reported that she was a new kid—calm, patient, not fidgety, and having minimal emotional outbursts. The patient reports that it is easier to think and easier to sit still in class and focus on what she is doing. And she is proud that she is able to easily follow directions now. The patient's teacher is impressed and reports that this is the most dramatic behavioral improvement she has seen due to a change in diet. The child's bed wetting also stopped immediately with the diet change.

SINUS HEADACHES

After suffering from sinus headaches for more than 10 years, my doctor had me tested for the IgG antibodies. Earlier IgE testing (through the arm-pricking tests) had failed to identify any allergies, but the IgG panel did uncover some culprits. I now stay away from the chief offenders for me (whey, casein, kidney and black beans, cane sugar, sesame, and eggs) and have had no sinus headaches. The type of headache the foods caused also helped me identify other allergens, including the local anesthetic articaine, which was used recently in a root canal procedure.

WEIGHT LOSS AND SLEEP

I thought being a light sleeper was just part of my personality. I had no idea that food sensitivities were behind my sleep problems. In addition, I've also lost seven or eight pounds since I've stopped eating my reactive foods. I had been trying unsuccessfully to lose five pounds of postpregnancy weight for more two years. In the past two months, I was able to lose the weight without eating less or increasing the amount of exercise, so I think it must be related to the type of food I'm eating. Although being able to sleep is the top benefit, being able to lose the added pounds from the pregnancy is definitely a nice bonus.

CONSTIPATION

A 35-year-old man suffered from constipation, muscle pain, lingering infections, nasosinusitis, and chronic fatigue. A blood test revealed elevated antibody levels specific to egg. After two months of avoiding eggs, and following the dietary guidelines from the lab, he reported considerable improvement and relief from his symptoms.

MIGRAINE HEADACHES

Constant migraine headaches had plagued a 55-year-old woman, and at age 31 she had to quit her job because of the debilitating pain. At age 50, this woman became suicidal, and a psychologist diagnosed her as melancholic. Her food allergy test results revealed elevated antibody levels specific to dairy, gluten, honey, and coffee. She was advised to avoid the allergenic foods and was given essential fatty acid supplements, probiotics, and a hypoallergenic gastrointestinal restoration product. After one month, her debilitating migraines ceased and have not recurred since. Also, her psychologist noted a much improved mental status and outlook on life.

DERMATITIS AND HEADACHES

A serious case of dermatitis, mainly on the arms, had tormented a 14-year-old girl for many years. She also complained of "heavy" headaches and being in a state of near-constant fatigue. Dairy, cucumber, and strawberry were all associated with elevated antibody levels for food allergy testing. She was placed on a customized elimination and rotation diet guideline and supplemented with essential fatty acids. After two months, her headaches were completely gone. She began to feel strong and able again. After four months the skin on her arms had become smooth and bright.

EAR INFECTIONS AND DERMATITIS

A five-year-old girl with serious dermatitis and frequent ear infections was found to have immediate and delayed reactivity to dairy, egg, beef, lamb, and gluten through food allergy assessment by US BioTek. She was instructed to avoid the allergenic foods, treated with probiotics (*Lactobacillus acidophilus*), and supplemented with essential fatty acids. After one month the dermatitis resolved, and after three months the frequency of ear infections diminished significantly.

GASTROINTESTINAL DISTRESS

A 40-year-old woman presented with a nine-month history of intestinal distress involving diarrhea, nausea, gas, fatigue, backaches, insomnia, and periodic numbness of her fingers. She stated that her stools were like "mud." A full gastrointestinal investigation proved negative. US BioTek food allergy testing revealed a strong delayed hypersensitivity to almond—her favorite snack. Eliminating almonds from her diet resulted in the quick resolution of all symptoms.

ALLERGIC CHILD

A child who developed reasonably well for the first two years started to experience a series of frequent illnesses, including gastroenteritis, conjunctivitis, rhinitis, recurrent attacks of bronchitis, urticaria, and constipation. Food allergy testing revealed the presence of severe delayed and immediate allergies to dairy products and egg. After the offending foods were removed from his diet, the child regained his health.

ASTHMA

The parents of a child with asthma sought medical help for their son through food allergy testing. His food allergy report revealed serious multiple food allergies. After following the recommended elimination and rotation diet guideline, he was able to discontinue his asthma medication. (*Author's note:* discontinuation of medications should only be done under the supervision of one's prescribing health care provider.)

CONSTIPATION

A 38-year-old woman had suffered from chronic constipation of several years. Food-specific antibodies to dairy, egg, and baker's yeast were quite elevated, After one month on the customized elimination and rotation diet guideline provided, her bowel functions completely normalized.

HYPERACTIVE

A six-year-old boy had a history of serious hyperactive behavior and was more than a handful for his parents. He was often in trouble at school and had difficulty playing with other children without getting "too rambunctious." The allergy test showed elevated immediate and delayed reactivity to dairy, chicken, egg, cucumber, gluten, and citrus fruits. The parents were advised to eliminate the allergenic foods from the child's diet and supplement with essential fatty acids and probiotics. After three months, the child's hyperactive tendencies greatly improved. His teachers and classmates noted that he had become a more sociable little boy.

ECZEMA

A patient had experienced severe eczema on the face, arms, chest, and legs of one year's duration. Hydrocortisone creams provided no relief. Identifying and eliminating the patient's reactive foods brought complete resolution of symptoms.

ECZEMA AND DERMATITIS

A 44-year-old gentleman affected by chronic conditions of eczema of 25 years' duration, psoriasis of 15 years' duration, and severe depression of 10 years' duration. The patient had also experienced digestive upset over his entire life. The patient became 100 percent symptom free after identifying and eliminating allergenic foods from the diet as identified via antibody assay. Patient no longer takes antidepressants or other medications. (*Author's note:* discontinuation of medications should only be done under the supervision of one's prescribing health care provider.)

NOSE BLEEDS AND HEADACHES

A patient had been experiencing chronic headaches for seven years (since the age of six years), at least three or four times weekly. The headaches were accompanied by severe stomach pain and vomiting lasting up to 12 hours. He was too incapacitated to remain in formal school, and the mother had been homeschooling him. He had significant fatigue with a very rapid pulse (95–109 beats per minute resting). He had been seen by multiple physicians and prescribed multiple drugs. He had undergone chiropractic therapy and a neurological workup with no success. Three out of four of the foods he was eating showed both strong IgE and IgG reactivity as identified via antibody assay. After food elimination, the headaches completely ceased and the nausea and vomiting went from a near-daily problem to twice the first month and none thereafter. His energy levels have improved and his once- to twice-weekly nosebleeds have disappeared.

BACK ACHE

A patient presented with back pain, chronic headaches, depression, fatigue, and prior diagnoses of reactive arthritis, irritable bowel syndrome, and fibromyalgia. Food-allergy testing was ordered, and the results of the test were discussed with the patient. After eliminating the reactive foods her diet, implementing the rotation diet, and incorporating other nutritional interventions, the patient now feels and looks fantastic. The transformation was phenomenal with virtually complete improvement all previous symptoms.

Author's note: US BioTek offers the IgG and IgE food allergy testing that I use in my clinical practice. I have used their testing for years now and have seen remarkable results when a health-promoting diet is incorporated into an overall wellness program. Whether it is IgG, IgE, or some other allergen that is burdening the body, when the burden to the body is removed one's full potential is more easily attained.

Index

About the Author

CHRIS D. MELETIS, N.D., is an internationally known author, lecturer, and media personality. Currently executive director of a nonprofit, the Institute for Healthy Aging (http://www.theiha.org/), he has served as dean of natural medicine and chief medical officer at National College of Naturopathic Medicine, the oldest naturopathic medical school in the United States. Dr. Meletis was named 2003 Naturopathic Physician of the Year nationwide by the American Association of Naturopathic Physicians for his commitment to education and for starting 16 community clinics for uninsured families. To learn more about Dr. Meletis and access health and wellness educational materials, visit http://www.drmeletis.com/.

MediaSpeak

Three American Voices

ROY F. FOX

PRAEGER

Westport, Connecticut
London

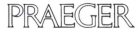

Library of Congress Cataloging-in-Publication Data

Fox, Roy F.
    Mediaspeak : three American voices / Roy F. Fox.
      p.   cm.
    Includes bibliographical references and index.
    ISBN 0–275–96193–1 (alk. paper)
      1. Mass media—Social aspects—United States. 2. Advertising—United States.
    3. United States—Social conditions—1980– I. Title.
    HN90.M3 F69 2001
    302.23—dc21   00—032372

British Library Cataloguing in Publication Data is available.

Library of Congress Catalog Card Number: 00–032372
ISBN: 0–275–96193–1

First published in 2001

Praeger Publishers, 88 Post Road West, Westport, CT 06881
An imprint of Greenwood Publishing Group, Inc.
www.praeger.com

Printed in the United States of America

The paper used in this book complies with the
Permanent Paper Standard issued by the National
Information Standards Organization (Z39.48–1984).

10 9 8 7 6 5 4 3 2 1

Copyright Acknowledgment

The author and publisher gratefully acknowledge permission to use excerpts from *An Artist in America* by Thomas Hart Benton reprinted by permission of the University of Missouri Press. Copyright 1983 by the Curators of the University of Missouri.

Every reasonable effort has been made to trace the owners of copyright materials in this book, but in some instances this has proven impossible. The author and publisher will be glad to receive information leading to more complete acknowledgments in subsequent printings of the book and in the meantime extend their apologies for any omissions.

For

Joe and Jeri

Contents

Acknowledgments

Some books are born by lightning, others by osmosis. This is one of the latter. I cannot remember a time when I was *not* intrigued by voice—first, in how individuals develop it, and later, in how voice applies to the whole of American culture. Hence, a long line of people have influenced my thinking in this book: family, friends, teachers, mentors, colleagues, and students. I am also indebted to those people whom I've known only through their work—their voices in word and image. Among many others, these include Walt Whitman, Thomas Hart Benton, Edward Hopper, George Orwell, E. B. White, and Rudolph Arnheim. I am especially grateful to Beverly Fox for her sturdy spirit and support. Finally, I thank Emma C. Fox and Joel F. Fox for not just tolerating my absences from their lives now and then, but also for reminding me, every day, that voice and heart go hand in hand.

Introduction

This introduction answers a few basic questions about this book. Readers have a right to know these things up front. First, what is this book about? Second, why did I write it? Next, who and what influenced my thinking on this fascinating but slippery topic? Finally, what are my assumptions and biases?

WHAT IS THIS BOOK ABOUT?

This book tries to describe and explain, as clearly as possible, three types of communication that dominate American discourse: Doublespeak, Salespeak, and Sensationspeak. Three chapters (3, 4, and 5) contain many examples of each voice, from all types of media and genres—print and electronic, verbal and visual. Along the way, my analysis of these messages focuses on how they are constructed and how they influence individuals, ideology, and culture. Sometimes, these analyses include the message's contexts and histories. I also explore how each voice connects with traditional American myths and values, including some emerging values of technology.

Chapter 1, "Whitman's Ghost: MediaSpeak and American Voices," answers some basic questions, such as, "What are voices and why are they important?" and "Why *American* voices?" The chapter also briefly describes how our Information Age has led us away from actual reality and toward a world inhabited by *representations* of reality. Chapter 2, "Making Sense of MediaSpeak," provides thirty approaches for how we can better understand and interpret media messages. The final two chapters (Chapter 6, "Voices Entwined," and Chapter 7, "Media, Technology, and Culture Entwined") offer conclusions and recommendations. Chapter 6 focuses on how these three voices, as a whole, influence American culture. The final chapter speculates on how these voices relate to their larger contexts, the "megasystems" of media, technology, and culture.

WHY THIS BOOK?

To understand any complex phenomena (from photosynthesis to clinical depression), it's natural to break it down into smaller parts. Therefore, much of this book analyzes public discourse—individual messages as well as their parts. These examples range from a politician's two-sentence utterance to a visual image on a Web site to a cover of *Time* magazine. However, exclusively focusing on smaller, discrete parts—especially with mass media and electronic technology—often causes us to forget to study the *whole* system. When this happens, we tend to ignore many things, including the message's overall effects, how we perceive and interact with messages, and how these messages function within larger systems. Therefore, this book also focuses on such questions as, What is the nature of America's deluge of public messages? What kinds of "larger" or dominant voices emerge from these messages? What are the effects of these voices? What might they have in common? How do the major systems of media, technology, and culture interact with these voices, as well as with each other?

HOW DID THIS BOOK EVOLVE?

This book was born in subtle, slow ways. Its roots run deeper than the summer of 1980, but I'll start there, when I began researching "Sensationspeak"—what I defined then as the verbal and visual language of tabloid journalism. This work resulted in a chapter for a book (Lutz 1989) commemorating (and updating) George Orwell's prophecies of "Newspeak" and "Doublethink" from his novel *1984*. After scouring old book and magazine stores in several states that summer, I learned that tabloid newspapers seemed to go out with each day's trash. One clerk gently told me, "Everyone throws them away."

The fact that texts so influential could be so uniformly expendable testified not just to their commonality, but to their importance. Tabloids were so common and so consumable that it never occurred to anyone to take them seriously. This situation paralleled what S. I. Hayakawa said about language more than forty years earlier: the last thing that fish would want to study is the water in which they swim. I realized that this was now true of Sensationspeak and electronic media in general;

that we are now in the same place with electronic and visual media as we were with language in 1941. In fact, today we are surrounded by more language and images than ever before. Consequently, language, images, and other symbols fuse to create far more complex messages than ever before. That is why I wrote this book.

During this period, I had been teaching writing, language, literature, and media, first in high school, then in college. At one university I served as director of writing, which included establishing a program in writing across the disciplines. At another university, I taught courses for students who would become English teachers, where I also directed a site of the National Writing Project and guided doctoral students' dissertations in literacy. Throughout these years, I collected thousands of examples of voices, as well as books and articles focused on the verbal and visual language of voices. In my writing, teaching, researching, and speaking, I played with how these voices related to the cultures and times that spawned them.

This work over the past two decades has essentially focused on the human voice: What is it? How do people develop it? What makes one voice effective and another one weak? How and why does one's voice change? How do writers develop voices that resonate with autonomy and trust? How does media alter our thinking, language, and behavior? By the early 1990s, I was teaching courses in media literacy and cultural studies and researching the ways in which TV commercials affected students (Fox 1996). I also explored how teachers developed their own voices to stay alive in their classrooms (Fox, in press).

Finally, all of this work convinced me that the voices of a *culture* were just as important as the voices of an individual—that our relationships with our culture's voices influence our own private ones, and vice versa. Along the way, I have learned that countless other writers, each in their own ways, have grappled with the same issues of symbols, voice, identity, and culture. These writers, to whom I am indebted, include George Orwell, Thorstein Veblen, H. L. Mencken, Walter Benjamin, Aldous Huxley, E. B. White, Jacob Riis, Walter Lippmann, S. I. Hayakawa, Harold Lasswell, I. A. Richards, George Seldes, Guy Debord, Rudolph Arnheim, and Marshall McLuhan. After all of this, when I decided to write this book, my learning started all over again.

WHAT DOES THIS BOOK ASSUME?

Once while waiting in a hotel lobby, I shuffled through the pages of a chamber of commerce brochure, a glossy booklet promoting the host city. The brochure was chock-full of toothy couples smiling over plates of red lobster. I stopped at a full-page ad that showed a woman's bare legs as she stood, spread-eagle, over the city's night skyline. The tallest building (and the antenna atop it) pointed to, and nearly touched, her crotch. The large caption promised, "We'll show you Atlanta's most interesting parts" (*Atlanta Quick City Guide* 1990). This ad doesn't directly or vigorously lie, or sell, or stimulate; however, most readers know what it *suggests* or implies visually, and this visual subtext seems to be the primary message.

Some readers will be offended by the fact that the woman's face is not shown—just the back side of her spread-apart legs—that the ad-makers focused on body parts and not a whole human being. Other readers would view the same ad as "normal" and natural. They could even agree with the ad's verbal claim, that it's "interesting," and maybe even enticing. These are only two simplified readings of this message, and many more exist. But regardless of how you perceive the ad, distinguishing the crude promise of "interesting parts" from the human being whose legs fill the page is a complex task. And so is separating these things from our own perceptions and lives, as well as those of our culture. Therefore, one assumption behind this book is that media often looks simple, but seldom is.

Even isolated images can wield great power: a single photograph (Jackie Kennedy waving from an open car) or other image (a golden arch) can become a national icon that communicates volumes to millions of people over many years. But when technology fuses layer upon layer of sounds, motions, images, smells, and words—and then multiplies them when creating new messages—the intricacy of the message itself, and the difficulty of understanding it completely, increases exponentially. Media messages are prevalent and complex.

I also assume that democracy will be healthier if we think more critically and analytically about these messages—that we'll make better choices of candidates and policies if we can cut through to the dominant or competing ideologies that reside within and behind many of these messages. We can live saner lives if we sometimes sever ourselves from that long train of inchoate desire pulled by media's shimmering illusions. A more critical evaluation of media messages cannot help but temper America's torrent of consumption, thereby slowing the rate at which we diminish our natural environment.

Also, I believe that just as our thinking and experience affect our symbols, our symbols, in turn, shape our thinking and experience. We can manipulate them, and they can manipulate us. This holds true for individuals as well as groups, communities, and cultures. Overall, the images and symbols of electronic media dominate language. However, language is our most effective means for mediating and negotiating these images and symbols. More than ever, we must rely upon language to control them, lest they control us.

Finally, media and our relationships to it are certainly not all bad.

Although this book often analyzes certain messages and the ways in which voices are often used, it is not critical of media itself. We depend upon media to communicate, to get things done in the world. We use symbols and images to learn, to construct meaning out of the chaos of everyday life. We use them to envision alternatives. We use media to bond with other people, as well as to entertain ourselves, to relieve the pressures and anxieties of our too-fast and too-fragmented lives. Indeed, I have always been awestruck by images, regardless of how I encountered them—in media, in language, in art, in music, in nature, in mind. I have long regarded images and imaging in the same ways that scientists view DNA—as the most fundamental element of human life, representing the most basic unit of thought and communication. The image is the single-most common thread in all of life's variety. The driving force behind my analyses of media, technology, and culture is an unshakable optimism that, ultimately, they will advance our thinking, communicating, and culture making in humane ways. We don't have any other choice.

1

Whitman's Ghost: MediaSpeak and American Voices

In 1848, Walt Whitman ventured from his home in Brooklyn to New Orleans and back. He traveled 5,000 miles across countryside and cities. He described America as "space and ruggedness and nonchalance" (Kaplan 1980). Those who traverse the landscape of today's media may reach the same conclusion: our electronic landscape resonates with space and ruggedness and nonchalance. This alone is worthy of inquiry, if not celebration. However, Whitman's passions for his native land also naturally led him to articulate its shortcomings. He described America's main traits as "rushing and raging," "indomitable energy," and "chainless enterprise" (Kaplan 1980, 111). Whitman reflected that if these characteristics are remembered, "it will be bad for us," because "posterity surely cannot attach anything of the dignified or August to a people who run after steam-boats, with hats flying off, and skirts streaming behind!" (111).

Americans are no longer running after steamboats, but we *are* rushing and raging after electronic media. Our world is soaked with messages from print and electronic media. What used to be called "The Information Age" is now often referred to as the age of "Data Smog," "Information Glut," "Analysis Paralysis," or "Electronic Alzheimer's Disease." Before we enter this hot-wired world of MediaSpeak in the pages ahead, let's briefly consider our journey here.

HOW THE FIRST UNCLE HOWARD DISAPPEARED

The media voices explored in this book are, of course, linked to the voices of human beings. Over time, human voices have changed for many reasons. These changes, often brought about by technology, have altered how we perceive reality. Not so long ago, our first-level or primary reality was the actual, physical world around us. If we wanted to talk to Uncle Howard, we'd saddle up our horse and clip-clop over to his house, knock on the door, and talk. And when we went to work each day, we might nail down planks on a new bridge, plant corn, or fix a gas furnace. That is, we did something. Direct and unfettered physical experience was our basis, our anchor to existence. Our fingers, noses, hands, eyes, and feet told us about our world. These actual, sensory experiences reaffirmed for us that we were alive.

Not long after this, if we wanted to talk to Uncle Howard, we could mail him a letter or call him on the phone. These activities removed us from the actual person and place—from Uncle Howard's gap-toothed smile, from smelling the melting creosote in the railroad ties that bordered his flower bed of irises and tiger lilies, not to mention the vaguely spicy aroma of chrysanthemums rooted in clay pots on his porch. Instead, we had to rely on representations of person and place—not Howard in his own true skin, in the home we could smell and see and touch. Instead, we relied on the sound of his voice, filtered through the phone's bad connection. We might have thought he said "pig," when he really said "dig." Or we relied on the letter he scrawled on a napkin in dull pencil. When his letter stated that "she fell over dead," we weren't sure if Howard was referring to his tractor or to his dog, Pearl, both of whom were mentioned in the previous sentence.

One day a TV reporter from a nearby city interviewed Uncle Howard about how the drought affected his soybean crop, and the person we saw on the news program the next night seemed like someone else: Howard looked heavier and darker, and his voice sounded slower than he normally speaks. And when Howard himself saw the program, he also found himself changed, because his words had been cut and spliced together in the newsroom, resulting in an entirely different message than Howard thought he had communicated. In short, these new representations of Howard could not only "remove" him from his own voice, but alter the message and how we perceived him.

Today, we have even more layers and filters between us and the actual Uncle Howard. We don't see his pencil scrawl on a napkin with a coffee stain. Instead, we see his e-mail message or a representation of a mailbox on our computer screen. Today we know our world mainly through representations of it—through multiple layers of representations, each one ever further removed from primary reality, each one bearing the direct and subtle imprints of many people. The further removed we are from first-order reality, the more layers of symbols and filters there are between us and Uncle Howard. And the more "artificial stuff" there is, the more things can go wrong. In more ways than one, the first Uncle Howard has disappeared forever.

If we were alive when a new technology became a part of everyday life, we may appreciate its benefits but also know its shortcomings. But if we were "born into" this same technology, then we have nothing with which to compare it. In such cases the new technology is the status quo, the normal world. Hence, reality for such people, their beginning frame of reference, is mass media—the unreal reality, or at least a reality several times removed from direct experience. Uncle Howard in flesh and blood has given way to representations of Uncle Howard. And each representation of Uncle Howard is modified—by various technologies, as well as by the people and ideologies behind these technologies. These many representations and changes can produce an Uncle Howard—indeed, *many* Uncle Howards—who differ from the first, original man.

WHAT IS "VOICE"?

I define "voice" as not just the meaning of the message, but also as the whole feeling or overall tone of the message. We recognize voice when we detect an authentic human being behind the message. We recognize voice when we sense some qualities of personality, values, attitudes, or beliefs that somehow ring true for us, that somehow connect with our own experiences. The communicator's voice—those qualities of tone, persona, character, authority, or sincerity—help us determine how much or how little we trust the person and message. Today, messages rain down on us in many forms—print and nonprint, and in genres of all kinds, intended for many purposes and audiences. Accordingly, in this book, message, content, and information all refer to discourse conveyed by any means—e-mail, television, Web sites, handwritten post-it notes, films "at theaters near you." However, I emphasize electronic texts because of their power and continuing growth. This book describes and explains three of America's most powerful public voices: Doublespeak, Salespeak, and Sensationspeak. In a collective sense, these function as archetypes.

What Is "Doublespeak"?

The first voice, Doublespeak, is any kind of communication that *pretends* to tell us something but doesn't. Doublespeak tries to hide something, to make it seem better than it really is. Doublespeak tries to shift responsibility away from real people, or tries to avoid responsibility altogether. For example, in Doublespeak, people are not killed, they are "terminated with extreme prejudice."

In 1984, the U.S. State Department decided that it would no longer use the word "killing" in its annual reports on human rights in other countries. Instead, it would use the phrase "unlawful or arbitrary deprivation of life." This phrase allowed the agency to avoid the embarrassment of supporting foreign countries that routinely engage in government-sanctioned murder (Lutz 1989). And in 1978, in order to obtain more insurance money, National Airlines reported the crash of one of its airplanes as the "involuntary conversion of a 727." Double-speak tries to sweep the grit of truth under a thick carpet of words and other symbols. What results are lies. Increasingly, though, communication consultants (Doublespeak for "spinmeisters") artfully micromanage the situation to produce half-truths and partial truths. And a message that is, for example, 43.5 percent accurate, becomes downright hard to evaluate for truthfulness.

What Is "Salespeak"?

The next voice explored in this book, Salespeak, consists of any type of message surrounding a transaction between people. Salespeak includes all those voices that demand, connive, and subtly suggest that we buy products, services, policies, ideas, attitudes, and ways of life. Salespeak can present us with facts, where logic, language, and numbers dominate the message. More often, though, it persuades by massaging us with a synthesis of language, imagery, sound effects, and music. Salespeak can also function as a type of entertainment or escapism—as an end in itself, where we are more focused on the experiences surrounding consumerism (e.g., browsing through a J. Crew catalog) than we are on actually purchasing the products themselves.

Today, Salespeak rarely depends on "testable" verbal claims. Instead, it focuses on people's attitudes, values, and dream-wishes, tapping into these through emotions. A growing trend is "transformational advertising." In this approach, within the confines of a single, largely visual message, advertisers first try to arouse emotions, then change them. The point is not so much that these are pleasant or unpleasant emotions. Rather, the point is for readers and viewers to engage in an internal experience in which our emotions literally move or change—in short, that we take a brief, inner journey from one point to another (Fox 1994).

What Is "Sensationspeak"?

Sensationspeak, the final voice examined in this book, is any print or electronic message in which the content or form stimulates or shocks the senses more than it does the mind. The term "Sensationspeak" also applies when even more neutral messages occur rapidly or in great volume, jarring us with as many "jolts per minute" (JPMs) as possible. For instance, mainstream television now routinely employs individual camera shots that last for only eight frames, or one-third of a second, or less. The shots used in commercials, music videos, and news segments often occur at or below our threshold of perception, which is about one twenty-fourth of a second, qualifying them as subliminal (Gleick 1997).

Although Sensationspeak *can* stimulate rational thought and activate humane instincts, it often does not. The extreme speed typical of Sensationspeak compresses time and represents reality in smaller and smaller units, fragmenting our lives more than ever before. Sensationspeak often occurs in quick montages that rely more upon metaphor, analogy, and slogans than logical sequence or even narrative. Sensationspeak can distract, crowd out, and even explode our memory, relegating us to live in the perpetual present. Overall, Sensationspeak is unconnected to larger concerns for order, beauty, truth, or a desire to change the world for the better. It mainly aims for the gut.

In terms of its prevalence and power in America today, Sensationspeak is second only to Salespeak. Yesterday's Sensationspeak often turns into today's mainstream journalism. When I first researched Sensationspeak in the early 1980s, it was still thought of as fringe journalism, and only a few tabloid newspapers were sold in supermarkets. Now it's everywhere, in all media, from the standard violence and gore of computer and video games to shock radio talk shows to mainstream television. How sensationalism gained such a foothold in American culture is a long story, but let me note only one key episode.

In the early 1960s, the tabloid *National Enquirer* boosted its circulation by giving out free subscriptions to the wives of food store executives and major advertisers. Once these women were hooked, it was easier to place those racks of tabloids in the grocery stores. The *Enquirer* also made a promotional film narrated by respected TV newsman Chet Huntley. This film contained endorsements from Joan Crawford, Bob Hope, Billy Graham, and presidential candidates from both parties, Barry Goldwater and Hubert Humphrey (Abrams 1982). With politics, Hollywood, and God on its side, the *Enquirer* brought Sensationspeak into the mainstream.

THE MAN BEHIND THE CURTAIN

Doublespeak, Salespeak, and Sensationspeak now dominate public discourse and shape our culture. Doublespeak manipulates us and hides the truth. Salespeak implores, massages, and connives us to depend on material items as substitutes for internal and spiritual values. Sensationspeak titillates us with verbal, visual, and aural jolts per minute, trivializing nearly everything it touches. Also, one of these voices often fends for another. Or, one voice will pave the way for the others. And, like all voices, these voices are generative: one can evoke another.

However abundant and varied these voices are, they have one element in common: they come to us disembodied from real, individual human beings. The illusions of media are so great that we often accept the spokespersons and actors on the screen as being the creators of the message itself. In *The Wizard of Oz*, the wizard commands Dorothy and her friends to "pay no attention to the man behind the curtain!" They expose him anyway. Most of us, however, are dazzled by Oz, and "the man behind the curtain" remains hidden.

In 1966, Walker Gibson also believed that voices dominated America. These voices included the laconic, swaggering, and "tough" voice from the hard-boiled detective fiction and movies—here, think of films based on the novels of Dashiell Hammett and actors such as Humphrey Bogart and James Cagney. Walker also identified the "sweet" voice of the innocent cheerleader, and the "stuffy" voice of pretentious bureaucrats, academics, and others. Today, though, things are different. Today we swim in information, both electronic and tangible. What we increasingly forget is that every shred of information has a human being behind it.

After centuries of published books and newspapers, human utterance became known as "text"—disembodied words on a page. The nuances and subtleties of meaning that were formerly produced by a person's vocal intonation and gestures were reduced to printed words that followed the rules of space and sequential order. Hence, voice became not what we heard or saw an individual human do, but what we read on a page, removed from the human being.

Because of its sheer volume, speed, and accessibility, electronic information can be even more anonymous than hard copy, more divorced from one human talking directly to another, even though it can create the opposite illusion. When we are not connected directly to our words, certain things invariably happen. We become used to thinking of symbols (on a page or on a screen) as pure meaning—as something unmoored from real people, as something untouched by human bias. Consequently, we feel less moral responsibility. We might wonder, "Why not tell a lie here and there, since my name will not be attached to this text—or at least my real name won't be." On the other hand, some technology allows us to shift easily from voice to writing to image and back again—to the point that we kind of think through it, which we find wonderfully fun and efficient. But every technology introduces its own problems, too. On my telephone's voice mail system, whenever the recorded woman's voice clips me off with, "That is not a valid pass code. Good-bye!" and hangs up on me, I often interact with her. But she can't hear me. Again we have two humans actively engaged in the *illusion* of communicating with each other.

This trend of divorcing human beings and human-ness from words and symbols did not arise because of Internet chat rooms. It has been building for centuries, as printing became more common. For instance, the concept of "ethos," the Greek term for a person's sincerity and honesty, is shifting in meaning. As the disembodied printed page has become the norm, ethos has come to mean not honesty, but merely the *appearance* of honesty—as marks that can be manipulated with technology to convince receivers that the message is sincere. Most textbooks don't even address the concepts of voice, tone, or ethics in discourse. And when they do, it's regarded not as truth or responsibility, but as "how to make readers believe what you want them to believe."

We have drifted away from the concept of honest voices and toward an acceptance of the appearance of honest voices, away from something that used to be inherently present (or not) within a human being and toward the belief that we only need to manipulate our style and appearance to get us what we want. Speakers and writers can now assume very little moral responsibility. The concept of one's voice as one's true identity dissolves, instead we play one different role after another, depending on who we're communicating with and what we want. Hence, the idea of a "true voice" that comes from our one true self vanishes. Of course, the self is quite complex. Many people believe we have many selves and many voices, all of which are true. Others agree with this notion of multiple selves and voices, but interpret it more skeptically, viewing the self as merely a trunk full of roles that we play, putting on one hat after another, manipulating appearances, to get what we want. The central issue at work becomes not honesty and accuracy, but appropriateness and appearance.

Although most of us, myself included, thrive on technology, this separation of voice from ethos and moral responsibility parallels the development of technology. I continue to believe that our selfhood consists of both the use of multiple voices and the single, true voice, but we too often diminish the latter. As Richard Lanham notes, whereas print text "fixes" things and seems authoritative, electronic text "unfixes" them and is "changeable and antiauthoritarian" (Lanham 1992, 86). This is often a good thing. The fluidity of electronic text lends itself to our playing more roles more effectively. But it also enables us to fake more roles more effectively—often at the expense of the single, true voice within us.

WHY ARE VOICES IMPORTANT?

Every day we face an avalanche of messages, most of which *appear* to have sprung from no identifiable creator. We are then left to determine the message's trustworthiness in a relative vacuum. When our culture was dominated by spoken and printed words, it was broadly true that the content of a message could not be separated from its voice—that words could not be conceived apart from their speaker. From the time of Plato, people have taken for granted that "listeners and readers get a sense of the real speaker and his or her real virtue (or the absence of it) through the words on the page" (Elbow 1994, xvii)—or, I might add, through the words spoken or the pictures drawn. Throughout history, we have accepted the notion that one's voice was very close to, or identical with, one's identity.

In other words, it was easy to identify the source of the stories and messages that surrounded us. If we read an essay by E. B. White, we recognized his voice and "knew" him. If our grandparents told us a story, we could link the message to the source and evaluate its trustworthiness. We knew that an uncle or grandmother told us a story for purposes of information, or to teach us something about work or life, and maybe even to entertain us in the process. These storytellers had nothing of material value to gain from such messages. I believe that this paradigm of assuming that one's voice is very close to, or identical with, one's identity, holds true today, but mainly in our personal, direct relationships with other people. However, this assumption cannot be applied to today's electronic messages, even though television, for example, mimics this direct relationship by beckoning us with voices and images rife with intimacy, lush with warmth.

Today, most electronic messages are manufactured by corporations for wide consumption. These messages do not flow from a single, identifiable source, but from multiple layers of people and technologies. These messages are highly mediated. Today, instead of detecting singular personalities behind messages, we are left with perceiving their tone—that "invisible persona" that lurks behind electronic media's highly crafted representations of reality. The common purposes of these voices are to manipulate, sell, entertain, and stimulate; their ultimate goal is to garner profits. These media voices *appear* to be very personal and close to us. In reality, though, they are produced, like other manufactured products. Nonetheless, many of us continue to regard these voices in terms of one-to-one, personal communication.

This book does not employ the usual categories to talk about media. Such traditional approaches include focusing on the electronic vessel that carries messages (radio, computer, TV); the genre (TV sitcoms, cop shows); the issues (film violence, racial stereotyping); the types of viewers (children, elderly women); the research method (statistical, ethnographic); and the time period (the "Golden Age of Movies" or "Early Radio"). Instead, this book conceives of media in terms of its three most dominant voices, employing descriptive labels that carry judgments not just about their meaning, but also about their overall tone, characteristics, and effects. There are many reasons for this, but I'll note only a few here.

Voices Are Not Peripheral to Real Actions—They *Are* the Real Actions

Many people dismiss language, media, and culture with a cavalier wave of the hand: "That's just all peripheral or secondary stuff," they say. "Actions are more important than words or images—what people *do* matters more than what they watch on TV." Today, however, our actions—what we do—often involves viewing media and manipulating information. These once "peripheral" activities are now primary—our main work, our main play. Quietly watching TV may not seem like doing anything, but by today's standards, it *is* action.

Voices Are Just as Crucial for a Culture's Health as They Are for an Individual's Health

A culture's dominant voices are just as important for that culture's well-being as your own voice is for you. An individual's voice—the fluency, uniqueness, intelligence, flexibility, strength, clarity, authenticity, and compassion with which one thinks and communicates—is a private as well as a social construct that develops over time. Our voice is cultivated, vulnerable, and ever changing. Our voice not only reflects who we are—it *is* who we are, and it helps shape the person we will become. An empowered voice helps us develop constructive, positive relationships with family, friends, and peers. It helps us gain confidence and independence. It helps us find meaningful work, helps us better navigate life. The words, images, and other symbols that make up voice cannot be conceived apart from people. The same holds true for a culture—its voices not only reflect what it is, but help fashion what it will become in the future.

If an individual's voice is somehow diminished, that person suffers definite consequences. For example, one's voice can become controlled by others, such as the American servicemen who were brainwashed by their captors during the Korean War. Or, one's voice can become artificially distorted, such as those who abuse drugs and alcohol. Or, one's voice can become diminished or stunted, such as those who are raped, battered, or psychologically abused. Unfortunately, there are myriad ways for one's voice not to develop to its full potential.

In the same vein, a culture's media voices can wreak just as much havoc—on individuals as well as on the culture as a whole. After reviewing three decades of psychological research, David Shenk identifies the following effects that information overload can exact on people: increased cardiovascular stress; weakened vision; confusion; frustration; impaired judgment; decreased benevolence (i.e., desensitization to people needing assistance); and overconfidence (Shenk 1999, 37–38). An entire culture can experience similar effects—confusion, frustration, desensitization, and impaired judgment. These effects stem mainly from overload, or the amount and speed of information, and not from the more complex (and hence more powerful) elements of media voices: their content, tone, attitude, or values. In short, an entire culture's relationship with its voices may function much like an individual's relationship with her own voices. And for either to survive, they must serve humane ends.

The More Soaked in Information We Become, the More We Need to Think about Voices

Over the past several decades in particular, the megasystems of media, technology, and culture have grown and changed drastically. And in the next few decades this rate of change will accelerate even more. The result will be more people having greater access, more quickly, to more information than ever before in history. We will add to what Shenk (1999) calls our "Data Smog." It may grow so thick that we could call it an information "White Out." If this is the case, it will be impossible to deal with the multitude of categories and subcategories of messages floating about the atmosphere. Nor will it suffice to apply one-dimensional generalities to the condition, such as "Information Glut." Rather, using a few "handles" that communicate judgments, such as "Sensationspeak," may prove more useful in coping with the situation.

Overall, the best-case scenario for living in a media-driven world is that we always take our time and exercise deliberate rationality when responding to media messages. On the other hand, the extreme volume (and serious threats) of so much information warrant our avoiding the paralysis that can accompany neutrality, "objectivity," or a slavish adherence to political correctness. As desirable as objectivity or neutrality are, in the face of a blinding overload of information they are relatively useless. Consider an analogous situation. Assume you are trapped in the world's largest art museum—more floors, corridors, galleries, and mazes than you could ever hope to navigate. In your first few hours, your responses to the art you view are likely to be at least somewhat objective or balanced. Eight hours later, if you are still wandering the corridors, anything you bother to look at will likely elicit an immediate and definite judgment: "That's trash! Next!" The stimulus overload makes cutting corners necessary.

A Culture's Voices Can Displace the Voices of Individuals

The cumulative effect of our culture's dominant voices (Doublespeak, Salespeak, and Sensationspeak) is to appropriate or displace the development of the individual voices of average people—especially kids, who are trying to discover their own voices. This is fundamentally important, because helping kids discover and nurture their own voices is our only hope for cultivating strong identities—which in turn beget honesty and sincerity, our main indicators of humanness and civility. A few years ago, I researched how the required in-school TV commercials affected students' voices—the ways they used language to think, talk, and behave. I worked with students attending schools that subscribed to Channel One, a commercial network that broadcasts an eight-minute news program, with two minutes of commercials each school day—for M&Ms, Snickers, Gatorade, Nike, Donkey Kong, Dorritos, and other brands. One day, I asked several ninth-graders sitting around the table with me, "What's advertised on Channel One?"

"Cinnaburst," replied Eric. "You know—that gum with those little red dots and—"

"No," injected Lisa, "those are *flavor crystals*."

Eric paused, muttered, "Oh yeah, flavor crystals." He then quickly continued describing the other ads he'd seen on Channel One. When Lisa corrected her classmate with the commercial's exact wording, the other students nodded in agreement. In their world, nothing strange had occurred. Of course, these students, captive to the Salespeak voices of daily TV broadcasts, did not know that their own voices were being appropriated by larger, dominant voices.

Not All Voices Should Be Communicated Visually or Electronically

Our most powerful voices are visual. They depict real people, places, and objects. They must rely on these same things even when they communicate about values and other abstractions. That is, visual voices such as TV rely on *showing* just as much as or more than they rely on *telling* its audience about, say, honesty or courage. A film can *show* us Sergeant York capturing enemy soldiers, instead of lecturing us about the abstractions of courage. On the other hand, someone speaking about, say, death or spirituality, merely constitutes a "talking head." And a pope or a brilliant philosopher may be passionate in person or on the printed page—but deathly dull on TV. In popular film and television, talking heads are often considered boring, and do not attract sufficient numbers of viewers and hence profits. The nature of the communication medium itself restricts the types of topics, people, and modes of delivery. In many ways, then, the most valuable qualities of a human voice have great difficulty translating into electronic media. Some legendary stage actors and silent film stars fell on their faces when talkies came along—they just weren't suited to that medium. The sustained time, focus, and subtleties that occur when speaking face to face are modified and sometimes don't survive in electronic media.

People who have grown up in an environment that privileges electronic voices have little basis for comparison. Most of us believe there is nothing that cannot be translated into electronic and especially visual media. We believe that if anything exists, and if it is at all worthy, we should be able to see it on TV. So we are surrounded by representations of concrete objects—things and faces that the largest audience will recognize, believe, and buy. These people, places, and things are invested with values and emotions—all promising far more than they could ever deliver. We hear the values of real voices, but they come to us through objects and the right faces, so we "purchase" those values by putting the objects they sell into our shopping cart. These representations and the objects they sell are made so appealing and beautiful that the act of consuming them becomes even more appealing and beautiful than the products themselves. Visual media, especially, has succeeded so much that this process of consumption has eclipsed the actual product (even though consumption of the product does not suffer; indeed it's increased). Lagging far, far behind is the individual human voice, with nothing tangible to sell.

Making the abstract or unknown visual resides at the core of art and culture, but it also has a downside. We are left, then, with communicating everything through the representation of objects—even those topics that can hardly be dealt with in this manner. For example, an abstract notion such as God is, by its very definition, impossible to represent in concrete terms, impossible to personify. Whoever or whatever is cast in this role will automatically fail—whether it's Charlton Heston or Whoopi Goldberg; God may not be a person who can be represented by an actor. Nor do things like abstract and conceptual thinking lend themselves to concrete representation. However, decades of visual media have convinced most of us, most of the time, that everything in life can be represented on a screen; if we don't see it on screen, maybe it just doesn't exist. Therefore, nobody thinks about or aspires to such unseen and unknown things. But life, to paraphrase Shakespeare, is far more than screens allow us to dream.

Dominant Voices Can Help Us Understand the Megasystems of Media, Technology, and Culture

This book focuses on our three dominant voices, because simplification in a crowded and fast media environment has to be our first priority. Of course, these three voices overlap, sharing certain characteristics (see Chapter 6, "Voices Entwined"). I hope that by reducing and simplifying to three the vast numbers and types of media voices that lure us every day, we will more easily understand the qualities and effects of each major type, as well as their cumulative effects. In other words, when faced with 153 brands of cereal in the grocery aisle, it's easier to judge them when we consider only the three most basic types, such as those high in sugar, those high in chemical additives, and those high in nutrients. Although I have concluded that our three most basic types of media voices are Doublespeak, Salespeak, and Sensationspeak, many readers will have sound reasons for disagreeing with me. However, we are at a point in our history when reasonable people cannot and should not avoid making such judgments.

Second we forget to study the relationships among the largest components of our environment. This is why I wrote this book—to avoid fragmenting media into smaller parts, such as print versus nonprint, TV versus film, music versus language, or soap operas versus sitcoms. Although these pages contain plenty of analysis of individual media texts, I have also tried to address the larger contexts of these messages—from the responses that people have to them, to the American myths and values from which these voices evolved, to the larger, enveloping systems of media, technology, and culture.

WHY *AMERICAN* VOICES?

The voices described in this book cannot help but be voices of the U.S.A. The voices of Doublespeak, Salespeak, and Sensationspeak are not fringe or competing ideologies nipping at the heels of some dominant discourse. Instead, they *are* the dominant discourses. There are many reasons why these voices are mainstream, but I will note only one here: Americans love electronic media. Because America is a land of action, of builders and movers and doers, we love being part of the show. We can never seem to get our fill of rich, vivid, powerful media, from the encompassing screens of Imax theaters to DVD, Surround Sound, and virtual reality games. We've been hooked ever since that day, a century ago, when a movie audience viewed a locomotive train coming at them and ducked. In this book, then, the exploration of each voice concludes with an inquiry into its "Americanness"—how and why it constitutes part of the American grain, how it is woven into American history, mythology, and ideology.

A note of caution. Some readers may be tempted to see this book as a validation or legitimation of Doublespeak, Salespeak, and Sensationspeak, since it acknowledges them as "normal" due to their deep traditions in American life. This is to some extent true: the voices fashioned from our history directly bear on who we are today. But I am not implying acceptance of these voices as future codes of behavior or rules by which we should live. Nor do I believe I am unduly cynical in focusing on these particular voices. Rather, I simply view an inescapable presence in our everyday lives for better or worse. My purpose in exploring them is to help improve our lot. This, I might add, is one of the deepest American instincts of all—to take what we've got and make it better. This is the spirit in which I hope you'll view this book.

Other reasons compel me to focus on dominant *American* voices. First, they not only reflect our national identity, but also perpetuate it. These three voices regenerate themselves, as well as each other, creating a wall of our "normal reality." Second, this book's brief illustrations of American history, mythology, and ideology boil down to values. These episodes of fact and fiction embody the essential values that guide our actions. Also, these three chapters not only look backward, but forward as well, to speculate on the roles these voices may play in America's emerging myths of technology, our largest frontier. Throughout our history, our newest and largest frontiers have generated our grandest, most potent myths and values, in turn influencing our actions. Thinking about how today's dominant voices relate to technology and its myths can help us better plan for the future. Overall, a culture's dominant voices are its DNA.

Third, this book focuses on American voices because we currently have little to hold us together. A crazy-quilt of religions, colors, beliefs, and languages, we are short on moral codes broad enough to gather most of us under one tent. Religion no longer serves this purpose. Nor does the camaraderie and banding together that was necessary for settling unknown territories. Nor do art or literature or even the English language provide much national cohesion.

What has filled this void? The media. Specifically, the dominant voices of Doublespeak, Salespeak, and Sensationspeak. These voices are bred within a collective consciousness that is unanchored to the codes, rules, customs, or habits that help guide us when the ground shifts beneath our feet, or when we face our own incoherent desires. A society that has somehow become unmoored understandably turns to those voices that are most readily available and attractive to fill the vacuum—Doublespeak, Salespeak, and Sensationspeak. At the least, these voices must be acknowledged head-on before we can address them effectively, before we can aspire to what Walt Whitman laid out for us in his preface to *Leaves of Grass*:

This is what you shall do: Love the earth and sun and the animals, despise riches, give alms to every one that asks, stand up for the stupid and crazy, devote your income and labor to others, hate tyrants, argue not concerning God, have patience and indulgence toward the people, take off your hat to nothing known or unknown to any man or number of men, go freely with powerful uneducated persons and with the young and with the mothers of families, read these leaves in the open air each season of every year of your life, re-examine all you have been told at school or church or in any book, dismiss whatever insults your own soul, and your very flesh shall be a great poem and have the richest fluency not only in its words but in the silent lines of its lips and face and between the lashes of your eyes and in every motion and joint of your body. (Whitman 1965, 714– 715)

These codes of selfhood, by which Whitman himself lived, are harder to find in millennial America, now rampant with the tangled wires and blurred airwaves of public voices, now faster and thicker with illusions of desire, beamed from unknown people and places. What we shall do, then, is best realized through the heart of our own voices.

2

Making Sense of MediaSpeak

> A democratic civilization will save itself only if it makes the language
> of the image into a stimulus for critical reflection, not an invitation
> to hypnosis.
>
> —Umberto Eco, 1976

OVERVIEW

How do we survive in a world saturated with messages? How do we make sense of our deep sea of images, words, and music? This section contains thirty suggestions to help you navigate these messages—to control them, lest they control you. The media situations described here can occur when these four elements interact: (1) people—receivers and senders of messages; (2) the medium or "vessel" that conveys the message; (3) the message or information itself; and (4) the context or environment surrounding the above elements. It's all messy, but natural. These guidelines apply to any type of print or electronic media. They should help you understand how the voices described in the chapters ahead work and don't work. Also, these guidelines should help you understand the daily messages you send and receive.

All voices have inherent pitfalls, because voices depend on symbols, which are, by their nature, biased. Neither words, nor pictures, nor music are "objective" in and of themselves. Also, the medium or vessel that carries words or pictures predisposes us in certain ways, as does the information it carries. They become even more subjective when we put our human prints all over them, as we select, craft, and deliver symbols that match our aims and purposes. Whether or not the senders intend it, symbols and the media that convey them invariably tilt our perceptions. It's easy for voices to confuse and scare us, to create realities where none (or very different ones) may exist.

A note of caution: reading, interacting with, and interpreting media is a highly complex, idiosyncratic process. Whether through reading a newspaper article or evaluating a virtual reality program, processing information involves the reader, the text, the context or communities to which we belong, and all the interactions among them. Therefore, the following suggestions cannot account for the many idiosyncratic ways in which we filter information through our own life experiences and psyche at any given moment. These sometimes overlapping guidelines are based on this notion: that flimsy symbols often bend, fold, twist, collapse, melt, shrink, expand, and do other weird things when held up against actual reality.

UNLOAD FIRST RESPONSES

"That's disgusting! She's nothing but a ruthless manipulator of men!"

Is this an appropriate or effective way to begin rationally responding to and evaluating a film or TV program or some other media text?

Most of the time, yes.

No matter what the information, genre, or medium, if a message elicits a quick response within you, then quickly acknowledge it—voice it, get it outside of you and onto the table. Whether you're reading Toni Morrison's novel *Beloved*, viewing the film *Saving Private Ryan*, or scanning through the Web site of the Ku Klux Klan, it's natural for first responses to be emotional, especially if the text in question involves emotions. TV commercials and other media are often crafted to elicit emotional responses. When this happens, a door swings wide open, exposing our attitudes and values, fears and dreams.

This advice does not mean that emotional responses are isolated from critical analysis. On the contrary, emotional responses are necessary for effective critical analysis. Because emotions play such a large role in our processing of media, it's important to place them on the table so we can begin to gain critical distance from them. If we keep the feelings inside, they simmer (or fester) as an integral part of our own selves—as content or ways of thinking that are undifferentiated from our private lives. In a sense, they become part of our private selves. However, if we get them out, these emotions begin to become objectified. Then we can more rationally ponder, manipulate, and analyze them. If such emotions remain hidden, however, they are more prone to confusion, misinterpretation, partial belief, or wholehearted belief.

Media messages that employ and elicit emotions from us create a kind of internal but active transaction or experience. Often, a media text creates an emotion and then changes it, thus creating an internal action or journey. Such internal movement helps us remember and like the media text. With ads, this mental activity may help us remember and feel positive about the product. Although giving voice to initial responses might undermine the suspension of disbelief necessary for becoming immersed in media, it's healthier to get it out. Doing so helps us separate inner reality from outer reality.

SEPARATE INNER REALITY FROM OUTER REALITY

A man down the street thinks he's Elvis Presley. Nearly every day, he dons the big hair, the white, sequined bell-bottoms, and purple-tinted aviator glasses. Something inside Jim has convinced him he's the King. Putting on the *Viva Las Vegas* outfit helps him align his outer reality with his inner reality. But if Jim checked his outer reality a little "further out"—to his mailing address, to his job at the fiberglass plant—he'd find discrepancies.

However, when Jim holds a mike and lip-syncs to "Blue Hawaii," or watches *Jail House Rock*, the vague line separating inner and outer reality nearly vanishes. In other words, although media messages are a definite part of our outer reality, they speak more powerfully to our inner worlds, and the parts of Jim that are non-Elvis become more Elvis. Jim is an extreme example, but my point is that people and animals naturally adapt to or mesh with their environment. The shepherd who lives with his sheep for long periods of time is more likely to talk to them, to be more like them. Similarly, people who spend long periods of time with media will adapt to this environment.

Granted, suspending disbelief is what makes much media meaningful. But the more media we have, the more messages must compete with each other to break through our perceptual defenses—those barriers we naturally raise in the face of such onslaughts, to safeguard our sanity. And heavy media competition breeds increasingly powerful entertainment. If Elvis is everywhere (and evermore vivid), then non-Elvis has a harder time surviving.

THINK OF MEDIA, CULTURE, AND TECHNOLOGY AS A FIGURE VERSUS GROUND RELATIONSHIP

Imagine the smiling face of Leonardo da Vinci's painting of the Mona Lisa. Now imagine that the background is a busy paisley print. Her winsome face is the foreground and the paisley print constitutes the background. We naturally pay more attention to the foreground than to the background. Rather than thinking of media in terms of a specific message, such as a TV program or a song, think of it in terms of *all* possible media—from books and newspapers to computer screens, films, pagers, cell phones, and laser discs. Consider the prolific output of all of these products and processes to be what, in reality, they are—the American foreground. Also, consider our background to consist of the megasystems of culture and technology.

Foreground of media messages, then, get all the attention, whereas backgrounds often remain submerged and hidden—but background issues affect our lives more powerfully. For example, during the media blitz of the O. J. Simpson murder trial, Americans were greatly focused on the foreground, the media messages surrounding the celebrity, the car chase, and the trial. Few people were concerned with the background of culture and technology—how the foreground was interacting with and affecting the background. Media is incredibly distracting. In my lifetime, the background has rarely become the foreground. Culture and technology have seldom overshadowed media. The culture of youth—the issues and problems and contexts of being young in America—never held sway over images of Eric Harris and Dylan Klebold wielding guns during the news coverage of the Columbine school shootings. Finally, consider the increasing number of instances in which media operates in both foreground and background, taking up our entire perceptual field. For instance, some visual and verbal ad messages on the Internet and elsewhere (foreground) reveal a huge logo as background or as wallpaper. Another example occurs during "product placement" in films, when we spot a particular brand of cereal on the table in a scene dominated by Kevin Costner or Meryl Streep. Overall, thinking of media in the context of technology and culture helps give us perspective.

SEPARATE SIGNS FROM SYMBOLS

When we drive, a red, octagonal piece of metal bearing the letters S-T-O-P is a sign for us to depress the car's brake pedal. For most of us, through agreement, it means one thing. On the other hand, the Vietnam War Memorial in Washington, D.C., means many different things, depending upon who you talk to: patriotism, blind patriotism, joyous celebration of life, subdued acceptance of needless death, our friend or sister killed in Cambodia, our own faces and selves staring back at us. The possibilities are endless. Signs mean one thing; symbols mean many things.

The confusion of signs and symbols—and how we react to each—is a major reason that we sometimes fail to separate outer reality from inner reality. Media messages can roughly be divided into two types: signs and symbols. Signs have a direct and natural connection to what they stand for. For example, if you touch a woodstove and it burns your fingers, this tingling is a sign that a fire burns inside of it. Similarly, the word "cat" is a sign that points toward the furry, four-legged creature purring in our lap. Signs point us toward concrete, observable things that usually have only one meaning upon which we have agreed.

Media messages can also be signs, or at least signlike. The billboard that displays a huge arrow, with the words "Turn right in 300 feet to eat at Dino's Steak House" is a sign. A direct relationship exists between the sign and that to which it refers (the cafe down the road). So, too, is a documentary film about Harry Truman, because the still photos, archival footage, and text-screens of Truman's famous quotes all point us back to Truman, the man. Signs usually point to something outside ourselves for their meaning.

On the other hand, symbols point inside us for their meanings. Symbols are open and can have multiple meanings. An abstract painting titled *Eating at Dino's* might elicit feelings of isolation and despair in one viewer, whereas another might perceive it as whimsical. When a political candidate uses the term "the American way," a female volunteer at a Planned Parenthood office may interpret this phrase to mean, "This candidate believes in a woman's right to abortion." A male bricklayer may take this same phrase to mean, "This candidate believes in legal marriages between same-sex couples." What symbols mean depends on the people who use them. Most media messages are symbols, though we often accept them as signs.

DON'T MISTAKE THE WORD FOR THE THING ITSELF

The marks you see on a road map—the dotted lines, the black dots, the labels of towns and highways—only represent reality. They are not reality itself. They look nothing like the actual land, the hills, curves, gas stations, and pastures. In other words, the map is not the territory itself. The word "smoke" does not smell, and the word "ton" weighs about as much as the word "feather." The problems come when we mistake the word for the thing itself—when my neighbor Jim has the word "Elvis" embroidered across the back of his white, sequined vest and then wonders where his pink limo is parked.

One main culprit that leads us to confuse words with things are labels—our human and useful habit of naming things. We name things to make sense of the data that floods our senses every day. Naming means categorizing and classifying phenomena. Creating fewer elements helps us manage information more efficiently and effectively. Naming is natural.

But too often we take labels to heart. When I directed a university writing program, students were required to pass a writing exam before they could graduate. Many middle-aged adults came to my office and informed me, with downcast eyes and in hushed, apologetic tones, that, as children, they had been "diagnosed as dyslexic." This handicap, they told me, meant that they could "never pass this exam." At this point, they'd look up to me for signs of understanding and sympathy. I learned to question their dismal self-confidence. When I sat down beside them and asked them the exam questions, or had them write something, I often found nothing abnormal about their literacy skills.

Other students I've worked with were labeled as "gifted" when they were in school. Now in their early twenties, many of these students can well articulate the effects that such labeling had on their lives: teachers expected more—and less—of them than they did students without the label, and they learned to behave in snobbish ways because they were convinced they were special (or at least like the children from Garrison Keillor's Lake Wobegon—"above average").

Worst of all, these labeled people often experienced rude awakenings when their lack of eternal giftedness was made plain to them in a single incident. Other students recount similar experiences with different labels: the athletically inclined live with being "jocks," the bookish kids labor as "nerds," the skateboarders slide through as "slackers," and the Islamic students suffer as "towel heads." Labels are hard, if not impossible, to erase from people. The point is that we are jocks only some of the time, not all of the time, as the label, the stereotype, makes it seem.

The problems with labels that we experience in everyday life also spill into our interactions with media. Creators of film and television texts can stereotype characters, just as viewers can dismiss entire texts by stereotyping characters or actions. Viewers can even dismiss entire genres through stereotyping: "Oh, another chick flick. Let's see something else." Such labeling can occur overtly or subtly. Labeling can be an actual part of the plot (an episode of the TV drama "Felicity" included a character referred to as a "rapist"), or it can merely be suggested, such as when Jill, Tim's wife in the TV sitcom "Home Improvement" talks with her husband while she, not Tim, puts all the groceries away.

DON'T MISTAKE THE IMAGE FOR THE THING ITSELF

When earlier generations were surrounded by words, it was almost inevitable that they would mistake the word for the thing itself. Today, we are not only more surrounded by words, but we're also swamped in images—from computer screens, films, TV, or advertising. Never before has a culture been so steeped in imagery as modern America. This makes it easier for us to mistake the image for the thing itself.

Because most media messages meticulously synthesize words, pictures, motions, sounds, and graphics, they are hard to ignore. When a

TV commercial about old friends "reaching out to touch someone" makes a lump in our throat, who can deny that what we feel isn't there? Because we tend to perceive wholes rather than parts when we engage with media, we accept most pictures as true. And even if we were skeptical about images, they occur in a flash and rob us of needed reflection time.

We also have trouble questioning or negating media messages because our culture still equates seeing with believing. This occurs for two main reasons. First, the link between seeing and thinking/believing is deeply ingrained in our language. Witness such words that refer to perception, including "foresight," "insight," and "hindsight." Witness common phrases indicating understanding and believing, such as "I see," "I just don't see it," and "From my point of view."

Second, we equate seeing with believing because imagery—especially electronic imagery—often parallels how we think, how we represent experiences to ourselves. When you try to recall the floor plan of a house, you'll probably place yourself at the front door and then walk from room to room, visualizing as you go. When you lose your keys and attempt to "retrace your steps," you'll visually reconstruct your earlier actions, replaying them in your mind's eye. Because photographic images are closer to actual or first-order reality, we trust them, even when we shouldn't. Even when actress Ann Margaret's body appeared with Oprah Winfrey's head on the cover of *TV Guide*, hardly anyone noticed.

DON'T MISTAKE MOVING IMAGES FOR THE THING ITSELF

When early movie audiences viewed a locomotive chugging down the tracks, they ducked in their seats to avoid being hit by the train. We continue to embrace such immersion and involvement. Americans found great delight in being "tricked," and have since loved being part of the show.

On the other hand, most of us can recall a time when we've blurred what happened on a screen with what happened in real life: "Hmm . . . Did Jack tell me about that, or did I see it on TV?" Former president Ronald Reagan was reported to have told stories that he represented as true but which in fact were based on plots from old Hollywood films. The more common media becomes and the more vivid and realistic, the more common such experiences will become. We often represent reality to ourselves in ways much like TV and film—and TV and filmmakers use camera techniques to mimic common thought processes. A friend wanted to have her dog groomed, but she mistakenly took the animal to her own beauty salon. She walked in and didn't realize her error until she stopped and looked: everything in the shop blurred—except the woman sitting under the hair dryer, who came into quick and sharp focus. In the movies, this is called "rack and focus."

The point is that media makers (especially creators of film and video) use their own creativity as well as increasingly advanced technologies to mimic how we think, perceive, and remember—as well as how we believe we experience actual life. The name of this game has always been to reduce the differences between reality and make-believe—which is why "talkie" films and Technicolor were invented, why Imax theaters, virtual reality, and interactive media have been created.

Such blurring between the real and unreal means more profit for media makers. Sometimes the blurring of reality and the unreality of media results from the complex web of an individual's psychology and environment, such as the growing number of "copycat crimes"—those unlawful acts committed by people who witnessed them in the media before acting them out for real. Other times this blurring is intentional, such as TV commercials crafted to look much like documentaries or public service announcements (Fox 1996). When our experiences with media outnumber our experiences with real life—and when those media experiences are nearly as vivid as real life—then it's easier to blur one with the other.

DON'T LET EMOTION TAKE YOU FOR A RIDE

If you think of a single image, such as Van Gogh's painting *The Starry Night*, you may have feelings of youthful intensity and first love. The fact that it's a picture—a whole representation—predisposes us to perceiving it in an all-at-once fashion. Images are mainly emotional from the get-go because their general absence of words and numbers means we don't have to think about them immediately to understand them. We merely encounter images and seemingly have an instant response—often an emotional one.

Television and film are especially evocative of emotions since they integrate words and music into images to craft even more powerful messages. Many media texts aim to evoke emotional responses from us—and then, somehow, to change those emotions. Television commercials try to accomplish this in thirty seconds (researchers call this transformational advertising). The idea is to move us from one point to another within our internal landscape.

In the first scene of a television commercial for greeting cards, we may see an older woman sitting by herself next to a telephone. Her facial expression, the background music, and the dark room all communicate loneliness. As a lump grows in our throats, the camera slowly pans to the window, where her kindly mailman, wearing a grin of pity mixed with hope, places a greeting card into her mailbox, rings the doorbell, and hurries away. The final scene shows the woman reading the card, teary-eyed but smiling, with fingers against trembling lips. Within seconds, we have moved from pity and sadness to relief and joy.

An emotional ride like the one created by this ad can proceed in any direction: from cool emotions to warm ones; from warm to cool; from loud to quiet; from confusion to order; from joy to despair. Regardless of the continuum traveled, such movements constitute symbolic experience. And if we experience movement, then we actively participate in the message. Active participation in messages may help us to remember them better and longer. It may even affect our behavior in some way, especially our consumer behavior. However, if we're somewhat aware of internal movements, we're less likely to be taken for a ride.

GET A GRIP ON HYPER INTERTEXTUALITY

Consider the TV program *The Simpsons*. Homer makes a joke about the town's mayor. For viewers to fully understand its intent, they have to know something about former president John F. Kennedy and to recognize that the mayor's voice sounds much like Kennedy's. Or, the mayor could give a speech that imitates former president Richard Nixon's vocal, facial, and nonverbal gestures, without directly mentioning Nixon. Using direct or indirect references to other texts outside the immediate story is called *intertextuality*. In short, we have to read one text in terms of others, current as well as past.

When information is so plentiful and moves so many places so quickly, it's inevitable that we often interpret a new text in terms of the old, in terms of what's already known. Such echoes can come from any type of text, from any time period, and appear as spoken allusions and references, imitated voices and gestures, similes and metaphors, editing style, genre, or medium. Homer and Marge may appear in another episode dressed in old-time farm clothing, holding a pitchfork, gazing, expressionless, straight ahead, as the couple portrayed by Grant Wood in his painting *American Gothic*. Or, the entire show can be presented as a 1940s movie musical.

Such echoes can be obvious or subtle. The TV program *Friends* may employ a character whose appearance, name, dialogue, and attitude, are similar to those of a character on another program, such as *Beverly Hills 90210*—or even to an earlier program, such as *Charlie's Angels*. In 1976, capitalizing on Americans' distrust of politicians in the wake of Richard Nixon's resignation from the presidency, Jimmy Carter announced his candidacy for president in a manner that evoked former president Franklin D. Roosevelt, widely acknowledged as one of our most trusted presidents. Carter did this by broadcasting his speech from Warm Springs, Georgia (a favorite place of Roosevelt's) and by sitting beside a lit fireplace (which evoked memories of Roosevelt's famous "Fireside Chats").

Fully understanding any media message taps into our knowledge of previous media. Because we now have so much information, moving to so many places so quickly, we live in a world of hyper-intertextuality. In many respects, media messages no longer refer to any underlying reality—but just to each other! We therefore have to sort through these uses of other texts to decide which echoes are relevant and what they state or imply, before we can fully comprehend and evaluate the message.

DON'T ASSUME THAT THINGS PLACED NEAR EACH OTHER ARE ALIKE

The main problem of hyper-intertextuality is that we can believe that two items are similar merely because they are physically positioned next to or near each other. It's a well-demonstrated principle of gestalt psychology (the law of proximity) that if two items appear close to each other, we may well perceive them to be the same thing, regardless of logic. It's natural to lump things together, even very different items.

Jimmy Carter's evocation of Franklin Roosevelt does not mean that Carter is like Roosevelt. However, we have a natural tendency to associate, transfer, or graft the qualities of one thing onto that which is near it. Former President George Bush, during the 1988 election, was filmed visiting a factory that manufactures American flags; the television footage showed him surrounded by flags. His opponent, Michael Dukakis, was filmed riding atop an army tank. Former Speaker of the House of Representatives Newt Gingrich was photographed surrounded by circus clowns; only the heads of the smiling speaker and clowns are shown in the photo. In the Red Scare of the 1950s, the major league baseball team the Cincinnati Reds briefly changed its name to the Cincinnati Redlegs to avoid being associated with Communists (Fariello 1995).

One of the most serious abuses of association has been the inclusion of violence and sex within the same scene—or violence and sex depicted in scenes close to each other, often achieved by rapidly cutting from one scene to the other. Such a presentation suggests that the two go together or even become the same thing. Park Dietz, a forensic psychologist and media violence researcher, believes that "a vulnerable youngster may watch a sexy slasher movie and become conditioned to sexual arousal through such images. When that boy becomes a man in his 20s or 30s, society runs the risk that he will seek sexual gratification through actual, not fantasized, brutality." Dietz has worked with many violent offenders who have been "inspired, instructed, or otherwise influenced by mass media" (Kieger 1994, 19). Transfer or association is one of the simplest yet most powerful techniques of media because the image seems to have been "born" with its elements positioned together.

SEARCH FOR WHAT'S MISSING

One day the *Washington Star* newspaper published three photos of Senator Edward Kennedy, in three editions. Each photo created very different impressions, even though they were cropped from the same photo (Ritchin 1990, 86). The first picture showed Kennedy leaving a building with a young woman, clearly suggesting that Kennedy was cheating on his wife. In the paper's second edition, the same photo was altered to show Kennedy by himself, and the third version in the final edition of the paper captured Kennedy with a priest, an old family friend. This photo suggested the opposite of the first one—that Kennedy was religious and family oriented. However, the version of the photo that did not appear at all was the uncropped, original shot, which revealed Kennedy leaving the building, flanked by several people—the young woman, the priest, and several others. The fuller context of this larger photo illustrated nothing as dramatic as the first two suggested— and certainly nothing as simple.

In each instance, it was easy for viewers to assume that everything within the boundaries of the photo was included—that each picture was a complete representation of reality. When we view media with obvious borders—whether the thin lines around a photo or the opening scene to the final fade-out of a movie—we tend to think that everything that matters has somehow been gathered into the corral. Not true. All media texts are mere abstractions from reality and bear the prints of the many people who decided what's left in, what's left out, how it's shaped, and how it's presented.

KICK THOSE KNEE-JERK REACTIONS

Once in a photography shop, the customer next to me picked up a camera, looked at it, dropped it onto the counter, and yelled to the clerk: "The krauts made this camera! I don't want it!" Such knee-jerk reactions occur when we respond to something automatically, without thinking. This is fine if we're responding to signs. There's no problem in automatically yelling, "Ouch! That fire's hot!" But there are problems in knee-jerk responses to symbols.

Aside from this man's use of labels and issues of context (addressed later in this chapter), he responded as if all German people were alike, all the time—as if there were a one-to-one relationship between Germany and all that it has ever contained and produced, for all time. He responded as if "Germany" were a sign. In reality, of course, "Germany" is a symbol that represents multiple meanings, not just the one that surfaced in the customer's head at the time. This man reacted to a symbol as if it were a sign. Such responses stop thinking before it even starts.

On the other hand, a symbolic response occurs when we slow down and think about the symbol and that to which it refers—when we think about the circumstances and conditions that surround the situation. A more deliberative, measured response simply acknowledges the fact that the world outside of us also determines what something means as much as the world inside of us. The man at the counter was being jerked around by the world inside his head.

BYPASS BUSINESS WITH *IS-NESS*

Another culprit that helps us confuse the word with the thing itself is that common, innocent, little verb "is." (Actually, all forms of the verb "to be"—am, is, are, was, were, etc.—work hand-in-hand with labels to wreak havoc on unsuspecting people). The word "is" is used not just to describe the present, but to make judgments for all time. If we say, "Mark is a great ball player," we usually take it that Mark is always a great ball player. And if this is the case, then all debate is cut off. If this is the way things really are, then there's no point in talking further. "Is-ness" and labels cut off further thinking and communication.

Is Mark always a great ball player? Probably not. He may have hit two home runs on September 8, 1998—but he may have struck out in every at-bat on September 7. The reality changes, but the language used to describe and define Mark remains the same, in effect "freezing" a label on him. Problems arise when, through habits with language and other symbols, we expect Mark to be a great player all the time, no matter what. No human can live up to this unrealistic expectation. A more rational statement would be, "Mark was a great ball player on September 8, 1998."

AVOID "ALLNESS" AT ALL COSTS

The title of this section is an example of "allness" orientation—our habit of not qualifying or specifying what we're talking about; our tendency to make blanket generalizations, relying on such words as "all, never, always, every time, forever," etc. An allness orientation describes the present situation—but it also makes judgments for every situation, all the time!

When dealing with information, it's fairly easy to fall into an allness orientation: about medium ("I don't believe in watching television" or "I never write letters, only memos"); about genre ("I hate poetry"); about time ("I always catch the news in the mornings"); about key people ("We go to every movie starring Leonardo DiCaprio") and about social and cultural context ("I never watch the Super Bowl alone," or "All new French films are about directionless, self-absorbed people"). Breaking the allness habit is important because the more media messages you receive, the greater the need for distinctions.

DEMAND MORE THAN TWO OPTIONS

"Either/or-ness" means we sometimes fall prey to thinking and communicating in polarized ways. We are led to believe—or we have convinced ourselves—that only two options exist for us. Our language conditions us to expect two options, often regardless of the situation: we vote either Republican or Democrat, liberal or conservative. Our water is hot or cold. We work days or nights, at jobs which make us happy or sad, rich or poor. Our economy is either feast or famine, where, regardless of income, our bread comes in either wheat or white. In the late 1960s, a popular bumper sticker, "America: Love It or Leave It," often drove a wedge between parents and children.

Either/or thinking also can result from a deeper dynamic at work in media messages. When you look closely, you'll often find tension or conflict created by opposing forces within many media texts—forces that tend to have two dimensions. Such dichotomies often fall along the axes of gender, age, class, race, motivation, values, and environment. Consider the TV classic *I Love Lucy*. Ricky Ricardo and Fred Mertz have jobs, but the women, Lucy and Ethel, do not. This opposition creates various conflicts. For instance, Lucy takes a job without telling her husband, and the fun resides in Lucy's efforts to keep him in the dark. Here's another opposition, this time related to class status instead of gender: Fred's job as an apartment manager is less glamorous than Ricky's job singing in a nightclub; it also may pay less. This opposition creates conflict when Fred wants a job in one of the club's acts, but Ricky doesn't think it's a good idea. In a sense, then, oppositions or conflicts are the building blocks or deep structure of many media messages. This fact, along with our habits of using polarized language, often steer us toward thinking in black and white terms. To accept the view that only two choices exist, when multiple options are usually available, creates grief—multiple shades of grief.

BEWARE OF TOO MUCH BACKGROUND

Too little context is a problem, but so is too much. If too much data (background) accompanies the central piece of information (foreground), it's easy to become buried in an "information dump." Floundering in too much background information (including only perceiving too much background) can create at least four problems. First, it requires much time and energy, even before we realize we are submerged in too much context. Second, it can deflect our attention (and goals) away from our original focus. Third, it can divert our attention to a new topic altogether. Fourth, it can simply make us throw up our hands and walk away.

Having too much background information can be intentional, accidental, or the result of someone's oversight, laziness, or both. As a juror for a grisly murder trial, I observed the prosecution lawyers build a convincing case by submitting one small piece of evidence after another. When you added it all up, the information pointed in the same direction—toward the defendant's guilt. The defense lawyers, on the other hand, had much less of a case. Hence, their strategy was to dump a lot of irrelevant information into the trial. On the surface, their "red herrings" appeared important, but they didn't hold up to scrutiny for very long.

Depending on the entire environment of any message (the information, the medium, the context, and the sender and receiver), either foreground or background may dominate in how the receiver makes meaning from the message. Especially in long-term and high-profile media events, the foreground usually dominates: the central people hold center stage, and the details of the background swirl about them. As viewers and readers, we focus most on the people.

O. J. Simpson and President Bill Clinton remained as foreground during their respective investigations and trials. In such cases, the background "feeds" the foreground. It's true that focusing on individuals "puts a face" on the news, and media makers use this to boost revenue. However, as audiences and consumers, we often "retreat" to the personalities involved because of the acres of information that constitute the background. Simply put, it's easier and much less work if we focus on the face instead of sifting through the mountains of data. In reality, though, neither background nor foreground should be slighted; the truest picture comes with constantly matching one against the other.

RESIST THE WRONG BACKGROUND

In addition to too much background, another problem can hinder our understanding of media; what appears to be a sufficient and natural background can really be irrelevant or even wrong altogether. A candidate for the state senate ran a television commercial. As the candidate strolled about the statehouse, inside and outside, a voice-over quietly described the politician's virtues. Everything about this brief ad seemed normal; it was a low-key, straightforward ad. In fact, what seemed most normal is the background—it was a natural, even clichéd location for such a message. However, in this video, the background was wrong. The candidate was not a member of the senate while he was running for office, yet the context led viewers to believe he was. The message makers wanted the audience to view the candidate as an incumbent, since they often attract more votes than challengers. Such discrepancies are found only by questioning that which appears to be most normal, as well as by matching background with foreground.

DETECT THE TONE

Are *you going to the movies?*
Are you *going to the movies?*
Are you going to the movies?

In these three statements, the content or information remains the same, but the tone or emphasis makes each mean something different. We often unconsciously pick up on the tone of a message—not what it's communicating, but how it communicates. Tone is referred to in different ways—as attitude, voice, persona, feel, and even style. Media and discourse tones have been described in many ways: sweet, tough, and stuffy; fast, angry, and psychotic.

If we can alter meaning with vocal inflection, media makers can accomplish the same thing through all the tools at their disposal—editing, sound, framing, camera angle, and so forth. To give a fair shake to media messages, we often must get beyond their overall tone. Some people dismiss the entire genre of rap music because they perceive an angry or cynical tone. If they merely read the lyrics, they might detect other sides. Similarly, the overall tone of *Star Trek* and other science fiction texts is often perceived as quiet, civilized, intelligent, even somewhat formal—qualities that help us accept whatever violence such texts portray. Likewise, it's easy to dismiss the TV program *South Park* as another kids' cartoon show because its overall tone or feel communicates this: the cut-out, flannel-board appearance of the show, the animated figures, the characters' squeaky cartoon voices, the bold, solid colors, the distorted bodies. However, if you focus on the content, on what the characters say and do, you'll find something quite different.

Sometimes tone becomes very tricky and is used to mask intentions. The late 1990s film *Starship Troopers* was criticized by some people because of its seemingly pro-Nazi messages. Critics observed that the movie glorified Aryan storm troopers—that their uniforms, insignia, and physical appearance, as well as their attitudes, beliefs, and actions—closely resembled Hitler's army. In the film, the storm troopers eradicate aliens. In short, the movie celebrates the power of white human beings over all else. However, other critics argued that the film is merely a satire or parody of Nazism. Although the best satires are straight-faced, this one, to me, did not feel like a satire, especially given that its primary appeal was to young audiences. My son, for example, who was eleven, certainly did not view it as a movie poking fun at anything. The point is that media makers can create any type of text they want and, if criticized, simply defend it by labeling it as satirical.

To better understand some media, disengage yourself from the context and return to the overall tone—or vice versa. In doing so, you may find contradictions or other ambiguities, intentional or not. Try to match up any differences you perceive between *what* the message is stating and *how* it is being said.

DON'T CONFUSE REPORTS WITH INFERENCES AND JUDGMENTS

A basic type of message is the report—a statement that tells of something we've seen, heard, touched, experienced. "There's only one parking space left at the Yum Tum Diner" is a report that we can verify pretty easily: we can drive out there and see for ourselves. We seldom doubt reports, nor do we often question "reports of reports," such as, "Louise heard on the radio that the parking lot at the Yum Tum Diner was full."

Inferences are guesses—hedged bets—based on what you know at the time. Pulling up to the restaurant, you might note that the parking lot is nearly full of cars. Then you spot a clutch of people gathered outside the doors. Inside, you might see another group of people waiting, as a man with a notepad writes down their names, as waiters dart to and fro. You might hear the hum of chatter, the clinking of plates. You could reasonably infer that it might take some time before you could eat and that you should therefore find another restaurant.

But this inference could be wrong. It's possible that the people waiting outside the restaurant have already finished their meal and are waiting for the rest of their party before getting back on the tour bus (which you didn't see, parked in the back). Inside, all of the remaining tourists could quickly rise at once and leave. The man with the notepad could be figuring the total bill for the tour's guides. Inferences can be carefully calculated, based on a meticulous review of evidence, or they can be wildly sloppy, based on rumor, or based on what is mistaken for evidence, or what might be masquerading as evidence.

Finally, a judgment is a statement of your opinion. The problem is that judgments can make us leap to unwarranted conclusions. Consider, then, these three statements: (1) "Only one parking space remains at the Yum Tum Diner"; (2) "Wow. It's too crowded to eat here very quickly!" and (3) "I have rotten luck." The first one is a report and easily verifiable.

The second one is an inference. The third one is a judgment—an evaluation that goes beyond the circumstances and applies more to the speaker than to an external situation.

The problem is thinking of inferences or judgments as if they were verifiable reports. Making judgments and evaluations often stops thought. The speaker's jump to "I have rotten luck" applies not just to the Yum Tum Diner at 6 P.M. on February 28, 2002, but to all areas of life, for all time. "If my luck is rotten," the speaker might reason, "then why pursue it further?"

In terms of media messages, we can view a film or TV production as a report—as a straightforward documentary or direct recording of reality. First, regardless of its documentary label, and regardless of how authentic the scenes shot on location appear, and regardless of the use of "real people," we still have to view such programs as inferences and judgments. Why? Because directors, camera operators, producers, script writers, and others have selected, sequenced, framed, edited, and shaped the material—to the point that it can hardly be considered an unfettered report, free of bias.

Even the so-called reality-based shows, such as *Hard Copy* and *A Current Affair*, sometimes use film not from the event being recounted, but from stock footage, film shot during another situation, in a different place and time (Seagal 1993). A scene of a burn victim from a gas explosion in Amarillo, Texas, on November 4, 1999, may actually be a car accident victim in Hanover, Vermont, from three years earlier. The events depicted in both shots are verifiable (but separately), but splicing one with the other creates something nonverifiable, a near work of fiction. What's more, viewers can mistake such "reports" for inferences and judgments: "Those Texans get pretty careless." In modern America, one falsehood can verify and substantiate another.

SLIP PAST THE SEDUCTIONS OF STORY

Narrative, a sequence of actions and descriptions, has enchanted human beings down through the mists of time. Narrative remains our most versatile, powerful tool of communicating and learning. Narrative is found everywhere—in TV commercials, political speeches, stained glass windows, soap operas, history, fairy tales and myths, grant proposals, conversations, comic books, video games, e-mail, Internet chat rooms, and contracts. Narrative can function as a single anecdote to illustrate a point, or it can shoulder the work of the entire message. Narrative helps us make sense out of the chaos of life. Like an opiate, though, narrative can seduce us. Becoming immersed in Samuel Taylor Coleridge's *The Rime of the Ancient Mariner* is not terribly different from becoming engrossed in the Jon Benet Ramsey murder investigation. The general pathway of most narratives is predictable: (1) the world goes awry, and (2) the world is set straight again. It's the journey in between that beguiles us.

Narrative also works in rational ways by placing information into some kind of an order. A narrative can occur as a straight chronology of events—from bed to breakfast. This is a logical, linear, rational approach. Or the narrative can "jump-cut" from past to present to past again. This approach is more irrational and nonlogical. Narrative can exert even more irrational powers by creating moods through the use of camera angles, background music, and pace of editing. These elements color our perceptions of character, setting, plot, and hence, overall meaning.

Of course, in media messages, you'll bring your own backgrounds and agendas to interact with these powers of narrative as you negotiate a text's meaning. Constructing meaning from media should be a back-and-forth tussle between message and receiver. Rather than evaluating narrative by "translating" it into more distanced and "objective" language (though this is very helpful and often necessary), you might begin by simply comparing the media text's story to stories of your own and others—stories you know to hold truth. Doing so gets us a half-step outside of the message, and is quicker than full-blown analysis. If we initially respond to media by analyzing it, we often don't go far enough fast enough, so we stop trying.

QUESTION WHAT'S PRESENTED AS NORMAL

With visual media in particular, our habit is to focus on the foreground, especially people. The same holds true with the foreground of narrative, which can be thought of as the main events of a story. These events are usually out of the ordinary for the world of the story being told—they are ruptures, abnormalities, or disruptions in normal life. Outside of these events is the background or "normal life" that characters return to—a story's wallpaper. It's not so much the unfolding of the dramatic events that count. Instead, it's the normalcy of what's depicted before and after the disruptions occur in the story. The background to which the story returns may be most emphasized, more deeply communicated—not the events that disrupt it.

In media messages, what we begin with and then come back to constitutes what the message maker presents as the norm, the calm, the constant, the natural, the universal. For example, in a TV commercial, two men are eating a bag of junk food snacks on a city street when two beautiful women slowly walk by. The men stop, stare with open mouths, change expressions, look at each other—and then return to eating their snacks. Consuming these chips is the natural, normal state of affairs here. It's also what the advertiser is selling.

However, it may not be *your* norm. Nor may it be the average reality of most people you know. But it's presented as such. And because it's mere background, we hardly question it. If we're out of the loop, then we'll feel abnormal or subnormal. A teenager living on a bleak reservation in New Mexico may feel that she's unlike or inferior to most other teens because, after resolving each of their weekly traumas, the characters she watches on TV's *Beverly Hills 90210* and *Dawson's Creek* drive off in their Mercedes convertibles or frolic in their backyard pools. It's hard to be aware of such background or wallpaper when the foreground— the beautiful people doing nasty and violent things—is so magnetic.

You can even think of TV commercials themselves as disruptions to the "normal" programs—which then makes it "natural" to watch TV— which of course leads you back to the ads! In another approach, one that is fast becoming reality, advertising itself functions as the background, the wallpaper. Procter and Gamble is considering the use of background ads on the Internet. Such ads would fill the computer user's entire viewing area; the information or noncommercial message would appear on top of that.

CREATE YOUR OWN CATEGORIES

For purposes of selling as well as communicating, makers of media texts must "cut up" information, label it, and package it, so that it fits into neat categories. This is necessary for sheer efficiency: newscasts cannot present the whole river of each day's life and must dip into the stream and show us only a handful. However, we often forget that what we see on the screen is a world more orderly and controlled. News anchors sit quietly at big desks and look us straight in the eye and speak in rational, measured tones. Newscasts also communicate that reality is neater, more logical, prone to causes and effects, and yes, more black and white, than it really is. This creates an illusion of objectivity. Consequently, we invest far more authority in media newscasts than they deserve. The tidy categories and classification systems presented to us invariably favor those who create them.

Another problem is that such prefab categories encourage us to think only in terms of those groupings presented to us. The neat boundaries tied around news stories often lead us to believe that the problems inherent in the story can be solved within the bounds of that category— that the problems are irrelevant to larger social and political structures. The Jon Benet Ramsey murder investigation, for example, has been routinely categorized by the media as a murder mystery. This imposed category tends to focus our thinking for us. Consequently, most of our thinking seldom gets beyond wondering who the killer could be. This category does not usually lead us toward related, larger social issues, such as our culture's obsession with appearance, our exploitation of children, and even our economic system, which reinforces values of materialism and appearance over everything else.

Humans have always depended on categories supplied by others to view the world, to help us fix objects clearly against the blur of incoherent experience. In 1927, Walter Lippmann wrote, "When we find a pattern which works well, in that it allows us to feel that we have made a large area of reality our own, we are grateful, and we use that pattern until it is threadbare. . . . As a mere matter of economy in time and trouble, we demand simple and apparently universal stereotypes with which to see the world" (Lippmann 1962, 88). Because we are now engulfed in information and symbols, we have become far more dependent on categories supplied by others. When reading any message, we should question the accuracy and appropriateness of categories, labels, titles, and other names.

SHUN SAVAGE SURPRISES

Many messages have more than one purpose—to inform, to persuade, and so forth. However, media makers usually subordinate these to a larger purpose—to entertain, to snatch attention. A basic building block of entertainment, humor, and fiction is the surprise. The unforeseen twist arouses emotions, and bingo—we're having an internal experience or journey, trying to reorient ourselves, trying to figure out just why or how the knife ended up in sweet Mrs. Baker's hands. In cruising through a Web site describing a mundane sales service, I spotted a little button labeled, "Press here for the love of your life." I was surprised—not just because I was conducting business, but also because of the compelling command. Usually, surprises are intended for one reason: to make you remain with the message, at least a little longer—you won't change the dial to another station, make a sandwich, leave the theater, or daydream. If you stay engaged, then media makers make money.

Sudden and often violent changes in our equilibrium are measured as "JPMs," or "jolts per minute." Unfortunately, loud bangs, explosions, screams, funny lines, name calling, and loud music have become the primary ways for media makers to attempt surprise. Over the past twenty-five years, writers and directors have continued to up the ante of violence in commercial media. The film *The Godfather* produced twelve corpses, *Godfather II* killed off eighteen people, and *Godfather III* killed fifty-three. In 1990, the children's movie *Teenage Mutant Ninja Turtles* displayed "133 acts of mayhem per hour" (Gerbner 1994, 134–135).

Accepting and tolerating such cheap surprises in media can make us impatient for more JPMs, hence perpetuating the cycle. Also, it can desensitize us to violence. Further, the more JPMs become expected, the more we are robbed of the time necessary to provide the psychological and social context that surrounds violent acts. Without this context, what's left is mere visceral spectacle—jump-cut scenes of mayhem, explosions, flickering lights, groans, and gore.

The result of all this is that, yes, media violence can make us act more violently. One of the best-kept secrets in America is the fact that we have accumulated massive evidence—more than 3,000 studies *before* 1971— that links television watching and aggression (Stossel 1997). However, most of us simply become anxious and scared, demanding more law enforcement, more prisons, more capital punishment, more isolation, as we try to survive in what we perceive to be a mean world. Consequently, many average people are more likely to assume the role of victim, not of victimizer.

DEMYSTIFY METAPHORS

First, metaphors (and similes) are not mere ornaments or decorations. They are not geegaws to slip on when we want to prettify our words. Far from it. Instead, we use metaphors when we want to express strong feelings, as well as when we want to influence how receivers think about our message. Indeed, metaphors generate new thinking. That is, when one idea or image is juxtaposed with another one in a sequence, a new idea surfaces. When yellow is juxtaposed with grief, producing as yellow as grief, then a third or new idea emerges.

Metaphors, whether expressed in words, images, or music, are double-edged swords. From "as fat as a pig" to "as yellow as grief," from the fresh to the stale, metaphors seem so clear, so up-front, so apparent. That's their job—to carry the weight of meaning, to find a fast track toward communication by comparing one thing with another. They can be windows into our thinking. I once heard a state legislator say that devoting more state money to education was like "pouring water down a rat hole." Whether you're holding the bucket or ore one of the rats peering up from the hole, you have a pretty good idea about the value this man placed on learning. The other side of this sword is that metaphors can become a prison—hard to break out of. That is, calling Bob a jackal doesn't leave much room for articulating the differences between Bob and the jackal. A comparison is a whole package that drops on the porch of meaning with a single loud thud.

Metaphors are common to all types of media and discourse. Fiske (1987) describes one study of television news that found that 165 metaphors were used to report six political stories. Of these, the thing most often compared to politics was war (followed by sports or games and drama). For example, "The President fought a hard battle today" and "The President took center stage today." Fiske concludes that "[m]aking sense of politics by metaphors of war or sport constructs politics as a conflict between parties and not as a public sphere serving the good of the nation. Using the metaphor of drama makes sense of it as a 'stage' upon which talented individuals 'perform' as stars" (Fiske 1987, 291).

Also, we're not always aware that we're inside a metaphor, especially large ones generated in film and television texts. Terrence Malick's 1999 film *The Thin Red Line* runs nearly three hours. It depicts American soldiers attempting to capture a hill held by the Japanese on Guadalcanal during World War II. Many scenes portray the horrors of battle: soldiers with gaping wounds, moaning and screaming in pain; soldiers trembling with fear. However, an equal number of other scenes capture the beauties of nature—solo birds in flight, colorful wildlife, sunlight dancing on ocean waves, and tall grasses undulating in the breeze. And some scenes capture both, as the atrocities of battle rage within the waving, sunlit grasses. Flawed and violent humans meet peaceful, perfect nature. Stark documentary footage of death meets *National Geographic* layouts of paradise. Howitzers meet Thoreau. In this film, two dissimilar concepts are juxtaposed in a sequence to create a third reality. Everything that happens in this film is influenced by the metaphor that frames it. Metaphors, then, guide the ways we perceive ourselves, and hence help us determine our actions.

MAKE THE FAMILIAR STRANGE, THE STRANGE FAMILIAR

America sails in a sea of famous faces. Also common are not-so-famous faces. It stands to reason that the more media we have, the more faces we see. Most message makers are well-versed with the phrase "put a face on it." Regardless of the medium, message, or context, linking points to a specific face or personality or anecdote helps communicate the point. We live in a cult of celebrity, a country where "fandom" is a legitimate field of academic research.

Overall, Americans have intimate, up-close relationships with their media, especially with television, which is extraordinarily warm and personal. Compare beeps over a telegraph wire to Oprah's expressive tones and extreme close-ups, as she and her guests chat with us. They subtly raise their eyebrows toward us, nod and smile at us, envelop us into the intimate ring of the conversation. Witness how a turned-on TV set transforms a lonely hotel room.

On the other hand, we easily forget that Oprah doesn't have a clue who we are. Our greatest paradox at the millennium is that media, the greatest influence on our culture, is so very intimate and friendly—yet so utterly impersonal. Over time, we haven't so much improved our relationship with machines as we have improved the appearance of our relationship with machines. TV and other media—as common as dirt and as chummy as your best friend—desperately require some distance, some balance. Simply put, the heavy media we live with daily is not from inside us. In worst cases, media displaces what's inside us. It can also displace (or replace) people near us.

So, you can make familiar media strange merely by ignoring it, by turning it off. Our exposure to that glut of unconnected voices, images, numbers, and noises demands that we make periodic withdrawals from it, because we become robbed of reflection time to quietly sort out what we're doing, what we want, and who we are. If you can't stop everything for a while, try limiting yourself to just one medium: drop TV for a week and use only the radio. Another option is to lower the volume of radio or TV to just below your threshold of hearing everything. Even better, turn the TV volume all the way down or leave it on mute. At the least, tape programs and edit out commercials.

DON'T GO WITH THE FLOW

On November 1, 1997, I watched a TV program with my 11-year-old son. The show was called *Dreamwalkers* and depicted scientists who research dreams. These scientists and their subjects, fully wired with electrodes taped to their foreheads and data gloves on their hands, climbed into glass, cockpit-like compartments, slid a shield over themselves and dreamed themselves away into strange worlds. By studying computer screens, the two lead researchers monitored the brains of these people, as colorful graphics flickered, beeped, and changed shape during their REM-sleep aerobics. My son and I watched the sleeping people's dreams, interspersed with lab shots of concerned technicians, one of whom wore an unbuttoned flannel shirt with a black tee shirt.

In one character's dream, we watched him alone, in a dark train tunnel. As a huge train barreled down, he leapt out of the way in the nick of time. The tension mounted. Soon, he was again on the tracks, heard the loud noise of the locomotive, and looked up in terror. This train plowed right into his forehead. The TV screen went all white, as the small figure of the man tumbled head over heels backward, through the air. I turned to my son and said, "Ouch!—what a bump on the head."

The white on the screen faded, and the very next scene showed two men walking through a busy hospital interior, talking to each other. One of them looked very much like the character from the program we had just been watching—same build, same curly hair, same unbuttoned flannel shirt and dark tee shirt. The only difference was that this man now wore a large Band-Aid on his forehead. As they exited the hospital, they spoke of how lucky the bandaged man was. However, this man was not the man from the program. We were instead watching a Band-Aid commercial. We had watched several seconds of the commercial before we realized that it wasn't the program. A very deliberate blur between the program and the commercial had "delivered" us to the ad.

Other types of flow are more common. As the credits roll near the end of the TV show *Dateline*, you may hear a voice associated with the following program begin speaking. Or, very near the end of the TV program, *Law and Order*, the anchors of your local evening news show may chime in with a "preview," promising a feature story on the same topic (e.g., child abuse) as the episode of *Law and Order* you just watched.

Every message has its junctures, its boundaries between one element and another. For instance, a TV program is a sequence of opening credits, opening scenes, internal scenes, closing scenes, and commercials. A block of TV time is a sequence of programs, news, commercials, and public service announcements. To sustain interest, media makers craft these elements to create an easy flow from one element to the next, just as my son and I were "delivered" from the traumatic program to the saving graces of products. Being aware of how flow operates may help you break the stream, allowing you a greater chance to view a segment in isolation. This, in turn, can sharpen your evaluation of the segment.

ASK WHO THE MESSAGE IS AIMED AT

Even before Sigmund Freud legitimized the unconscious, writers and artists explored it by crafting messages that tapped into our "shadow side"—our emotions, attitudes, values, and dreams. As Freud (and Carl Jung) brought such concepts to light, advertisers and filmmakers also began to appeal to our irrational sides. Today, identifying, describing, researching, and targeting our values, attitudes, beliefs, and lifestyles is the business of marketing. Marketers are no longer satisfied with knowing only what year and model of car we drive, or the highest level of education we've attained. They also want to know if we are externally motivated: Do we feel rewarded by a salary increase? Do we look to the church and the law for authority? Conversely, they want to know if we're internally motivated: Do we look inward to ourselves for authority, not outward to other people or institutions?

Early on, try to size up the intended audience of the message. Begin by asking questions of the text itself: Who are the people in the message? What level of income or lifestyle do they display? What are they doing? What is the message emphasizing—the people themselves? Their actions? Their ideas? How are they like or unlike you and people you know? Why and how do things happen? That is, what causes or motivates these people and events? Which group of people do you think would like this message? Which groups would not like it? Forgetting about the conflicts and tensions for a moment, ask yourself, what in the message is presented as normal, natural, and universal? What is life like in the absence of conflicts and disruptions? Speculating about the intended audience of a message can help you become more objective and analytical.

IDENTIFY VALUES

If we use Bright Bite Toothpaste, the ad shows us, more people will gather about us at a party. This must mean we'll be more popular. This ad is selling something invisible—the intangible lure of popularity—as much or more than it's selling toothpaste, the actual product. Are toothpaste and our desire for popularity the same thing? Are they even remotely connected? Why would the toothpaste people sell popularity? Who is most concerned about social acceptance?

Although we may not be able to answer all of these questions, it's important to ask them. If we go straight to the values we perceive in media messages—especially those related to conformity, materialism, instant gratification, spirituality, nature, violence, family, patriotism, work, technology, and gender—we can sometimes then work backward to determine the validity or appropriateness of the message. If we can identify some values stated or implied within the message, we can evaluate if or how they align with the intended audience and purpose.

It's very hard for media messages *not* to communicate values. It happens directly (e.g., a camera shot of a mourner weeping at Princess Diana's funeral) as well as indirectly (e.g., the camera lingering a little too long on a mourner who had recently made headlines by her criticism of the royal family). Values in media can be communicated implicitly through the decisions made by its creators—judgments about setting, camera shots (long, short, extreme close-up, panning), background music, the characters' sex, age, race, and class status. Even smaller elements communicate values, such as facial expressions, nonverbal behavior, dialogue, dialect, soundtrack, and setting. Even the simple act of labeling a value we observe in media texts imposes some critical distance between us and the text, a necessary first step.

STOP STEREOTYPES

Media stereotypes—whether of gender, race, age, or socioeconomic class—can chip away at how millions of people perceive millions of other people. Such unfounded perceptions become visible in political and social debates. Stereotypes are born when a single character on TV, for example, can "stand for" or "come to represent" an entire, large group of people. During the days of early television, *Amos 'n Andy* embodied many white people's ideas of what African Americans were like, just as

Michael Jordan and Bill Cosby did decades later. Hence, there are negative and positive stereotypes, though we may not always agree on which is which.

The National Association for the Advancement of Colored People (NAACP) has fought against racial stereotypes since the debates over D. W. Griffith's film *Birth of a Nation* in 1915. In 1951, the NAACP leadership objected to the *Amos 'n' Andy* TV show, just as it had opposed the earlier movie stereotypes of Steppin' Fetchit. The NAACP leadership rightly argued that, because of segregation, television was the sole means that many white Americans had of knowing blacks. Walter White, the NAACP executive secretary, observed that this program "tends to strengthen the conclusion among uninformed and prejudiced people that Negroes are inferior, lazy, dumb, and dishonest." White also concluded, "Every character in this one and only TV show with an all Negro cast is either a clown or a crook. Negro doctors are shown as quacks and thieves. Negro lawyers are shown as slippery cowards, ignorant of their profession and without ethics. Negro women are shown as cackling, screaming shrews, in big mouthed close-ups, using street slang, just short of vulgarity. All Negroes are shown as dodging work of any kind" (1951, 31).

Consider more recent TV stereotypes: Jed Clampett of *The Beverly Hillbillies*, Alexis of *Dynasty*, and the title character of *The Fresh Prince of Bel Air* are all wealthy, yet we never see them work. In the same vein, the disproportionately small number of mature and elderly Americans portrayed on TV—Archie Bunker, Maude, Lou Grant, Grandma Walton, Detective Lenny Briscoe—are cranky. Young women on TV—from Ginger on *Gilligan's Island* to Charlie's Angels—function as sex kittens. And during the 1980s and 1990s, most film and TV villains appeared to be from the Middle East.

Media stereotyping occurs in more subtle ways. A once-popular cigarette ad depcited two jeans-clad men in the country, carrying a long pole. Each end of the pole rested on each man's shoulders. A young woman was suspended from the center of the pole, hanging by her hands and feet. Everyone in the ad was laughing. It's just that the woman was situated like that of a slain deer—a prize being hauled out by hunters (Moog 1994). Another subtle way in which media stereotypes people is through "framing"—how a text introduces an issue or theme, as well as how it concludes it. Introductory segments, such as the first paragraphs of a document or the opening credits and first scene of a film, influence how we interpret what follows. Similarly, concluding segments influence how we interpret the material we just experienced.

Research on various texts (stage productions, television newscasts, single sentences) has demonstrated that the most powerful positions in a message—those parts we recall most vividly and after the longest time—are beginnings and endings. If we listen to a radio broadcast about a recent murder, the first slot may be an interview with a neighbor of the woman who has confessed to the crime. The neighbor describes what a wonderful mother the assailant was to her children and to the other neighborhood kids. Next come the middle two slots—facts about the gun and knife used and the brutality involved. The final slot may be another interview, this time with the assailant's husband, who also praises his wife's dedication to their children. This text, then, is framed, at either end, by a stereotype of motherhood—that mothers can do no wrong. Regardless of what we heard in the middle, we'll often put most weight on either end.

ENJOY MEDIA

Most of the advice in this chapter asks you to become more conscious of media—to question it, to actively use language in probing it. This is what we need to do most of the time. But there are times when it is appropriate to leave agendas behind, to rest our critical eye, and not just for the usual reasons of enjoyment and escapism.

First, for some people, the more deeply they become immersed in a media text, the more likely they are, after the fact, to see how media separates from reality. Second, surrendering completely to some texts can help us be fresher, more critical with others. Third, for some messages, we cannot become critically aware until we first allow them to "wash over us."

CONCLUSION: THE CONVALESCENT FISH

The late U.S. senator from California S. I. Hayakawa devoted much of his life to general semantics, which focuses on the roles of language in human behavior. Several of the principles in this chapter are derived from Hayakawa's work, which popularized (and extended) the theories of Alfred Korzybski, the founder of general semantics. Both men believed that a knowledge of semantics would make the world a saner, more rational place. I agree.

When Hayakawa's *Language in Thought and Action* was marking its fifty years in print with a fifth edition in 1991, I talked with him at his home. I asked him if he had applied the principles of general semantics to his own life—if he'd carried them around and used them every day. He replied, "No. To do that, you'd have to be recovering from something."

Later, I remembered his analogy from the late 1930s—that most people are about as interested in knowing how language affects their behavior as fish are interested in examining the water they swim in. We're too close to it. Today, it's not just language we're swimming in, but all kinds of electronic and visual media as well. Then I realized that, in postmodern America, we are often recovering from something every day.

3

Doublespeak

If falsehood had, like truth, but one face only, we should be upon better terms; for we should then take for certain the contrary to what the liar says: but the reverse of truth has a hundred thousand forms, and a field indefinite, without bound or limit. The Pythagoreans make good to be certain and finite, and evil, infinite and uncertain. There are a thousand ways to miss the right, there is only one to hit it.

—Michel de Montaigne, "Of Liars," 1580

THE DAY THE CANDY MACHINE BROKE

Scene: *First-time visitor to city enters hotel lobby and walks up to desk.*

Visitor: Excuse me, sir, but I'm a little lost here. Could you please tell me how to get to the Riverport Casino?

Clerk: You mean the multidimensional gaming facility?

Visitor: What's that?

Clerk: It's an interactive environment that supports a variety of recreational diversions focusing on amusements dependent upon serendipitous outcomes.

Visitor: Uh, right. Will a cab or bus get me there?

Clerk: I can contact an urban transportation associate if you like.

Visitor: Thank you. And one more thing. While I'm waiting, where's the nearest place to grab a quick snack?

Clerk: Just down this pedestrian corridor you'll find an immediate disbursement channel for confectionary consumables, but you'll need the required monetary units in order to finalize your purchase.

Visitor: Fine. I've got enough quarters.

Clerk: Good, because my most recent interaction with that mechanism precipitated a series of dysfunctional behaviors.

Visitor: It doesn't work?

Clerk: At that point in time, the signal transform unit in question appeared to engage in a series of internal performance miscalculations.

Visitor: Does it work?

Clerk: Well, it's perfectly understandable that someone in your situation would conceivably pose the same inquiries with regards to that unit's disposition to perform at or near some predetermined level of satisfaction.

Visitor: But does it *work*?

Clerk: For all practical purposes, when I eventually retrieved my rectangular refreshment unit, its contents far exceeded the odor threshold.

Visitor: The "odor threshold"?

Clerk: This particular type of consumable could possibly be considered an inhalation hazard. Therefore, I tried to rescind my metallic resources, but to no avail. From all informal observations, the internal reciprocation mechanism seemed not to fully integrate the operations initiated by its external signal device.

Visitor: Oh?

Clerk: Then, experiencing a variable degree of serenity dissonance, I actively participated in a series of consecutive verbal defilements, which, at a later time, elicited considerable resistance.

Visitor: Resistance to what?

Clerk: Resistance to the attempted behavior-altering discourse initially communicated with a moderate degree of brio.

Visitor: What happened then?

Clerk: I communicated this consumer misadventure—what some individuals would refer to as an involuntary conversion of personal capital into a corporate financial domain—to the corporate divisional unit responsible for the maintenance of this mechanism. Another viable option, which I did not elect to act upon at that point in time, was to attempt to reconceptualize my irretrievable resources as mere customer capital cost reduction.

Visitor: What did you tell them?

Clerk: My communication basically outlined a consumer scenario in which personal investments were deposited within an element of that corporation's infrastructure but which were never in turn credited to the initial level of expenditure, to an approximate amount of $3,800.

Visitor: Wow. Did you really lose that much?

Clerk: The financial losses incurred within the confines of that pedestrian corridor, over approximately the same length of time as indicated in my earlier communication, could not necessarily be assigned to the same category of financial attrition as was indicated at some previously predetermined point in time.

Visitor: So you lied?

Clerk: At that point in time, my internal psychosocial environment operated within the realm of semidysfunctional behavior.

Visitor: So you lied?

Clerk: Individuals who have actually manifested various elements of E.F.D.S. or "Episodic Fictitious Disorder Syndrome" have, in the past, experienced some degree of reality augmentation.

Visitor: You lied.

Clerk: In most circumstances, it's relatively safe to assume that the essence of terminological inexactitude has the ability to correlate in a positive manner with an individual's self-concept, at least in the *faux* domain of that perspective.

Visitor: Gotta go. My urban transportation associate is here.

WHAT IS DOUBLESPEAK?

> The present era of incredible rottenness is not Democratic, it is not Republican, it is *national*.
>
> —Mark Twain

The previous conversation is Doublespeak. Not only is the candy machine broken, but so is the communication itself. Broken communication can fracture ideas and even people and cultures. Doublespeak is the first type of voice explored in this book because it often serves as a foundation for the others. Doublespeak is any print or electronic message that intentionally tries to change how we view the world. Doublespeak *pretends* to tell us something, but doesn't. Doublespeak tries to hide something, to make it seem better than it really is. Doublespeak tries to shift responsibility away from real people, or tries to avoid responsibility altogether. Sometimes, Doublespeak may be just plain contradictory, *if* you know the facts. For example, in its coverage of the Clinton-Lewinsky affair, the *Washington Post* ran this headline: "Ex-Prosecutors Uncomfortable with Starr's Tactics" (February 13, 1998, A1). The same day, this headline appeared in the *Wall Street Journal*: "Ex-Prosecutors Defend Starr's Handling of Clinton Probe" (February 13, 1998, B2). The ex-prosecutors appear to approve and disapprove at the same time.

The term "Doublespeak" combines two labels from George Orwell's novel *1984*—"Newspeak," the official language of the controlling government, and "Doublethink," the ability to believe, simultaneously, in two contradictory things—to have your cake and eat it, too. For example, the mayor of Lt. Colonel Oliver North's hometown stated, "I think he

[North] is a hero. He lied to Congress, but he was a true American to admit he lied" (Kehl 1988).

Doublespeak, whether intentional or unintentional, is communication that is obscure, pompous, vague, evasive, confusing, and deceptive. Doublespeak can make something bad sound good: "low-income housing" sounds more livable than "ghetto." And if a pit bull completes a dog training course, it can become a "St. Francis terrier," and sound gentler, if not more saintly. Doublespeak can enhance or puff up something: "pasteboard receptacle" sounds fancier and cleaner than "cardboard box," and "customer retention specialists" may snub those lowly salesclerks. Doublespeak can also turn objective, common knowledge upside down and state it as a truth: "poverty is wealth," "life is death," "man is woman," and "liars are heroes."

Statements such as "Abortionists are murderers" illustrate a more subtle form of Doublespeak, which tends to shut down our thinking. Why? Because nobody can reason with it: the label wholly asserts what abortionists "really" are. Such strong judgments allow no alternatives. There is no room in "abortionists are murderers" for people to sit down and talk it over. Identifying Doublespeak is complicated because you have to analyze language within its rhetorical context: the speaker, the audience, the reasons for communicating, the occasion, and the consequences of communicating versus remaining silent. Today, Doublespeak means dishonest and even destructive uses of symbols, including print, images, graphics, and statistics.

Doublespeak is slippery. Although it often communicates a big fat lie, it more often nips at or shades the truth rather than telling obvious, black-and-white lies. Instead, it evades, suggests, implies, wiggles, weasels, slides, and slithers here and there. In the candy machine scenario, you likely noticed that the vague clerk never directly answered questions. And if you noticed any hint of a real answer at the beginning of his responses, you probably soon forgot about it as you wandered deeper into the dense fog. This clerk uses plenty of pure Doublespeak, saying "urban transportation associate" instead of "cab driver," or "terminological inexactitude" instead of "lie." Although this conversation is fiction, I did not invent most of these examples of pure Doublespeak. Indeed, they are direct quotes from real people who have used them quite purposely (see, for example, Lutz 1996).

Our hotel friend mucks up his message in other ways, too. First, the clerk employs as many syllables as possible, for example, using "mechanism" instead of "machine," when the shorter word does the same job. But it gets worse: the phrase "E.F.D.S.," or "Episodic Fictitious Disorder Syndrome," sounds, to many ears, learned or educated, but it simply means the habit of lying. Such puffed-up language is sometimes called "word magic" because of the spells it can cast on the unaware. Also, many of the clerk's sentences are unnecessarily long. Sheer, brute length alone can wear down the receivers of the message, usually ensuring that they give up before they even get started. Third, the clerk qualifies his language when it's not needed, thereby diverting and confusing his audience: "The financial losses incurred within the confines of that pedestrian corridor, over approximately the same length of time as indicated in my earlier communication, could not necessarily be assigned to the same category of financial attrition as was indicated at some previously predetermined point in time."

There's no need to remind the visitor that the hallway (not corridor!) is intended for pedestrian use; aren't they all? And who cares about the length of time here? That information wasn't even requested. And who cares about assigning things to categories? You get the idea. To paraphrase Mark Twain, when we listen to this guy, we feel like we're killing time at a train station, just waiting for the verb to arrive. But verbs should not travel in the caboose of a long, slow train to nowhere. By the time a glint of comprehension finally rolls into the station, we have mentally checked out. This is one evil of Doublespeak: it only pretends to communicate, through the use of long sentences, polysyllabic words, jargon, euphemism, passive voice, and inflated language. It benumbs the receiver, halts thinking, and wastes time and money. Unfortunately, Doublespeak works evil in other ways, too.

When Doublespeak, like novocaine, numbs our minds, people react differently. Some are awestruck at how sophisticated and smart Doublespeak sounds. Every squeak, whine, puff, groan, and clatter of the engines of verbosity can make us feel stupid and small—somehow far removed from the expert's celestial realm of knowledge. Such visitors would have obediently nodded toward the clerk's supreme intelligence, then quickly gone about their humbled way.

By the end of his conversation with the clerk, the visitor is not only beginning to understand Doublespeak, he is using it himself. This is another evil of Doublespeak: it can be highly contagious. We swim in a sea of symbols, and it's becoming increasingly common for us to survive in this sea by adapting to it—by tolerating and using Doublespeak. This is a common response to immersion in propaganda or any common type of message. Even if we fight them, we become overwhelmed and drift along with the current.

An equally unsuitable response to our immersion in Doublespeak is to ignore it entirely, as Noam Chomsky observed:

When I'm driving, I sometimes turn on the radio and find . . . a discussion about sports. People call in and have long and intricate conversations with a high degree of thought and analysis. They know all sorts of complicated details and have far-reaching discussions about whether the coach made the right decision yesterday and so on. They don't defer to sports experts; they have their own opinions and speak with confidence. These are ordinary people, not professionals, who are applying their intelligence and analytic skills in these areas and accumulating quite a lot of knowledge. On the other hand, when I hear people talk about, say, international affairs or domestic problems, it's at a level of superficiality that is beyond belief. I don't think that international or domestic affairs are much more complicated than sports. . . .

It does not require extraordinary skill or understanding to take apart the illusions and deception that prevent understanding of contemporary reality. It requires the kind of normal skepticism and willingness to apply one's analytic skills that almost all people have. It just happens that people tend to exercise them in analyzing what, say, the New England Patriots ought to do next Sunday instead of questions that really matter. (in Barsamian 1991)

So we ignore the Doublespeak surrounding social and cultural issues— "questions that really matter"—because we find a distraction that not only entertains us, but stimulates our analytical skills. Although both football and social issues can stimulate thinking, one of these topics seems a tad more entertaining than the other. When we have a choice between two such activities, we too often opt for that which moves, flashes, and makes noises. To boot, there's a larger reason for ignoring Doublespeak—we're too close to it. Just as moles would not question the earth in which they burrow, we don't question information.

None of this means we should roll over and die. In the age of data glut, it's more important than ever for individuals to critically evaluate messages, applying the types of strategies described in Chapter 2, "Making Sense of MediaSpeak." Ever-increasing information necessarily means more fragmented information. We often only comprehend bits and shards of information and these can contradict each other. Hence, the greater the amount of fragmented information, the more normal contradiction and Doublespeak seem to us. We've become used to it. And when something becomes "the norm," our power to make fine distinctions can diminish.

Further, the instantaneous flow of news and information robs us of the reflection time so necessary for rationally evaluating Doublespeak (Gerbner 1994). The stronger that mass systems become (i.e., the ever-faster technological explosion of information), the more crucial it is for individuals to make their voices heard, with the hope that many small changes will lead to qualitative changes in the information culture.

Although our hotel visitor became delayed, confused, and irritated, and although most of us may engage in white lies, such as choosing a softer word to spare someone's feelings, or mildly overstating our job qualifications, these are trifles compared with what real-world Doublespeak *can* do, especially when it's generated by large, well-financed groups such as the government, corporate America, or the entertainment industry. Doublespeak has often misled and harmed large numbers of people. This, then, is the ultimate test for Doublespeak: How much bodily and psychological harm is done? To how many people? For how long? If I told you that you "may experience an enhanced radiation device," you might think that you had just won a new microwave oven, not a nuclear bomb.

OVERVIEW

The next two sections focus on the broadest types of Doublespeak: that which occurs mainly through language and that which occurs mainly through images. Both approaches manipulate readers in similar ways, although visual Doublespeak relies more heavily on readers' emotions. Following these, "Doublespeak in the American Grain" explores some of Doublespeak's roots in American history, and the next section, "Doublespeak and Traditional American Myths," examines how Doublespeak relates to such enduring beliefs as "rags to riches" and "rugged individualism." The next section, "Doublespeak and Emerging Myths of Technology," speculates how Doublespeak plays a role in shaping current and evolving myths, such as our widely held belief that technology is omnipotent. In addition to providing some ways to combat Doublespeak, the conclusion explores how technology and nature will affect future Doublespeak.

DOUBLESPEAKING IN WORDS

Like the other voices explored in this book, Doublespeak occurs not just in spoken and printed words, but also in pictures, sounds, music, graphics, and even smells. In the past, Doublespeak appeared as language only—when a speaker or writer deviated from actuality, she was heard or read or talked about in words. This language could be general and abstract in nature or it could be highly imagistic. As technology advanced, printed Doublespeak integrated words *and* pictures, although one might dominate. Today, Doublespeak communicates increasingly through visual means alone, as well as through the multisensory media of computers, film, and television. The following sections illustrate Doublespeak that's mainly communicated through language. Next, the section "Doublespeaking in Pictures" focuses on the primarily visual Doublespeak of magazines, television, and film. Our information excess almost ensures that a variety of constructions will continue to flourish.

The Big Bang

Reporter: Can you explain what happened?
Nuclear Plant Spokesperson: Under a plethora of moderately routine circum-

stances, were those to occur, such a situation as an *uncontrollable power surge to the point of criticality* indicates at least some moderate possibility of *thermal enrichment.*

Reporter: So—there was an explosion?

Spokesperson: Precisely what I'm saying is that, in general circumstances, *abnormal occurrences* such as those that have *taken up residence* at various points of time in facilities such as this one may have included various *energetic disassembly situations.*

The Doublespeak that appears in italics was actually used by the nuclear industry to explain nuclear-related accidents or "misadventures," as the nuclear industry has referred to them (Hilgartner et al. 1983). Similarly, during wartime, when lots of people and property suffer massive damage, Doublespeak runs amok.

Boys Will Be Psychos

Like most kids, Marty Wolt liked to play. At his school in Fort Myers, Florida, Marty once followed some of his peers around and scrawled what they said onto a notepad. This seems part of a long tradition of boyhood detectives—from Tom Swift to Junior Brown or the Hardy Boys. (Every day when he got up in the morning, my son used to don a trench coat and old felt hat; in his pockets were the requisite notepad, pen, plastic magnifying glass, and plastic handcuffs.) Marty soon tired of the gum shoe's life and turned his energies to organizing a student strike in response to his math teacher's homework assignments (Brent 1997). After all, boy detectives are eminently resourceful and rational.

How should the school have responded to curious Marty? A talk with the teacher, school counselor, or principal? A parent-child conference? Sorry. Instead, Marty's mother was called into the school and told that he suffered from "attention deficit disorder," or ADD, and should begin taking psychoactive medication—chemicals. Marty, they thought, was not a normal boy, but instead suffered from a chemically treatable disease. This is one example of the type of Doublespeak used to describe normal boy behavior. Diane McGuinness, a psychology professor at the University of South Florida, states that "schools have pathologized what is simply normal for boys." The incidence of slapping kids, mostly boys, with the ADD label nearly doubled between 1992 and 1997 (Zachary 1997). Other kinds of Doublespeak occur when schools and parents rush to saddle kids' normal behavior with language formerly reserved for the organically and mentally ill:

The U.S. Department of Education admits that things are getting out of control, though it continues to speak in nebulous terminology. James Bradshaw, a spokesman, says, "We've had a problem with over identification." Nonetheless, the tendency to "remediate unproductive behaviors" through labeling kids as "disabled" (and sometimes suggesting drug "therapy" for them) goes on. In Largo, Florida, a mother was told that her son should be "evaluated for disabilities" because he mischievously bent a fork while eating lunch. The mother refused and believed her son's explanation: "I saw other kids doing it. I thought it was cool." In Oregon, a mother was summoned to the school, surrounded by six teachers and administrators and told that her son was probably autistic and needed to undergo testing. The evidence? He tended to stare out the window and made "limited eye contact" with others. The mother refused. (Brent 1997, 7)

Before we prescribe chemicals, we should at least consider another possible reason for kids' lack of ability to concentrate, their restlessness, their tendency to engage in several activities at once, and their tendency to feel bored and distracted. Such symptoms could also indicate "information and stimulus overload" or "culturally induced ADD" (Shenk 1999). That is, kids may be conditioned to be restless because of their long exposure to electronic media. It's bad enough to saddle kids with any kind of self-fulfilling label, no matter what it is—gifted, behaviorally challenged, or low-track. However, when a label also carries doses of chemicals that a kid must swallow night and day, then things are clearly out of hand.

That Disarming "Armed Situation"

The following phrases in the left-hand column were used by the U.S. Department of Defense during the Persian Gulf War. The right-hand column explains what each phrase really meant to a group of English teachers.

U.S. Department of Defense	English Teachers
armed situation	war
efforts	massive bombing attacks
weapons systems, force packages	warplanes
visiting a site	a bombing mission
airborne sanitation	jamming enemy radar and radio, blowing up anti-aircraft guns and missiles, shooting down enemy airplanes
disruption	bombing
hard and *soft targets, assets*	human beings and buildings that were the targets of bombs

degraded, neutralized, attrited, suppressed, eliminated, cleansed, sanitized, impacted	destroyed
collateral damage	civilians killed or wounded, and any "nonmilitary" targets that were blown up

The English teachers found so much discrepancy between reality and the language used by the Defense Department (or is it "war department"?) that they awarded it their annual Doublespeak Award (National Council Teachers of English Committee on Public Doublespeak 1991). However, as important as words are, it's still possible to engage in Doublespeak by using scant few of them, or none at all.

They Shoot Horses, Don't They?

Many ranchers in western states want their grazing land to be used by their livestock, not by wild horses. To solve this problem, we'll simply round up all the wild horses and put them up for adoption, right? Well, not necessarily. Language allows other things to happen, too.

Actually, ranchers can "adopt" wild horses—but then sell them at a profit to American or Canadian slaughterhouses, or even kill them. They can do this because of the language of the Wild Free-Roaming Horses and Burros Act of 1971. This law states, "It is the policy of Congress that wild free-roaming horses and burros shall be protected from capture, branding, harassment or death." However, when horses and burros are adopted, they lose this protected status. According to the Associated Press, the U.S. Department of the Interior has ruled that once a horse is "adopted," it's no longer "wild"—and the law applies only to "wild" horses. Therefore, ranchers are free to kill the horses they adopt (PeTA n.d.).

DOUBLESPEAKING IN PICTURES

The following sections illustrate how Doublespeak has "evolved" from words to images. Although Doublespeak was once constructed mainly with language, today visual elements often dominate. These forms of visual Doublespeak increasingly appear as synthesized, finely honed productions of language, visuals, music, and graphics. Those who create messages dominated by visuals understand that we think in pictures more than in language. As psychologist Rudolph Arnheim said, "We think by means of the things to which language refers—referents that in themselves are not verbal but perceptual" (1986).

The Two Emotions

More than just technology is responsible for the growth of visual Doublespeak. Another reason is that imagery is more efficient than language at eliciting and changing emotions. Some argue that images are also more effective than language in accomplishing these tasks. In the early 1960s, the Federal Trade Commission began cracking down on advertisers' false verbal claims about their products ("One bar of Zing soap is three times bigger than its competitor, for the same low price"). In response, advertisers used fewer and fewer words, to avoid being held accountable. Instead, they relied more and more on graphics, visuals, and packaging. Consequently, sales went up.

Since that time, marketing research has revealed a great deal about how our emotions interact with images. One type of this research is known as "transformational advertising," ads that first establish an emotion and then change it—all in a matter of seconds. In such research, warmth is defined as a "volatile emotion involving physiological arousal and precipitated by experiencing directly or vicariously a *love, family, or friendship relationship*" (Aaker and Stayman 1990, 54; italics added). The opposite of warmth is coolness—the absence of love, family, or friendship relationships. These two emotions are often used in visual Doublespeak.

Of course, most products, in and of themselves, do not elicit much emotion: a plastic bottle of dish soap quietly resides under your sink, and your car remains an ever-so-stoic chunk of metal. The same can be said of politics and politicians; they do not naturally arouse our emotions, nor were they ever supposed to. This is why media makers want to *transform* viewers—to help them see the object or person in question as somehow different from or better than it really is. And to make something appear better than it really is, or different from what is really is, Doublespeak does duty. For example, the three photos in Figures 3.1, 3.2, and 3.3 appeared in this same sequence in *Vanity Fair* (March 1992). Each image filled a double page.

The burning car, the refugees climbing aboard the ship, and the dying AIDS patient are three parts of a single ad from Benetton, a clothing company. Benetton invested $80 million in this campaign of news photos to promote its spring and summer fashions (*Columbia* [Missouri] *Daily Tribune*, February 14, 1992, 7A). Other than the company logo, "United Colors of Benetton," and a statement and phone number about the new catalog, no words appear with these pictures. A company spokesman did not refer to these as ads. Instead, he employed Doublespeak and called them "corporate communications."

Even a brief sequence of images, like this one, functions somewhat like film and video. First, the multiple scenes usually create some sense of

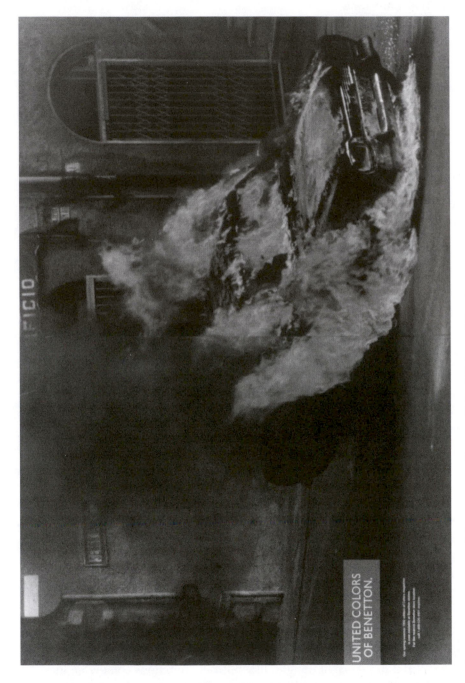

Figure 3.1. Benetton ad, burning car. Source: United Colors of Benetton.

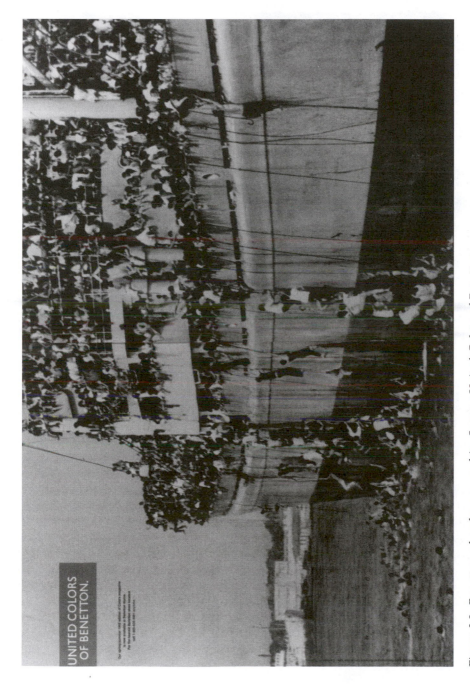

Figure 3.2. Benetton ad, refugees on ship. Source: United Colors of Benetton.

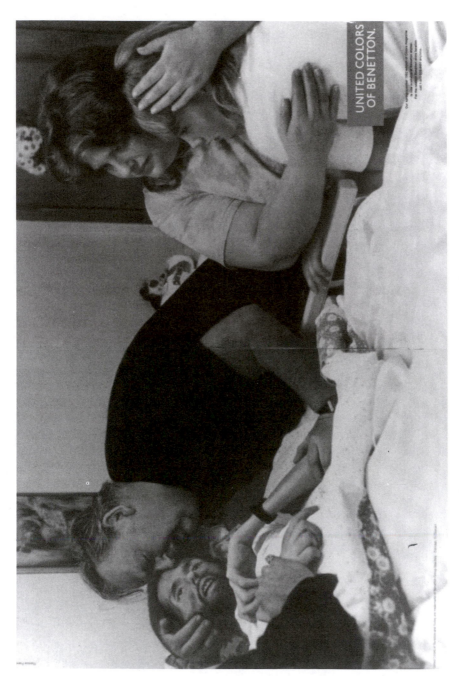

Figure 3.3. Benetton ad, dying AIDS patient. Source: United Colors of Benetton.

conflict or tension. Second, we naturally try to fill in missing information, providing our own links. This encourages us to actively invest ourselves in the scenario. Media makers know that we construct meaning in personal ways, so they often leave considerable ambiguity, allowing room for us to feed in our own associations and meanings. This internal activity is the whole point of transformational advertising.

We can begin to make some sense of this series of images by looking at it for warmth—the degree to which each scene evokes responses we normally reserve for family, friends, and other loved ones. For instance, do the scenes begin with warm ones and proceed to cooler ones? Or do they begin with cool emotions and end with warmth? This direction of emotions communicated in visual scenes is fundamentally similar to other types of messages. Shakespeare may have us feeling cool toward King Lear in the first and second acts, but regarding him with considerably more warmth by the final scene. The point is that, using no language at all, we can have our emotions aroused and directed in specific ways.

The flaming car (Figure 3.1) is a nonwarm or cool image. It communicates destruction and death—not the love, family, or friendship characteristic of warm images. As the first image in the series, the orange flames contrasting with the dark, urban streets somewhat arouse us. But we see no people, no faces of those who could be family or friends, so we are a little agitated but remain detached, viewing the scene from an emotional and physical distance—like seeing it on the six o'clock news. In this context, the burning car suggests an act of terrorism, coldly premeditated. Personally uninvolved, we are some distance away from warmth.

The second image of people clambering aboard a ship (Figure 3.2) is also mainly cool, but slightly less so than the car. This second image conveys disenfranchisement, poverty, and the struggle to survive—not the feelings of love, family, or friends evoked by warm messages. Here, we're still watching from afar, seeing boat people, foreigners, on the evening news. Also, this image is cool because we cannot see individual people, who would be more akin to our own loved ones. Instead we see only the faceless, foreign masses.

At the same time, though, this image moves us another step closer to warmth: unlike the previous burning car, where we can only imagine, not see, the victim, this image depicts people threatened, however faceless and unlike us. While eliciting an essentially cool, detached response, we at least see people—people we could more easily associate with the warmth of friends, family, and loved ones. Therefore, this image brings us nearer to warmth, but stops short.

Compared with the two images preceding it, the final double-page photo of a grieving family huddled around a dying AIDS patient (Figure

3.3) is highly emotional and warm, evoking strong feelings attached to love, family, friends. The human connections only hinted at in the burning car photo, and more strongly suggested in the boat people image, now hit us full blast. The angle of the older man's back and of the other people's hands and arms—including the patient's, as well as those in the religious painting on the wall—lead our eyes to the dying man's face and the person embracing him. These people, obviously close to one another, could easily be us. Unlike the previous two images, this is a close-up shot, positioning us not as a detached viewer of the evening newscast, but as another member of the family, closing ranks around the hospital bed. The hand extending from the foreground, grasping the patient's hand, could be our own.

In merely three scenes we undergo a transformation: from far-away to up-close; from the impersonal to the personal; from an absence of people, to faceless foreigners, and finally, to a family like ours. We move from observers to participants—members of a family, silenced and encased in grief. In only three images, we complete an internal journey, from cool to warm emotions.

However exploitative these images may be, they illustrate the power of visuals to deliver Doublespeak—to represent something as being different from what it really is. These images are Doublespeak in nature because they pretend to be news or documentary, informing us, when they are actually entertaining and persuading us. More importantly these three images provide us with an active experience that differs from the ordinary event of buying and wearing a Benetton sweater. And this little internal movement is the kind that hits closest to home, closest to the heart of our emotional lives.

The Two O. J.s

Both pictures and words can communicate negative messages as well as positive ones. Consider two of the magazine covers that depict O. J. Simpson at the height of his murder trial for the deaths of his ex-wife Nicole Brown Simpson and Ronald Goldman: for example, one from *Time* (June 27, 1994) and another from *Newsweek* (June 27, 1999). These covers demonstrate how words and pictures interact in a somewhat complex way.

Both magazines use the same police mug shot of Simpson, although *Time* (as it later admitted) darkened Simpson's face, thereby dealing the "race card." Such manipulation of images should be considered Doublespeak, too. Dark, shadowy, and unshaven, Simpson becomes "just another black man behind bars." The word "Time" even comes down low upon his face like jail bars. The implied message of this visual is clearly negative. However, the words are more positive: "An American Tragedy" suggests sympathy—the notion that Simpson himself cannot be held completely accountable for the crime—even though the verdict was not yet in when this issue appeared. Overall, the negative visual and the more positive words even out; the cover's words and image appeal to a wide range of the magazine's readers. People who might have some sympathy for Simpson will invest their belief in the headline about an American tragedy. Those who think he's guilty will have their beliefs confirmed by the sinister face behind bars.

The *Newsweek* cover employs the same strategy, only in reverse. Unlike the *Time* cover, Simpson's image is more positive: he doesn't appear nearly as dark and shadowy; nor is his head behind the bars of the magazine's title. He even looks like the proverbial deer in the headlights. However, the verbal portion, "Trail of Blood," is certainly more negative than *Time*'s "An American Tragedy." "Blood" is cast in a type size larger than any other words on the cover. These words strongly imply that Simpson is guilty. Both covers employ Doublespeak through words as well as visuals. One combines a negative picture with positive words, whereas the other uses a more positive picture with negative words. (Neither *Time* nor *Newsweek* would allow me to reprint the covers here.)

With Doublespeak, then, both pictures and words can operate in tandem, or they can wear two faces, as the magazine covers demonstrate. Of course, Doublespeak works in an infinite variety of ways—a fact that seems more natural when we remind ourselves of how deeply Doublespeak and propaganda (as well as their opposites) are embedded in American history and culture.

The Two Histories

For every event, there seem to be two histories: that which we know for sure happened, and that which we don't know. Take, for example, the 1963 assassination of President John F. Kennedy. There are the facts (all of the public information related to the case) and there are endless speculations—from paranoid scenarios to educated guesses. In the 1991 film *JFK*, director Oliver Stone exercised meticulous care and technology to fuse actual archival footage with docudrama (dramatic reenactment of scenes known to have occurred). Stone also used "speculative reenactments"—totally fabricated scenes that have no basis in documented events (Doherty 1997). The film seamlessly glides between these three levels, fusing them into an undeniable truth for the person sitting in the theater. Many viewers, especially those born after Kennedy's assassination, cannot tell where actual footage leaves off and the reenactments of actual events and the totally fabricated material begin. Or they view the entire sequence as actual footage. In other words, Stone anchors his fiction to just enough reality so that viewers believe all of his version.

Further, Stone communicates that the Zapruder film (shot by an amateur photographer) and other network TV film shot that day in Dallas is not to be trusted. Stone communicates this by enlarging these videos to fill the movie theater screen—or by allowing viewers to see them play on TV monitors in the background of certain scenes. The enlargements motivate viewers to look closely (usually for supposed untruths), and the playing of the film on TV screens in the background demonstrates to viewers the repetition and universality with which officialdom spread its lies. These techniques prod viewers to trust Stone's full-color narrative and to distrust the black-and-white, official film record. The larger point here is that images are hard to deny or negate—especially fictional images that are meticulously blended with actual ones.

The Two Lovable Phonies

The film *Primary Colors*, based on Joe Klein's novel and set during the 1992 presidential campaign, depicts candidate Jack Stanton, played by John Travolta. In the film, Stanton is accused of having an extramarital affair, just as Bill Clinton was accused by Gennifer Flowers in 1992 and by Monica Lewinsky in 1998. Stanton and his wife go on television to explain, just as the Clintons appeared on *60 Minutes* back in 1992.

After the Watergate scandal unfolded, President Richard Nixon resigned, after which we got the book and movies on the subject. This time around, though, we knew little about the actual events (Clinton's alleged behavior and possible perjury), but a whole lot about the movies. In the absence of facts, this film served them up for us, all vivid and concrete and realistic and ready to digest. This constitutes a new form of Doublespeak, because this message preempted the truth: it vividly illustrated what happened before anyone really knew what the truth was. Of course, fictional films do not claim to tell the truth; they claim the opposite. However, in the absence of truth, such expensive, vivid, high-voltage productions can fill the void more effectively than anything else. Although *Primary Colors* is fiction and set in 1992, how could we not have interpreted the film in the context of its release? To varying degrees, this film defined the truth for us—in those immediate, active, concrete ways of cinema—before this truth was ever known. It's like releasing the film *Titanic* before the real ship even leaves the dock.

The media has begun to report on this blurring (thereby allowing it to perpetuate itself). However, in so doing, it blurs things even more. *Time*'s March 16, 1998, cover featured actor John Travolta as Clinton, smiling straight-on, with an American flag behind him, his large head eclipsing most of the magazine's title at the top. The large print, one word per line, proclaims, "Lights! Camera! Clinton!" Smaller print on the cover states, "*Primary Colors* is an uncanny take on his relationships with women, the truth, and America." Oh? When this magazine appeared, we had not yet learned about these things!

Inside, the cover story's title, "A Tale of Two Bills," is set against a full-page photo that splices the left half of Travolta's face with the right half of Clinton's face, a not-so-subtle form of visual Doublespeak. The next article contains several boxed features extolling the similarities between the film and reality, such as side-by-side photos of the movie's characters and their real-life counterparts. This article blurs film and reality in more subtle ways. Consider this description of Clinton as president: "Other Presidents had an anchorman aura: authoritative, a bit square. Clinton has the urgency of a talk-show host. Or guest . . ." (Corliss 1998, 66). Also consider the words describing Jack Stanton, the fictional Clinton: "In the book and movie, Jack is a guest star. His role is not so much supporting as hovering" (Corliss 1998, 67). The metaphors here are not from history or politics, they are from TV. The reference point here is not Washington, but Hollywood; not Gerald Ford, but Harrison Ford. Not long ago, using film and TV as a basis for comparisons happened only in the tabloids (Fox 1989).

Most of us would consider this cover story of Clinton as Travolta to be quite enough, thank you. But the article that immediately follows, "The People's Choice," presents Travolta as Clinton. The accompanying photo shows Travolta sprawled across a bed (of course). Here we learn that, like Clinton, Travolta (1) has responded to "prying" questions about his sex life, which he, too, shrugs off with "roguish charm"; (2) works long and hard; and (3) consumes massive amounts of food. Travolta himself states: "I'm good at schmoozing and being very caring and tolerant . . . It's that great P.R. thing" (Ressner 1998).

If that doesn't unsettle your breakfast, try the article's conclusion. It begins by itemizing Travolta's massive wealth: "Twenty-million-dollar paydays. Four homes, three jets, cool cars." Right at this gag point comes the final blow: "The only thing that might give him [Travolta] more power might be, well, politics. Is the world ready for Candidate Travolta?" John-Boy replies as the coy politician: "I don't have a natural or innate desire to run" (Ressner 1998).

Is this a great American drama, or what? Aren't these lunky phonies lovable? Two of our all-time favorite characters, a president and a movie star, merged for their greatest, epic role. We show our adoration by pushing the pollsters' buttons. And the actors and directors respond in kind.

DOUBLESPEAK IN THE AMERICAN GRAIN

Doublespeak has long been a basic part of American life. So have the forces that fight it, which I refer to as "Anti-Doublespeak," or resistance to Doublespeak and propaganda, including messages perceived as clear, direct, honest, and unpretentious. These opposing forces are not unusual for our governing system of checks and balances, not to mention special interest groups devoted to each tide of immigrants, social classes, always-good causes, and every other conceivable stake. As John Steinbeck once observed, "Americans seem to live and breathe and function by paradox." Our long and abundant uses of Doublespeak support Steinbeck's observation.

Americans, of course, did not invent Doublespeak. We only inherited a universal, genetic condition. We could blame Aristotle, whose *Rhetoric* remains a primer in how to persuade others. Or we could pin it all on religion. After the printing press was introduced, religious publications flourished, many attempting to persuade readers to take up a particular faith. In fact, the earliest uses of the term "propaganda" can be traced to the Catholic Church, in 1662, when it founded the Congregation de propaganda fide, or "Congregation for the Propagation of Faith" (Nelson 1981, 323).

Later, Napoleon carefully cultivated his own legend, using the printing press, the arts, and the church, similar to what the French king Louis XIV had done. Napoleon imprinted his own picture on countless medals because he knew they would be widely circulated, wouldn't wear out, and would be passed on to future generations. He favored metal over painting and sculpture because coins were seen by more people than just the rich and over a longer span of time. Although he printed many dramatized scenes from his life on paper (e.g., his victorious battles, his huge suffering), he knew that art was the province of the rich and that paper soon wore out. Coins enabled Napoleon to reach the commoners.

Throughout American history, we've freely practiced Doublespeak, as well as fought against it—not unusual for a democracy that must always be at odds with itself, must always try but not always succeed, to right itself. Doublespeak is embedded within our culture, beginning with the exploits of Columbus and his dogged pursuit of slaves and gold, resulting in the decimation of the naive but cultured peoples he encountered. When Columbus and his crew landed in the Bahamas, the Arawak Indians swam out to greet them. Once the group was ashore, these natives brought them food, water, and gifts. However, later, when Columbus made this entry in his log, his motives and values seem clear:

They brought us parrots and balls of cotton and spears and many other things, which they exchanged for the glass beads and hawks' bells. They willingly traded everything they owned. . . . They do not bear arms, and do not know them, for I showed them a sword, they took it by the edge and cut themselves out of ignorance. They have no iron. Their spears are made of cane. . . . They would make fine servants. . . . With fifty men we could subjugate them all and make them do whatever we want. (Zinn 1995)

A little later, Columbus described native Haitians: "[They] are so naive and so free with their possessions that no one who has witnessed them would believe it. When you ask for something they have, they never say no. To the contrary, they offer to share with anyone" (Zinn 1995, 6). After forcing the Arawak to bring him bits of gold, Columbus captured 1,500 Arawak men, women, and children, and selected the 500 strongest to be slaves, which he sent back to Spain. Upon their arrival, a local official described the Arawak as being "naked as the day they were born" and observed that they displayed "no more embarrassment than animals." Columbus then wrote, "Let us in the name of the Holy Trinity go on sending all the slaves that can be sold" (Zinn 1995, 6). When Columbus pledges to enslave others *in the name of God*, he engages in early American Doublespeak.

By 1620 in Plymouth, Massachusetts, the leaders of the English settlers were at least conscious of Doublespeak. William Bradford, for example, promised that he would describe this experience by beginning "at the very root and rise of the same. The which I shall endeavor to manifest in a plain style; with singular regard unto the simple truth in all things, at least as near as my slender judgment can attain" (Bradford 1901). At least in print, Bradford wanted to communicate clearly and truthfully. But within several years, commercial plantation owners were creating "misleading promotional documents" to entice new workers to the area (Nelson 1981).

By the mid-1700s, America's landowning aristocracy mainly feared that those groups they were exploiting the most—the poor whites, the Indians, and the slaves—would somehow unite against them. This indeed happened in Virginia in 1676, during Bacon's Rebellion, which pitted white frontiersman, black slaves, and white servants against the white ruling class. A white ruler in the Carolinas wrote that they needed a policy to "make Indians & Negros a cheque upon each other lest by their Vastly Superior Numbers we should be crushed by one or the other" (Zinn 1995).

The ruling class resolved this dilemma by creating a wondrous invention—not liberty and equality, but the *language* of liberty and equality—not the real thing, but a representation of the real thing. The flaming prose of Thomas Paine and others was perfect for keeping poor whites, Native Americans, and black slaves off the backs of the ruling class. The patricians' patriotic rhetoric galvanized just enough poor whites to fight against Britain. At the same time, in all the ensuing fuss, slavery and inequality were maintained. Hence, early American propaganda effectively manipulated symbols for purposes of persuasion, giving birth to American Doublespeak.

A few cherished lines from America's founding documents are resolute in their directness and elegance. Even now we harbor little doubt about the forthrightness of "All men are created equal." It leaves no wiggle room for interpreting who should be treated fairly. Nor does the phrase "life, liberty, and the pursuit of happiness" seem to include anything other than the good stuff—certainly not being lied to. On the other hand, such absolute phrases from our founding documents seem like set-ups for letdown, especially for Native Americans, women, poor whites, and slaves. The term "all" seldom holds true for anything. And much of America's history since that phrase was first ingrained in our collective psyche has been devoted to evening the score, to making the words match up more closely with our actual lives.

From today's perch, it's easy to view such hallowed phrases as Doublespeak. However, back then, these words must have seemed like honest truth from sincere people. The point is that truth and Doublespeak seldom hold still for very long. When the processes of technology and culture manipulate symbols, it is harder to reflect upon and identify Doublespeak. For example, during childhood, many of us learned a seminal moral lesson through the story of George Washington. As a boy, the story goes, Washington was asked if he had cut down a tree. George responded, "I cannot tell a lie. I chopped down that cherry tree." Generations of Americans have grown up knowing that Washington—the "father of our country"—could never consider lying. I was one of them. There's no way he could have done such a thing.

The Pursuit of Life, Liberty, and Doublespeak

In some children's books, this story of Master George and the cherry tree continues, unchanged. Other authors, though, explain that it never happened. The following writer assumes the voice of Washington to set the record straight:

I suppose you've heard the story about me as a child going up to my father and saying, "I cannot tell a lie. I chopped down that cherry tree!"

Well, a parson named Weems made up that story after folks started to call me "the father of our country." He did it to teach boys and girls to be as honest as George Washington. It would have been nicer if he had been just a little more honest himself, because I never did chop down that tree! (Weinberg 1988, 2)

Let me get this straight—the story about not lying was a lie, told by a preacher? By 1995, though, not even the U.S. Forest Service believed in this morale tale. This organization could not communicate clearly about "cutting down trees" or "clear-cutting." Instead, it referred to such stripped areas as "temporary meadows" (*Independent Record*, July 25, 1993, Helena, Montana, 2A).

Okay. So Washington never cut it down, never swore off lying. He did, though, grow up to lead troops during the American Revolution—an "uprising" that was not, as we often believe, a purely spontaneous act of oppressed people. Instead, as mentioned earlier, this war was largely motivated by propaganda which functions very much like Doublespeak. These messages intensified the colonies' good qualities while downplaying the king's good qualities, and intensified the king's bad qualities while downplaying the colonists' bad qualities. This was accomplished through a propaganda campaign waged by Samuel Adams, Patrick Henry, Benjamin Franklin, Thomas Paine, and others. "Give me liberty, or give me death," the statement attributed to Patrick Henry, employs a classic propaganda technique, the two-valued orientation, which forces us to choose between two extremes, enabling us to ignore the vast middle ground. Nearly 200 years later, during the Vietnam War, the slogan "America—Love It or Leave It" showed that such either-or demands had not lost their power over American minds.

Equally relevant today are Thomas Paine's *Common Sense* (1776) and *The American Crisis* (1776–1783), which are still studied by students of Doublespeak and propaganda. These authors taught us that persuasive messages require channels to get the word out, such as their group, the Sons of Liberty. They taught us that complex concepts such as democracy and revolution had to be drastically simplified into pictures (e.g., the Liberty Tree) and catchy slogans (e.g., "Don't tread on me"). Propagandistic artwork and slogans continued into the Civil War, when envelopes were printed with drawings of soldiers on them, along with the phrase "Death to traitors!" Our country's founders also taught us about the power of staging events for public consumption (e.g., the Boston Tea Party), as well as seizing opportunities to frame the agenda for debate before one's opponents do.

This band of men and women also demonstrated how to hammer home the same message over and over—for mass audiences, as well as for special groups of "opinion leaders" such as preachers. Their methods of propaganda seem precocious for the time, because we use them so much today. We forget that this group's practical methodology—*how* they achieved their goals—is just as important as the goals themselves. We celebrate their vision but not their ways of working. Had we focused on their methods a little more, we might be less susceptible to Doublespeak today.

Throughout American history, Doublespeak and propaganda led the way. Amos Kendall is not a household name today, but he has been dubbed the nation's "first presidential public relations man" for Andrew

Jackson. Harriet Beecher Stowe's *Uncle Tom's Cabin* (1851) sold a record-breaking 300,000 copies its first year out. This antislavery novel is often credited with fueling the passions that led to the Civil War.

Once begun, the Civil War was not entirely popular in the North, as evidenced by the 1863 draft riots in New York and the "Copperhead" peace movement. Hence, the Lincoln administration introduced several methods—Doublespeak—to control public opinion, working to convince the public that the North was doing better than it really was. These included the press conference and the press pass, which were set up to censor information about battles whose outcomes favored the Confederacy. Also, organizations in the North such as the Loyal Publication Society cranked out pro-Union pamphlets. What's more, in Watergate parlance, "the highest levels of the White House" were also involved: "Lincoln personally dispatched up to one hundred special agents to Britain, along with a boatload of foodstuffs for unemployed English cotton textile workers so as to counter propaganda gains made by the Confederacy" (Nelson 1981, 325).

In the late 1890s publisher William Randolph Hearst (immortalized as Charles Foster Kane in Orson Welles's classic 1940 film *Citizen Kane*) helped foment a war between the United States and Spain. Along the way, the circulation of his newspaper, the *New York Daily World*, quadrupled its circulation. Also during this period, films were used to heat up Americans' sense of patriotism, in effect liberating Doublespeakers and propagandists from exclusive reliance on language. For instance, *Tearing Down the Spanish Flag!* (1898) depicted Americans doing just that, and movie audiences leapt to their feet in patriotic frenzy. An entire series of films called *The Campaign in Cuba* (1898) showed battle scenes of this war. Never mind that these movies were filmed in New York and New Jersey.

America's two world wars also qualify as milestones in Doublespeak. During American participation in World War I (1917–1918), the new Committee on Public Information was freely acknowledged to be in the propaganda business. Headed by an advertising executive, this group collaborated with private filmmakers, newsreel companies, and the U.S. military to carry out its official charge—to "sell the war to America." Using artists such as Charles Gibson and Norman Rockwell, this office alone cranked out more than 100 million patriotic posters and other publications.

During World War II, newsreels and posters—especially Rockwell's warm illustrations for *The Four Freedoms* posters—continued to dominate America's perception of the war. This rich diet of slogans and huge poster images created the climate conducive for America's later acceptance of television sound bites. The fact that we won World War II helped convince us that image-laden, emotional information is valid and trustworthy (Robertson 1994).

DOUBLESPEAK AND TRADITIONAL AMERICAN MYTHS

Doublespeak and our resistance to it are deeply ingrained in America's myths—those collective attitudes, frames of mind, assumptions, values, and beliefs that help control what we think, say, and do every day. The following sections explore these myths: free speech and individualism; rugged individualism; newer is always better; manifest destiny; and rags to riches. These powerful, prevalent values are often embodied in cultural representations. For example, the value of patriotism shows up in the statue in Washington, D.C., of marines hoisting the flag at Iwo Jima. Patriotism is also embodied in popular films such as *Born on the Fourth of July, Independence Day*, and *Saving Private Ryan*. The following sections speculate about how Doublespeak functions within these dominant myths and values.

Free Speech and Individualism

Freedom of speech is an inalienable American right. It runs deep in our culture. Inextricably tied up with freedom of speech is our long-standing love of individualism—of being the person we most want to be, regardless of what others think, regardless of our own status. Self-definition, of course, is closely linked to language and communication. After all, how can we be an individual without somehow communicating?

Consider the case of candidates for public office. To win elections, politicians must set themselves apart from the pack. As voters, we must not only recognize the candidate (out of a gaggle of office seekers), but also believe that she is an individual, unfettered by links to special interest groups and ideologies we may disagree with. Herein comes the rub: political candidates must accomplish this feat with multiple types of voters. Enter Doublespeak. Governor Smith may omit or downplay the truth about his position on the death penalty when he speaks to a congregation of Quakers, but he may intensify his opinion when he meets with the state highway patrol commission.

Then Governor Smith's opponent, Senator Jones, calls him on it. Voila: we now have Anti-Doublespeak, as Jones assumes the stance of righteous truth teller and public servant. Next, Governor Smith counterpunches by accusing Jones of "taking his remarks out of context," accusing or implying that Jones is really the shady character. Here, Doublespeak breeds Anti-Doublespeak and vice-versa, creating an ongoing drama of leaks and sound bites, salted to taste for public consumption. The longer this tit-for-tat cycle continues, the harder it becomes for voters to know which messages constitute Doublespeak.

Televangelists, sports stars, media celebrities, and others who must differentiate themselves in the public's eye can engage in Doublespeak and Anti-Doublespeak in a different way. In this drama, no other people are needed. When the preachers/presidents/high profilers get caught Doublespeaking, they go on TV and 'fess up, as the cleansing tears of Anti-Doublespeak open the golden gates of ethical and spiritual rebirth.

The stars of such dramas become our models. They embody what "good and successful people" are like. And because the movement from Doublespeak to Anti-Doublespeak (and vice versa) takes place as a drama, we participate in it. And if we symbolically participate in it, then we better internalize it. Although we can construct opposing interpretations of messages, they can never be entirely denied or wiped clean from the public consciousness, even though this often appears to be the case. Instead, they are folded into the thick, doughy mix of other media messages, which gradually change the texture of the whole.

As consumers of these dramas pitting Doublespeak against Anti-Doublespeak, free speech is vividly demonstrated for us, as scripted as the whole thing may be. However, this cycle ends up hurting the individual's exercise of free speech. That is, in response to these cyclic, public dramas, individuals can respond by simply withdrawing or limiting their own voices. Because we have experienced it in media, we think we've somehow done it ourselves. Another group of people interprets these cyclical dramas mainly for their entertainment value. When the fun wears thin, it is replaced by a vacuum, if not cynicism. These scenarios apply to people who conscientiously follow media messages. Many others never get this far. The longer such dramas of Doublespeak/Anti-Doublespeak unfold, and the more common they become, the more people cease to participate not only in civic life, but in the information stream. In essence, this frustration leads to a kind of demoralization. This is the invisible but destructive fallout of Doublespeak.

Rugged Individualism

In American history and myth, our heroes have been more than mere individualists; they've been *rugged* individualists. Isolated by choice or circumstance, they have been perceived as single-handedly victorious: Natty Bumpo, Daniel Boone, and Davy Crockett (alone in the wilderness); Sergeant Alvin York (alone in capturing Germans during World War I); Charles Lindbergh (alone over the Atlantic); John Wayne (alone against the bad guys—from Bataan to the Alamo); John Glenn (alone orbiting the earth); Martin Luther King Jr. (alone in jail); Rosa Parks (alone on the bus); Forrest Gump (alone on a park bench). Although these people possess an abundance of stellar personal qualities, our tendency toward hero worship, intensified through media, exaggerates them.

What's left out of these pictures are all of the other people, events, and circumstances that helped our heroes to succeed. It becomes easy for us to assume that individuals instigate all actions and changes—that hard work through social cohesion and cooperation with many different groups and individuals has nothing to do with it. The effect is that we then believe that heroic actions and truth telling are rare; that only a few special and lucky people can ever attain them.

Also, the messages surrounding these heroes, as well as the secondary media texts around them, make it seem as though their generally clear and seemingly honest communication is a greater force than it actually may be. In short, these are heroes, yes, because they do great things, but also because they seldom evade the truth. The more heroes, the more vividly Anti-Doublespeak is represented. This resultant idealism contrasts even more with Doublespeak, when it turns up, thus enhancing the appeals of rugged individualism.

For example, O. J. Simpson was admired as an athlete and African American who succeeded on his own. As hero worshippers fed by media, we remained largely ignorant of the support system that helped him attain his success. We believed in him, not in his extensive support system. Then, after he was accused of murder, the ensuing Doublespeak and propaganda observed during his criminal trial created a razor sharp contrast, in turn motivating a countermove—an Anti-Doublespeak response, which took the shape of a civil trial, in which Simpson was found guilty. Once again, the Doublespeak/Anti-Doublespeak cycle perpetuated itself.

Newer Is Always Better

Ever since the colonies broke away from England and formed their own brand-new country, Americans have believed that newer is better and that progress is newness. This attitude became entrenched because of two events—the expansion of the frontier and the growth of a free-market economy. Both movements depended on large amounts of propaganda. Northern entrepreneurs who wanted to expand their markets needed people to move in, settle, and do the work.

Although many of these settlers chose to leave their homes to try for a better life, they were also prompted by the Doublespeak mill—from misleading promotional documents promising jobs and free or cheap land to dime novels featuring Western heroes in a romanticized land. This belief that something unknown or new is inherently better directly feeds a society rooted in a free-market economy, which generates the products and services to fill these very desires for something new (whether or not we need it).

Because Europeans settled a "new" land and kept pushing the frontier westward, Americans have come to believe that such expansionism—the push toward whatever is unknown, uncharted—is our destiny. Few people could ever resist the "romance of going," even when it failed to live up to their shimmering dreams, as was often the case. Thomas Hart Benton recalls his memories of people heading west during his childhood in the early 1900s—people who had sold their land for a pittance, sometimes receiving only the cost of a train ticket west:

I expect that the majority, nomadic and romantic rather than economic minded, with their sons and daughters, drifted into tenantry, moving from place to place, getting at all times worse and worse off and ending their lives and lineage in the bitter serfdom of the sharecropper. But however they ended or whatever happened in the meantime, they were, when I knew them, young and old, filled to the brim of their souls with the romance of going—of going places that were far away and unknown and therefore full of the "promise of heaven." (Benton 1983, 70)

Since our planes and cars have largely conquered time and space, it's hard for us now to imagine the intoxications that our forebears felt when they left everything and headed west. The "romance of going" is hard to shake. But since we've already settled the West, we have to embark upon new frontiers—of information. The Conestoga wagon and riverboat gave way to the six-horse stage, which yielded to the train, plane, automobile, and space shuttle. In the main, these have yielded to electronic media.

To satisfy these instinctive urges, we now roam the back roads of the Internet. Instead of boarding a train for Big Valley, Texas, we head for an Omnimax big screen. With authentic physical adventures a relic of the past, we now seek "the romance of going" by interacting with symbols. And if our roving ancestors' dreams often delivered them to the "bitter serfdom of the sharecropper," then Doublespeak can lead us to similar impoverishments. In this way, we are much like our forebears. The vehicles and terrain may differ, but the human spirit rises and falls in the same way.

Rags to Riches

The Horatio Alger story of the poor waif selling newspapers on the street corner, working hard and eventually achieving great wealth, runs deep in American mythology. If we work hard enough, achievement and success will be ours. The role of Doublespeak in this myth is not so much that people use it to achieve success and then to hold onto it (though they often do). Instead, Doublespeak and propaganda play a far more important role in perpetuating the myth itself by presenting us with images of shimmering affluence.

Most people portrayed on television are upper middle class or rich, but we rarely see them working for a living. Ozzie Nelson never went to work. The Cartwrights, even though they owned an enormous tract and called it a "ranch," were seldom seen hauling hay for their livestock. It's hard to imagine Bob Newhart as anything except affluent—as a successful Chicago psychologist or the owner of an upscale Vermont inn. Not even a "hipster dufuss" like Kramer in the *Seinfeld* program pays cheap rent. The plain folks of *Dallas* and *Dynasty* are off the gross income charts. Shows for younger viewers, such as *Beverly Hills 90210* would have us believe that everyone lives in a beachside mansion and tools around in red sports cars. Even when a film such as *Titanic* includes a poor boy (Leonardo DiCaprio's Jack Dawson) who contrasts sharply with the fur-clad passengers lolling about in first class, viewers tend to believe that Jack—because he is smarter, kinder, and more talented than the rich dolts—will eventually surpass them in material wealth.

Americans are drenched in images of wealth, but these images seldom show how these people obtain and keep their money. Average and especially low-income people, forever bombarded by such images, feel this disparity. (When I was a young man, penniless on the streets of Los Angeles, every gleaming luxury car and morsel of food—actual or represented—seemed far more shiny, more delectable, than they ever did when I had a little money.) Overall, we compensate by purchasing items we cannot afford, which ensures our substandard existence. In this situation, it's hard for Anti-Doublespeak to gain any foothold. Television programs that do feature lower–middle class characters often trivialize them. African Americans on television who live in "the projects" are often minstrelized or recast as Steppin' Fetchit, wearing clownish clothes, speaking loudly in exaggerated dialects, rolling their eyes and mugging. When television includes Hispanic characters, they're not only poor, but they're trying to gain wealth by stealing or selling drugs. Poor white people hardly appear on television at all. When the poor are trivialized or invisible in our mass media, it's easier to believe they can pull themselves up by their bootstraps. It's even easier to believe that they don't even exist. All of these Doublespeak issues in "representation" help perpetuate the rags-to-riches myth, simultaneously shutting out Anti-Doublespeak.

DOUBLESPEAK AND EMERGING MYTHS OF TECHNOLOGY

As America's traditional values continue to evolve, new ones emerge, such as those connected to materialism, entertainment, and cultural-social egalitarianism. The first two of these are explored in the chapters devoted to Salespeak and Sensationspeak. However, the richest source of emerging American myths is technology. The following sections explore how Doublespeak perpetuates some myths about technology: Humans (and God) Hum in the Hard Drive; Technology Is Anything But a Machine; The Web Will Connect Us; Technology Will Help Us Become Individuals; and Technology Will Free Us from Drudgery.

We continue to believe that technology can answer any question and solve any problem. For the past quarter century, technology's answers and solutions keep on coming, like clowns spilling out of a Volkswagen: fax machines, cellular phones, personal computers, laptops, calling cards, telephone answering machines, e-mail, interactive television, Nintendo games, VCRs, DVDs, CD players, modems, voice mail, and more. We continue to regard the language of technology and computers as smart and cutting edge. When we built our family's house and researched kitchens, most of them were referred to as "smart kitchens," if they housed a built-in appliance or two.

After the technological explosions of the past decades, everyone became a technician. Janitors became maintenance technicians and car mechanics became automotive technicians. The word "system" has functioned the same way. A suitcase is now a travel luggage system. Diapers are antileak systems, televisions are home entertainment systems, car radios are car audio systems, car brakes and antilock brake systems, air bags are supplemental restraint systems, shampoos are hair care systems, mattresses are Posturepedic sleep systems, and even friends are support systems ("Systems" 1997). "Technicians" and "systems" suggest cleanliness, intelligence, completeness, and complexity. The effect is to reassure us that all of our messy human problems are being efficiently and neatly solved. Such Cyberspeak has become holy scripture, and technology our savior.

The popular media, of course, is a major fountain of myths about technology. A popular magazine cover blares: "The Strange New World of the Internet: Battles on the Frontiers of Cyberspace" (*Time*, July 25, 1994). Its cover depicts computer monitors (with little orange explosions on their screens) soaring through the air over a rugged moonscape, into the silver light of a misty dawn. Such visual Doublespeak helps construct myths of technology's awesome powers, as surely as ancient scribes helped construct stories of Zeus and Appollo. The past twenty years of film and television have depicted people in front of computers, feverishly diddling on keyboards, as well as scenes showing the mystery unfolding on the actor's monitor. Computers starred in the film *Mission Impossible* just as much as its human star, Tom Cruise. And where would *The X-Files*'s Mulder and Scully be without computers? We are now a society of people watching screens that depict other people watching screens. In such self-reflexive ways, technology reproduces itself and perpetuates its myths.

Of course, nobody could argue with the myriad ways in which technology has improved and saved lives, from the use of laser surgery to restore someone's sight, to the use of software that determines which types of crops will grow best in Chernobyl's soil as it recovers from nuclear radiation. The problem is the by product left in its wake, machine worship. It's hard to say whether the myths that surround technology are growing faster than the technology itself. Either way, varied forms of Doublespeak are enmeshed within the following myths of technology.

Humans (and God) Hum in the Hard Drive

Consider computer ads from the 1980s, when personal computers were still being introduced to consumers. Such messages often consisted of Doublespeak because they promised and implied things that they could not possibly deliver. This approach remains a sturdy workhorse for selling technology and creating myth. A series of ads from Amiga computers, which appeared at a crucial time during the growth of personal computers, blur the lines between what humans can do and what machines can do (*Time*, October, 30, 1989). About two-thirds of one ad is composed of a photograph of a father and son, heads together, faces smiling with optimism, eyes cast hopefully upward. The father's hand rests upon that of his ten- or twelve-year-old son's, which rests atop a computer monitor.

The largest line of print, across the top of the photo, states, "He's using it to untrap his son." The smaller text beneath the photo explains that the boy is dyslexic. According to the ad, this boy responds to print with "incomprehension," "embarrassment," and "terror." With the help of a "talking" computer, the ad states, "His son and others are able, suddenly, to 'read' by listening; able to comprehend." This boy "can now learn as fast as he can think" and even faster than that, as the ad next clarifies: "The faster Phillip races to catch up with himself, the farther the Amiga can take him: from listening to comprehending to reading to . . . who knows?" All of this is a "small miracle," the ad tells us.

Other ads in this series promise additional human and superhuman feats. In these ads, close-up shots of people's faces appear directly next to the computer screen, as they physically embrace the machine or lean on it. Above a full-page photo of a young woman hugging her computer keyboard, we learn that "She's using it to write songs," and that a bearded, British archaeologist is "using it to stop destroying history." In another ad, an executive uses his computer "to give the Pentagon what they asked for: more realism." The point is that reading and interpreting printed language and composing music and lyrics are creative activities that only humans can accomplish. Computers can quickly retrieve information, move it around and manipulate it, and categorize it, using key words. But they can't divine a love song. Nor can they analyze and interpret archaeological artifacts unearthed on the island country of Dominica.

Eight years after these ads appeared, the same myth about technology was still going strong. The hoopla surrounding the chess game between Garry Kasparov and Deep Blue, the computer, had many people believing that Kasparov was indeed playing chess with a machine. Assigning the computer a name that suggests deeply introspective intelligence is, again, using Doublespeak to oversell computers. Actually, Kasparov was playing chess against the combined efforts of thousands of scientists, engineers, teachers, programmers, technicians, and others who constructed the machine and its software.

Today, we still believe that humans live inside of hard drives. Educational Testing Service has invented "e-rater," a software program to evaluate essays written by business school students each year, for the Graduate Management Admission Test (*New York Times*, January 31, 1999, 17). However, this program only identifies a writer's use of certain words (e.g., however, therefore) and certain clause constructions (e.g., subordinate clauses). Of course, this program is useless for detecting originality, coherence, logic, sequence, irony, insight, and voice, as well as the selection and articulation of main assertions and supporting evidence, to name only a few characteristics of an active human mind engaged in creating meaning in language. Nonetheless, Doublespeak kicks into gear when ETS sells this software as "the most highly developed, holistic electronic writing assessment application to date." What is more amazing, though, is that so many people can be sold on such a bogus package. Even more amazing (and damaging) is that each year 200,000 students will be at its mercy.

Granted, computers have long since passed us in the ability to *process* information—to retrieve it, move it, manipulate it, distribute it. However, these useful but mechanical abilities have been represented—labeled, packaged, and sold—as comprising *all* of human thinking—even superhuman thinking. However, human thinking, such as inventing ideas and solving problems, is far more complex, time-consuming, organic, and deep. "Deep time" or "flow experience" (Csikszentmihalyi 1991) is required for creative thinking—time to become immersed in what we're doing, to lose our awareness of surroundings, to be oblivious of the passage of clock hours.

This type of purely internal suspension of time is unharnessed from nearly all artificial constraints—what we're supposed to be doing, what our deadlines are, and so on. Instead, we heed only our senses, which are operating in sync with each other. Such thinking and time reside at the opposite end of the spectrum from what computers can do. However, this myth of technology—that computers that can do the work of humans and God—tells us otherwise. I once participated in an institute focused on teaching faculty members about the uses of technology. One chunk of the course was labeled "Using Technology for Critical Thinking." What was addressed under this heading was Internet search engines. None of the faculty members objected to this assumption that data collection is the same thing as critical thinking.

Technology Is Everything (Except a Machine)

A common type of Doublespeak is that which calls or names something differently from what it actually is. Labels and names are powerful symbols that often help determine the behavior of whatever they "govern." Labels and names create self-fulfilling prophecies. Of course, calling a zebra an elephant doesn't make it one. But if we do it often enough, for long enough, in some ways we'll eventually come to believe that the zebra is indeed an elephant. This is the way that symbols determine perception and behavior.

To sell technology, advocates have called it different things. They have often personified technology as people and animals. For years, we've lived with our computer's mouse and bugs. The cute little rodent with the tail (a grandchild of Mickey) is something to cup our hand around. Computer bugs, though, are often little more than an overlooked software option that should have been clicked on. Over time, we've realized that these "bugs" can be monsters, ranging from exploded hard drives to systemwide catastrophes. That's likely why Microsoft employees have been told not to use this term anymore when they speak to customers. Instead, they are supposed to refer to bugs as known issues, undocumented behaviors, and design side effects ("Technology," *Quarterly Review of Doublespeak* 1998). Here, as often happens, one type of Doublespeak is replaced with another type.

An early example of personifying technology is Hal, the computer in Stanley Kubrick's film *2001: A Space Odyssey*. Viewers soon learn, though, that the calm, eerily warm voice of Hal betrays a diabolical mind. Hal has been regarded as an antitechnology statement: "Beware of sneaky computers." In another sense, as satirical or scary as Hal might be, his character nonetheless perpetuates the myth that computers can have minds of their own—human or godlike minds. Other media machines that were humanlike and had minds of their own are much more likable. Indeed, the Tin Man from *The Wizard of Oz* and R2D2 and C3PO from the *Star Wars* films are more endearing than many of media's human characters.

Personifying technology, thereby promoting it, occurs not just in media, but in real life, too. When NASA landed a spacecraft on Mars, the agency orchestrated many details to enhance its image and hence sustain or increase its federal support. The craft touched down on July 4, 1997, as Americans celebrated Independence Day and had the time to watch television. More importantly, NASA scientists and administrators communicated these scientific and technological events with the clarity, accessibility, and warmth of an exhibit at Disney World. They even anthropomorphized the small roving robot named Sojourner. This machine became not a tool, not a probe, and not a vehicle, but a space traveler with human qualities. They even assigned a gender to this machine, and even provided a romantic interest:

Rover scientist Henry Moore bragged that "She is the robotic equivalent of Neil Armstrong." Then he announced that "she's your field geologist." Moore even said that she wanted to thank the taxpayers for her existence. . . . When she went picking her way some 16 inches to the rock dubbed Barnacle Bill, deputy project manager Brain Muirhead said, "Sojourner and Barnacle Bill are holding hands." Matthew Golombek went a bit further to suggest that Sojourner "nestled up and kissed affectionately Barnacle Bill." (Goodman 1997)

This type of Doublespeak tries to transform machines into cuddly humans or animals. Through the use of Doublespeak, it tries to close the gap between what is and what the message makers want us to believe.

The Web Will Connect Us

An Internet enthusiast wrote, "A recurring vision swirls in the shared mind of the Net, a vision that nearly every member glimpses . . . of wiring human and artificial minds into one planetary soul. . . . Distributed headless, emergent wholeness becomes the social ideal" (Kelly 1994).

This writer (breathlessly) echoes a common argument: that the Web is a grand and positive force because it connects everyone, regardless of our station in life. While this may become true in the future, it also constitutes pure myth, again fostered by Doublespeak. Yes, being connected via e-mail is highly convenient and useful. But the notion of a "planetary soul"—or any kind of soul, or any kind of creative, in-depth thinking—involves more than busy electrical circuits.

Rather, explorations of "soul" involve deep thinking, as noted earlier, about a broad range of complex topics and issues. It requires face-to-face communication, physical travel, and a large number of actual, lived-through experiences, not to mention the infinite hours devoted to deep, introspective thought and communion with a wide variety of other people and texts, across time and space. Such overselling of technology involves presenting external breadth as if it were internal depth. This is the backbone myth of technology. The Internet as a "planetary soul" can be considered Doublespeak, for it puffs up and tries to make something sound better than it really is. Of course, other metaphors can describe the same thing. Another option is to think of the Internet as "just a bunch of filing cabinets" (Reese 1997).

Technology Will Help Us Become Individuals

At the same time that technology advocates tell us that we're all connected with each other (and with every morsel of information), they're also telling us that technology is developing us into unique, individuated human beings. Can both be true at the same time? The computer ads discussed earlier try to sell such individuality: the machines are presented as helping each person do his or her own thing. Each illustration focused on a specific individual, with his or her job or profession also described. Again, computers will help with the mechanical work involved in composing music or filling orders, but certainly not with the subjective, in-depth experiences necessary for an individual's creative thought and expression.

What we never hear in the awe-inspiring messages about technology is its ability to flatten, to homogenize, to make us more like everyone else. Technology helps us develop habitual patterns of perception, expectation, and response, just as any other common element of our environment. If we are dropped suddenly onto a street, we will first look for moving cars, for purposes of avoiding them. Dropped suddenly into a Web site, we will first look for a menu of options, to move to another topic. Every medium encourages its own set of perceptions, expectations, and responses. We enter into a television sitcom with expectations that the characters will engage in verbal one-upmanship. We likewise enter an Internet chat room with the expectations that we cannot see the people we speak with, and we therefore view their comments with some skepticism. Most large forces in life, from institutions to transportation, are large forces precisely because of their "leveling" effect on individuals. Technology is no exception, yet its Doublespeak would have us believe the opposite.

Another way in which technology militates against our developing individuality resides in its increasing ability to publicize our private lives. In the past, our private sins, large and small, have been ours alone to deal with. They served as powerful forces that influenced our thinking as well as our future behavior. Within our private realm, only God or some other higher being really knew the score. Technology has modified this relationship. The impeachment trial of Bill Clinton focused on the publicizing of very private events, parading them about for all to see.

Clinton's investigators, and eventually the public, became the God that observed and passed judgment.

A less obvious way in which the Internet militates against the development of individuality is its increasing power to limit serendipity (Gup 1998). Finding that which we did not expect to find, and then celebrating it, learning about it, and learning from it, is a prime shaper of our uniqueness, a major process for differentiating ourselves from others. As a high schooler, I would aimlessly wander among the bookshelves of the Kansas City Public Library, where I first discovered the work of Sartre, Pirandello, Picasso, Gauguin, Scheeler, Chagall, Miro, DeKooning, Seurat, Pollack, Warhol, and others. As a college student, I would sit on the floor of the library's stacks for hours thumbing through old, bound volumes of *Life* magazine and the *Nation*. I did all of this for no class, no assignment, no purpose, no reason. Just pure wandering in the service of wonderment.

Stumbling upon things that excited me created its own internal, powerful narrative of learning. When I first encountered the painter Marc Chagall, I was enchanted that he made his dreams into artworks (or so it appeared to me). A little later, when I discovered the film directors Ingmar Bergman and Federico Fellini, I linked what they did to what Chagall did. This linkage formed a more powerful hypothesis about the origins of art—more meaningful, authentic, and vivid than any classroom could have accomplished. I was much less a student in a classroom than I was a kid in a candy store. These experiences were all homemade and completely serendipitous, so when I struck such veins, it was internally magical. I have also realized that these episodes were significant because they were answering questions that I had not yet asked—large, important questions such as "How will I spend my life?" "How does the imaginary connect to the real?," and "What's most important or good in life?"

Finding responses—especially multiple responses—to such unasked questions was a powerful elixir in defining my individuality. The people and ideas I found tugged at the edges of who I was, moving me a little further into my own selfhood, adding flesh to the vague form of the person I wanted to become. Finally, because I found some real victories in serendipity, I learned to trust it, a trust that helps us take risks in life, extending our boundaries, learning more than if we'd remained closed tight to randomness. The point is that, aside from surfing the Net, technology is increasingly discouraging serendipity, especially for the younger people who most need to experience and trust it. As the volume of information continues to explode, the technology for selecting and focusing that information will likewise improve. We will much more easily obtain exactly what we want. Filters on information will become increasingly sophisticated, removing the true romance of random reality.

Even with current search engines that bring us abundant irrelevant information, it's not the same as people, devoid of agendas, exploring for themselves. We are losing our ability to be completely open to new ideas.

Technology Will Free Us from Drudgery

The myth that technology will liberate us from grunt work also carries the promise of what we'll do with our extra time: think grand and sublime thoughts to advance humankind and renew ourselves in leisure activities. We instantly embrace each whiz-bang piece of new or improved technology because we've learned (and been told) that technology is just another part of *us*, what Marshall McLuhan called "extensions" of us, natural appendages that make us better.

We slap these onto our lives but never ask how they change us. Is it good to own a pager so that I can see that it's Karen calling me and hence choose to avoid her? Will putting off Karen's phone call necessarily translate into additional time for relished activities? Or will not answering cause many more time-consuming dominos to fall? As Chris Ryan observes, "Faster airplanes don't mean that the businessperson has time to relax once she reaches her destination. Rather, she is simply expected to arrive sooner. And portable computers demand that she do work on the plane as well" (Ryan 1997). Does this technology make it easier to judge Karen based not on the present but on the past? The time we gain from technology is commonly offset by the large amounts of time needed for learning the technology, correcting errors we make with it, having it repaired, and, once we are skilled at using the technology for its primary purpose, learning technology for additional purposes that are not necessary.

We do these things (and more) because we're convinced that we cannot live without the latest and speediest technology. Doublespeak has often been used to intensify how fast computers are, to sell us on speed. The common term "e-mail," at two syllables, looks and sounds quick. Certainly faster than "electronic mail." If we want to make a lot of money fast, we'll engage in "e-commerce," where we can also use text that's hyper or frenetic. Metaphors of heat are increasingly applied to the Internet: from hot Web sites, to hot links, to hotbot, to flaming messages. This language implies that the Internet is smokin' fast.

We're also constantly reminded of the importance of "cyberspace." This term attempts to make electronic impulses into something real, into something they are not. Again, this is the puffery of Doublespeak. The common terms "going to" or "visiting" a Web site dramatically inflate what we actually do. We're not going anywhere, especially that quickly. We're sitting still—the opposite of going visiting—as we call up a screen on a monitor. That's all. When I played with a Viewmaster as a kid and held the circular, plastic slides of Disneyland up to the light, nobody told me I was "visiting" California, because this type of Doublespeak was not thick in the air then.

Of course, computers are fast, especially compared with, say, manual typewriters or adding long columns of numbers by hand. But beyond this now antiquated distinction, speed is of relatively little consequence: in everyday technology use, why do nanoseconds make much difference? The assumption behind all this Doublespeak is that the faster computers are, the more time we'll have for thinking great thoughts to benefit all of humanity and for enjoying ourselves in leisurely pursuits. At bottom, the appeal is to intellectual snobbery.

CONCLUSION: DOUBLESPEAK, TECHNOLOGY, AND NATURE

> Technology is the knack of so arranging the world that we don't have to experience it.
>
> —Max Frisch

When Doublespeak oversells us on technology (and Doublespeak is not the only culprit), the most serious consequence is that we increasingly distance ourselves from reality, from nature itself. Each new gizmo, each upgrade, adds another layer between people and what's real, what's natural. This is a basic process of abstracting, of taking a little bit from the whole and relying only on that, as if it were the whole. For instance, the experience of appreciating a wildflower's bright bit of color in the forest is "first-order" reality—natural. But if this experience is replaced (thanks to technology) with raising the flower in a greenhouse, we're already one step removed from the experience in the woods. If we replace this greenhouse experience with viewing the walk in the woods on a TV or computer screen, we further remove ourselves. None of these abstracted elements can stand for the entire experience of strolling in the woods: much is left out.

The further we distance ourselves from nature, the more we lose our relationships to it. For one, nature has always been our best model for how to live. If we surround ourselves with technology instead of nature, then technology becomes our model, hence perpetuating itself. Also, the further we remove ourselves from nature, the more we lose our sense of mystery about it—and there's plenty left to wonder about. The boy who is wired to a Nintendo game is less likely to become awestruck, wondering about his place within a black sky peppered with white stars. Such enigmas have always been our given, our root, our basis. Detachment from nature reduces our opportunities for asking the big questions,

questions that always need asking: Who are we? Where did we come from? Where are we going?

TOMORROW'S ROUGH BEAST

Doublespeak often "intensifies" something. Doublespeak might enable a political candidate to sound better than she really is by making much ado about her work with abused and needy children. By the same token, Doublespeak can downplay something. It can present the same candidate as not responsible for something she actually said or did. Her campaign, for example, may never mention that she owns a clothing factory in Venezuela that violates child labor laws. Therefore, here is one effective, simple way to combat such Doublespeak: if you detect that something is being intensified (through repetition, placement, choices of language, symbols, medium, etc.), your immediate response should be to downplay it. If, on the other hand, you believe that something is being downplayed (through omission, language and symbol choices, etc.), your first response should be to intensify and find out more about it (Rank 1976). However, larger, often ignored issues are involved in fighting tomorrow's Doublespeak. First, Doublespeak and Orwell's notions can seem old hat. His futuristic novel is more than a half-century old, and Big Brother never showed up in quite the guise that Orwell predicted or that readers imagined. Nonetheless, it's becoming easier to see ourselves in Orwell's characters.

To successfully combat Doublespeak, we have to do three things. First, we have to be aware of it. Second, we have to spot it before it does any damage; hence, we must have *time*. Third, we must have context to identify Doublespeak—the most relevant information surrounding it. At millennium's shift, when our need for awareness, time, and context meet continuous explosions in technology and information, we seem to be headed toward more, not less, Doublespeak.

Our collective awareness of Doublespeak occurs in cycles. History tells us that we'll pay attention to it only when major events finally grab us by the gut. The use of the "Big Lie" and other techniques by Adolf Hitler and Joseph Goebbels (the Nazi minister of propaganda) beginning in the 1930s alerted us to large-scale manipulation, leading to the establishment of the Institute for Propaganda Analysis in 1939. Other waves of interest in Doublespeak have followed—after the Korean War (because of the Chinese Communists' "brainwashing" of prisoners of war) and after the Watergate scandal during Richard Nixon's presidency (when burglary became "surreptitious entry"). We tend to forget all about Doublespeak unless it shows up as a crude, bloody beast, clawing at the door. And with so much information competing for our time and energy, Doublespeak, to get our attention, will have to come rougher and beastlier than before.

Second, Doublespeak is likely to thrive in the future because communications technology shrinks time faster than you can say "Huh?—what happened?" We live in a land with an infinite amount of words and numbers, all in perpetual motion at eye-blinking speeds. An event can occur in the Mideast and our country can respond to it in nearly the same time that the average American hears about it. We do not know whether these events and our government's responses to them have been planned ahead of time. And this question diminishes in importance when it all becomes a done deal—when it becomes "old news" within a few hours. Why would Jason write his senator, opposing the bombing of Istanbul, if it's already happened and five other events have followed on its heels, distracting him? With technology's shrinking of time comes a corresponding shrinking of public memory and participation.

Finally, Doublespeak will bloom profusely in the future because the basic structure of our information world has become much like the basic structure of Doublespeak itself. Let me explain. Doublespeak succeeds when we hold at least two contradictory notions in mind at once—what we believe something to be, and what the message is telling us it is. We'll get better at this for two main reasons. The first reason is that our culture, time and again, has accepted or tolerated doublethink. For example, O. J. Simpson can be declared not guilty by one jury, yet guilty by another. Marshall Applewhite and his Heaven's Gate followers can devote their lives to the rationality of computers on the one hand, yet make elaborate plans (including mass suicide) to reappear with aliens from outer space. Although there are great benefits to holding opposing realities in mind at the same time, tolerance for Doublespeak is not one of them.

A second reason we'll get even better at accepting the opposing realities inherent in Doublespeak is that our information glut provides us no choice. The sheer quantity of information, of context, guarantees that—no matter what the question or issue—we'll likely find answers that do not agree with each other. We have learned to accept contradictions as part of life. In many cases, this isn't a bad thing. It does, though, make it much harder for us to sort the shams from the other options, which is time-consuming, hard work. In short, the more information, the more options. And the more options, the more likely that assertions will contradict each other. Consequently, contradictions or fragmentation will become the norm. And if they're the norm, who will care? Said another way, if we find a part (an assertion about the world) that doesn't fit the whole (its information context), then we can either find another part that *does* match the context, or find another context to slap together with the part and make 'em fit. Technology makes this a breeze.

A third reason that Doublespeak will continue to rise is again related to having too much information. Under ordinary circumstances, more information and more options help us make sounder judgments. Faced with three brands of soap in the grocery aisle, we can compare and make a better decision than if we had only one or two choices. But faced with 564,873 brands, we give up. The greater the pile of information before us, the greater the amount of irrelevant information. The data glut—or too much context—can so overpower us that we close our eyes and grab one, for they have all become the same, even though they are not.

Another effect of data glut is that the information that "gets through," that pierces our selective perception, is that which is most carefully honed and crafted. Such messages are hugely expensive. So, swamped in information, we are likely to (1) pay attention to the well-financed message that has been crafted to break through; (2) focus on irrelevant information, because the odds favor this; or (3) ignore most or all of the information. All of these scenarios are conducive to Doublespeak, to the manipulation of humans by other humans using symbols.

THE CAT IN THE DARK

"I'm truly sorry about your cat," the man softly consoles. "We did all we could for her."

"Yes, of course. Thank you. But I do have a question."

"Yes?"

"When I got the news and went to pet her one last time, I noticed that both of her eyes looked like they had been sewn shut. I don't get it. What's going on here?

"Oh, yes, that. Not to worry. That was just binocular deprivation, an exploratory, health-effects procedure."

Doublespeak, the evil voice, often overlaps with the other voices described in the chapters ahead. Doublespeak is evil, or destructive, because, when all of the qualifications and complexities have been illuminated, most Americans cannot accept being lied to. We ultimately veer toward our internal sense of truthfulness. This is good. On the other hand, all of us engage in Doublespeak. It's a human impulse and depends upon context. We would not say to a friend, "Sorry that your grandmother is dead." Instead, we might whisper, "I'm sorry to hear about your loss," even though "loss" is a euphemism for 'death.' The use of the term "loss" is quite different from using "binocular deprivation," a phrase actually used to describe sewing a cat's eyes shut for purposes of animal experimentation.

Again, the best way to evaluate Doublespeak is to determine its effects on the public: "How many people will suffer and to what extent?" It often boils down to how people with power—social, cultural, economic, or political power—use symbols. Government and military leaders who use words such as "incursion," "protective reaction," "pacification," and "systems" to sell and wage war do so at a high cost to many people.

Most of the time, as long as Doublespeak breathes life, so, too, does Anti-Doublespeak. But not always. Some wars, such as the Persian Gulf War, can be so well planned, well packaged, well managed, and fast (thanks to high tech) that we're well into it before we are aware of even a few dissenting voices. And even then, such voices mainly serve to "inoculate" us from hearing more or louder voices. That is, if we hear a few rattlings, we figure that dissent has not been stifled. Thus reassured, we go about our easier, already-established ways. Most of all, though, fighting Doublespeak may depend not just on our ability to see it, but upon our own willingness to feel outrage, to cast light outside of us as well as within.

Salespeak

No profit whatsoever can possibly be made but at the expense of
another.

—Michel de Montaigne, "Of Liars," 1580

WHAT IS SALESPEAK?

Salespeak is any type of message surrounding a transaction between
people. First Salespeak is persuasive in nature. It can convince us to
purchase products and services. It can also persuade us, directly and
indirectly, to "buy into" political candidates, beliefs, ideologies, attitudes,
values, and lifestyles. Salespeak persuades by presenting us with facts,
where logic, language, and numbers dominate the message. More often,
though, it persuades by massaging us—entertaining and arousing us,
and changing our emotions with imagery, sound effects, and music.

Second, Salespeak can function as a type of entertainment or escapism—as an end in itself, where we are more focused on the experiences
surrounding consumerism (e.g., browsing through an L. L. Bean catalog)
than we are on actually purchasing something. Salespeak occurs when
messages are crafted so as to "hit" a specific, "targeted" audience.
Therefore, Salespeakers collect and analyze information about their audiences to help them shape their messages.

Third, Salespeak usually employs a systematic approach in targeting
its audience. A theme for Boltz laundry detergent, such as, "It's white
as lightning!" might unify different types of messages communicated

through different channels. The goal here is to create "overlapping fields of experience" (Ray 1982), hitting us from several sides in different ways, in short, to create an "environment" of persuasion. In this chapter, Salespeak also includes any type of message about transactions between people, such as a market report describing a specific group of consumers.

We live in a market-driven economy in which we consume more than we produce. It's little wonder, then, that Salespeak flows constantly—from television, billboards, print ads, and blinking Internet messages. Because Salespeak touches nearly every area of life, its infinite tones and painstakingly crafted imagery appear in an endless variety of forms. Salespeak ranges from the hard-sell radio pitch of the local Ford dealer to the vague, soft, amorphous TV commercial that merely wants you to know that the good folks at Exxon care.

Salespeak includes the envelope in your mailbox that states, "God's Holy Spirit said, 'Someone connected with this address needs this help.' " Salespeak ranges from the on-screen commercial loops playing on the ATM machine while you wait for your cash, to the plugs for car washes that appear on the screens affixed to the gas pump as you fill up your car. Salespeak even shows up in slot machines designed to entice children (Glionna 1999). These slots for tots now feature themes such as Candyland, Monopoly, the Three Stooges, the Pink Panther, and South Park. This is the gaming industry's attempt to promote a "family-friendly" image, which will help ensure that future generations will support the casino industry (Ruskin 1999). Salespeak also sprouts from the "product information" about a new computer embedded within the instructions for installing a software program, from the camera shot in a popular film that lingers on a bag of Frito's corn chips, and from the large sign inside Russia's *Mir* space station that states, "Even in Space . . . Pepsi is Changing the Script." Salespeak is indeed the script, on earth as it is in heaven.

A DAY IN THE LIFE

At 6:03 A.M., Mrs. Anderson's voice comes over the intercom into her teenaged daughter's bedroom. Mrs. Anderson asks, "Pepsi? It's time to wake up, dear. Pehhhp-si . . . are you up and moving?"

Pepsi answers groggily, "Yeah . . . I'm up. Morning, Mom." As Pepsi sits up in bed, she reaches over and hits the button on her old pink Barbie alarm clock, which rests on her old American Girl traditional oak jewelry box. As both cherished items catch her eye, she pauses and wistfully recalls those happy days of girlhood, rubbing her hand over the *Little Mermaid* bedsheet. If only she hadn't given away her favorite purple My Little Pony to her best childhood friend, Microsoft McKenzie, who lives next door.

Just then her mother's voice calls her back to reality, "Good deal, sweetie. Let me know when you finish your shower. I just got your Gap sweatshirt out of the dryer, but I couldn't get that Gatorade stain out of your Tommy Hilfiger pants, so I'm washing them again."

Once upstairs, Pepsi sits down for a bowl of Cap'n Crunch cereal. She peels a banana, carefully pulling off a bright yellow sticker, which states, "ABC. Zero calories." She places the used sticker onto her McDonald's book cover. Pepsi's younger brother, Nike, dressed in his Babylon Five T-shirt, places a Star Trek notebook into his Star Wars book bag as he intently watches the Amoco morning newscast on the video wall. The network anchor tells about the latest corporate merger as he reads from his perch within the "N" of the giant MSNBC logo. Then Mrs. Anderson walks into the nutrition pod.

Mrs. Anderson: Hey, Peps, what's going on at school today?

Pepsi: Nothing much. Just gotta finish that dumb science experiment.

Mrs. Anderson: Which one is that?

Pepsi: That one called "Digging for Data." We learned about scientific inquiry stuff and how to deduce conclusions. We learned that American settlers were short because they didn't eat enough meat and stuff like that.

Mrs. Anderson: Oh, yes! That was one of my favorites when I was in school. Those National Livestock and Meat Board teaching kits are wonderful! I liked it even better than Campbell Soup's "Prego Thickness Experiment." How 'bout you?

Pepsi: I dunno. Everyone already knows that Prego spaghetti sauce is three times thicker and richer than Ragu's sauce.

Mrs. Anderson: Well, yes, of course they do. But that's not the only point. There are larger goals here, namely, your becoming the best high-volume consumer possible. Isn't that right, dear?

Pepsi: Yeah, I guess so.

Pepsi's school bus, equipped with the latest electronic wraparound billboard, mentions that the price of Chocolate Cheetah Crunch "is being sliced as you read this—down to $48.95 per ten-pounder!" Pepsi takes her seat and discusses this price reduction with her locker partner, Reebok Robinson. They engage in a lively conversation about which of them loves Cheetah Crunch more. Next, the screen on the back of the seat in front of them catches their attention: a large dancing lamb sings, "Be there! Tonight only! At the IBM Mall! All remaining Rickon collectibles must go! Pledge bidding only! Be there!" Even Reebok cannot contain a squeal.

At school, Pepsi watches Channel One, the National Truth Channel, during her first three classes. The first news story documents the precise steps in which Zestra, the new star of the Z-5 Lectradisk corporate communication spots, went about purchasing her new video wall unit. Afterward, Pepsi and her peers receive biofeedback printouts of their responses registered during this program via the reaction console on their desks. Next, the students use voice-print technology to describe what they were feeling during the broadcast.

Then their teacher, Ms. Qualcomm, tells them to take a twenty-minute recess at the Commoditarium before they return for Tech Lab, where they will begin the unit "Product Scanning: Art or Science?" At the Commoditarium, Pepsi purchases one bag of Kwizzee sticks, one can of Channel One soda, and a One-der Bar, in addition to a pair of Golden Arch earrings she can't live without. The accessories for the earrings, which she also longs for, will have to wait.

Back at Tech Lab, Pepsi and her peers receive a half hour of AT&T ("Allotted Time & Testing," sponsored by AT&T, in which students are free to explore their own interests on the GodNet.) In the upper-left corner of her computer screen, Pepsi watches what appears to be an enlarged part of human anatomy, alternately shrinking and enlarging, as one of her favorite new songs beats in sync. The olfactory port of her computer emits a musky odor. In the background of this pulsating image, sticks of lightning flare randomly against a deep blue sky. Pepsi looks at them more closely and detects that each one contains three small letters: A, T, and T. She smiles, points, and clicks on the window.

Immediately, this message forms on screen in large, puffy blue letters: "A, T, & T Loves You." Then the message begins dissolving and enlarging simultaneously, so that the background is now the same blue as the message. Huge lips fill the screen. Pepsi is unsure whether they are the lips of a man or woman. The lips slowly murmur, "You, Pepsi . . . You're the one . . . Oh, yes . . . Nobody else. Just you."

Pepsi, mesmerized, half whispers to herself, "Me?" as the lips fade at the same time that the blue background re-forms into the previous message, "A, T, & T Loves You." Pepsi clicks again. Three golden books appear on screen. One is titled "A, T, & T's Pledge to You, Pepsi Anderson." Another one is titled, "Making Love Rich," and the third is titled, "Us . . . Forever." The lights of the Tech Lab dim, signaling students that it's time to begin their new unit. The lights slowly fade out until the lab is nearly dark. Pepsi hears muffled patriotic music from the opposite side of the room—a flute and drum, playing the tune of "Yankee Doodle Dandy." From the far end of the ceiling, an image of the traditional "fyfe and drum corps"—the three ragged soldiers in Revolutionary Army garb—come marching across the screen; above the U.S. flag flies a larger one, with a golden arch on it.

As the tattered trio exit via a slow dissolve on the opposite end of the ceiling screen, the room goes completely dark. Pepsi twists her head and limbers up, as her classmates do, almost in unison. Then, on instinct, Pepsi and her peers look upward to the neon green and pink Laser Note swirling above them: "To thine own self, be blue. And rakest thou joy into thine own taste sphere! Tru-Blu Vervo Dots: now half price at Commoditarium!" A laser image of Shakespeare forms from the dissolving lights. Next, the bard's face dissolves into blue Vervo Dots. Pepsi, feeling vaguely tired and hungry, saves her place on screen so she can return later to find out what's in the three golden books. Before she exits, she is automatically transferred to another screen so that she can input her biofeedback prints from the past half hour.

At home that night, Pepsi and her family gather in the Recipient Well. To activate the video wall, Mrs. Anderson submits a forehead print on the ConsumaScan. Before any audio can be heard, a Nike logo appears on the screen for two minutes. Mrs. Anderson turns to her daughter.

Mrs. Anderson: So, Peps, you were awfully quiet at dinner. Are you okay? Everything all right at school?

Pepsi: Fine. I just get tired of learning all the time.

Mrs. Anderson (sighing): Well, sweetie, I know. Things are so much different nowadays than when I was your age. You kids have to work harder in school because there are so many more products and services to keep up with.

Pepsi: Yeah, I guess so. . . .

Mrs. Anderson: But you've also got many luxuries we never had. Why, when I was born, parents were completely ignorant about giving their children beautiful names. My family just called me "Jennifer." Ugh! Can you believe it?

Pepsi: Oh, gag me, Mom! "Jennifer"?! You're kidding! How did you and Dad name me?

Mrs. Anderson: Well, let's see. . . . We first fell in love with your name when Pepsico offered us a lifetime membership at the Nova Health Spa if we'd name you "Pepsi." I thought it was so refreshing—not to mention thirst quenching and tasty. Besides—it's your generation!

Pepsi: And I'll always love you and Dad for bestowing me with eternal brandness . . .

Mrs. Anderson: It's just because we love you, that's all. Growing up branded is a lot easier these days—especially after the Renaissance of 2008, just after you were born.

Pepsi: What was that?

Mrs. Anderson: You know—*life cells*! We got them a few years after the Second Great Brand Cleansing War.

Pepsi: But I thought we always had life cells, that we were just born with 'em. . . .

Mrs. Anderson: My gosh, no, girl! When I was your age we had to stay glued to National Public Radio to keep up with the latest fluctuations of the NASDAQ and high tech markets.

Pepsi: Jeez . . . I can't imagine life without life cells.

Mrs. Anderson: Me either—now! Back then, it all started with Moletronics and the first conversions of Wall Street datastreams into what they used to call "subcutaneous pseudo-neurons." But that's ancient history for you!

Pepsi: Mom?

Mrs. Anderson: Yes, dear?

Pepsi: Can we set aside some special family time, so we can talk about that relationship portfolio with AT&T?

Mrs. Anderson: Well, of course! Maybe during spring break at the cabin? That's not the kind of thing we ever want to slight.

At this moment, the video wall's audio activates. The Nike swoosh logo forms into a running cheetah as a male voice-over states, "Nike Leopard-Tech Laser Runners. Be the Cheetah you were born free to be." Mrs. Anderson turns back to her daughter and asks, "Would you mind running to the Pantry Pod and seeing if there's any more of that Chocolate Cheetah Crunch left?" "Sure," says Pepsi, turning as she leaves the room, "*If* we can talk about those new shoes I need."

OVERVIEW

Is Pepsi's world already here? That's what the next section addresses. After that, "Notes from the World of Salespeak" provides a series of brief facts to illustrate the expanding boundaries of this voice. Next, "Zeroing In on Zippies: Salespeak and Audience Analysis" explores some of the approaches used by marketing research to influence human behavior. I next examine how Salespeak can affect our physical, emotional, social, and cultural health. Salespeak's deep roots in American history are explored in "Salespeak in the American Grain," before I consider how Salespeak relates to traditional American myths and values, as well those that are emerging. After discussing some major conclusions (ranging from "McCulture" to environmental concerns), I offer several recommendations, which include legislation, litigation, and education.

IS PEPSI'S WORLD ALREADY HERE?

Yes. Most of what happens to Pepsi in this scenario is based on fact. A few other parts are extensions or exaggerations of what already occurs in everyday life. Let's begin with a girl named Pepsi. In Pepsi's world of Salespeak, nearly every facet of life is somehow linked to sales. Pepsi, the girl, lives in a Pepsi world, where person, product, and hype have merged with everyday life.

Salespeak is all-powerful. As small children, as soon as we become aware that a world exists outside of ourselves, we become a "targeted audience." From then on, we think in the voices of Salespeak. We hear them, we see them. We smell them, taste them, touch them, dream them, become them. Salespeak is often targeted at young people, the group marketers most prize because first, they spend "disposable" income, as well as influence how their parents spend money (see the following section, "Notes from the World of Salespeak"); second, people tend to establish loyalties to certain brands early in life; and third, young people are more likely to buy items on impulse. For these reasons and more, Salespeak is most prevalent and vivid for children and young adults. Hence, most of this chapter focuses on the layers of Salespeak that surround these groups. The core issue is targeting kids in the first place, regardless of the product being sold.

What's in a Name?

At this writing, I've neither read nor heard of a human being legally named after a product or service (though I feel certain that he or she is out there). I have, though, heard that school administrators in Plymouth, Michigan, are considering auctioning off school names to the highest bidder. It's only a matter of time before kids attend "Taco Bell Middle School" or "Gap Kids Elementary School" (Labi 1999). Appropriating names—and hence identities—is essentially an act of aggression, of control over others' personal identity. Our practice of naming things for commercial purposes is not new. Consider San Diego's Qualcomm Stadium. Unlike St. Louis's Busch Stadium or Denver's Coors Field, the name Qualcomm has no connections to people or things already traditionally linked with baseball. In Pepsi's world, "AT&T" stood for "Allotted Time for Testing." To my knowledge, commercial or corporate names have yet to be used for identifying processes. However, they have been used to identify specific places where educational processes occur.

For example, the Derby, Kansas, school district named its elementary school resource center the GenerationNext Center. The district agreed to use the Pepsi slogan to name their new facility, as well as to serve only Pepsi products, in exchange for one million dollars (Perrin 1997, 1A). Even ice cream is now named so that it can advertise something else: the name of Ben and Jerry's butter almond ice cream is called "Dilbert's World: Totally Nuts" (Solomon 1998a).

Every time we see or read or hear a commercial name, an "impression" registers. Advertising profits depend on the type and number of impressions made by each ad message. Therefore, Pepsi Anderson and her friend, Microsoft McKenzie, are walking, breathing, random ad messages. (Similar important names) are now devised solely for purposes of advertising. Nothing more. Such names become ads. In earlier times and in other cultures, as well as our own, names were sacred: they communicated the essence of our identity, not just to others but to ourselves as well. To rob someone of her name was to appropriate her identity, to deny her existence. In *I Know Why the Caged Bird Sings*, Maya Angelou speaks of how demoralizing it was for African Americans to be "called out of name" by white people, who would refer to any African American male as "boy," "Tom," or "Uncle."

Similarly, several years ago, the rock musician and composer known as Prince changed his name to a purely graphic symbol. The result, of course, was that nobody could even pronounce it! By default he became known as "The Artist Formerly Known as Prince." In an interview on MTV, this musician-composer explained that the public believed he was crazy because print and electronic media had proclaimed him so, over and over. He therefore changed his name to something unpronounceable to halt this labeling. It worked. In effect, this man regained control of his own life because he found a way to stop others from controlling it for him, as they were doing by writing about him in the media. This man understands the general semantics principle that the word is not the thing symbolized—that the map is not the territory (see Chapter 2, "Making Sense of MediaSpeak").

The long-term effects of replacing real names with commercial labels (of important spaces, processes, and possibly even people) can benefit nobody except those doing the appropriating—those reaping revenue from increased sales. At the very least, this practice demonstrates, in concrete, definitive ways, that we value materialism and the act of selling above all else.

Celebrating Coke Day at the Carbonated Beverage Company

At century's end, the question is not "Where and when does Salespeak appear?" Rather, the real question is, "Where and when does Salespeak *not* appear?" Only in churches and other places of worship? (Not counting, of course, the church that advertised itself by proclaiming on its outside message board: "Come in for a faith lift.") Salespeak is more than a voice we hear and see: we also wear it, smell it, touch it, play with it. Ads on book covers, notebooks, backpacks, pencils, and pens are common. So are the girl Pepsi's Gap sweatshirt, Tommy Hilfiger pants, Barbie alarm clock, and *Little Mermaid* bedsheets. The bulletins that Pepsi and her classmates received about current sales are also authentic: Pepsico has offered free beepers to teens, who are periodically contacted with updated ad messages.

Salespeak is seeping into the smallest crevices of American life. As you fill your car with gas, you can now watch commercials on a small screen on the gas pump. As you wait for your transaction at the ATM machine, you can view commercials. As you wait in the switchback line at an amusement park, you can watch commercials on several screens. As you wait in your doctor's office, you can read about medicines to buy, as well as watch commercials for them. As you stand in line at Wal-Mart's customer service desk, you can watch ads for Wal-Mart on a huge screen before you. As you wait for the phone to ring when making a long-distance call, you'll hear a soft, musical tinkle, followed by a velvety voice that intones, "AT&T."

As your children board their school bus, you'll see ads wrapped around it. When you pick up a bunch of bananas in the grocery store, like our friend Pepsi in the earlier scenario, you may have to peel off yellow stickers that state, "ABC. Zero calories." When you call a certain school in Texas and don't get an answer, you'll hear this recorded message: "Welcome to the Grapevine-Colleyville Independent School District, where we are proudly sponsored by the Dr. Pepper Bottling Company of Texas" (Perrin 1997).

Salespeak also commonly appears under the guise of school "curriculum"—from formal business-education partnerships, to free teacher workshops provided to introduce new textbooks. Corporate-produced "instructional materials" are sometimes thinly veiled sales pitches that can distort the truth. The curriculum unit "Digging for Data" mentioned earlier as part of Pepsi's school day, is actual material used in schools.

For another "learning experience," students were assigned to be "quality control technicians" as they completed "The Carbonated Beverage Company" unit, provided free to schools by PepsiCo. Students taste-tested colas, analyzed cola samples, took video tours of the St. Louis Pepsi plant, and visited a local Pepsi plant (Bingham 1998, 1A). Ads have even appeared in math textbooks. *Mathematics: Applications and Connections*, published by McGraw-Hill, and used in middle schools, includes problems that are just as much about advertising as they are arithmetic—salespeak masquerading as education. Here's a sample decimal division problem: "Will is saving his allowance to buy a pair of Nike shoes that cost $68.25. If Will earns $3.25 per week, how many weeks will Will need to save?" Directly next to this problem is a full-color picture of a pair of Nike shoes (Hays 1999). The 1999 edition of this book contains the following problem: "The best-selling packaged cookie in the world is the Oreo cookie. The diameter of the Oreo cookie is 1.75 inches. Express the diameter of an Oreo cookie as a fraction in simplest form." It seems no accident that "Oreo" is repeated three times in this brief message; repetition is an ancient device used in propaganda and advertising. More insidious is the fact that such textbooks present the act of saving money for Nike shoes as a *natural* state of affairs, a given in life. Requiring captive audiences of kids to interact with brand names in such mentally active ways helps ensure product-identification and brand-name loyalty during kids' future years as consumers.

Some schools slavishly serve their corporate sponsors. After sealing a deal with Coca-Cola, a school in Georgia implemented an official "Coke Day" devoted to celebrating Coca-Cola products. On that day, Mike Cameron, a senior at the school, chose to exercise his right to think by wearing a T-shirt bearing the Pepsi logo. He was promptly suspended ("This School Is Brought to You By: Cola? Sneakers?" 1998, 11A).

This intense focus on selling products to a captive audience of students is illustrated by the following letter sent to District 11's school principals in Colorado Springs, Colorado. The letter was written by the district's executive director of "school leadership." In September 1997, the district had signed an $8 million contract with Coca-Cola (Labi 1999).

Dear Principal:

Here we are in year two of the great Coke contract. . . .

First, the good news: This year's installment from Coke is "in the house," and checks will be cut for you to pick up in my office this week. Your share will be the same as last year.

Elementary School	$3,000
Middle School	$15,000
High School	$25,000

Now the not-so-good news: we must sell 70,000 cases of product (including juices, sodas, waters, etc.) at least once during the first three years of the contract. If we reach this goal, your school allotments will be guaranteed for the next seven years.

The math on how to achieve this is really quite simple. Last year we had 32,439 students, 3,000 employees, and 176 days in the school year. If 35,439 staff and students buy one Coke product every other day for a school year, we will double the required quota.

Here is how we can do it:

1. Allow students to purchase and consume vended products throughout the day. If sodas are not allowed in classes, consider allowing juices, teas, and waters.
2. Locate machines where they are accessible to the students all day. Research shows that vender purchases are closely linked to availability. Location, lo-

cation, location is the key. You may have as many machines as you can handle. Pueblo Central High tripled its volume of sales by placing vending machines on all three levels of the school. The Coke people surveyed the middle and high schools this summer and have suggestions on where to place additional machines.

3. A list of Coke products is enclosed to allow you to select from the entire menu of beverages. Let me know which products you want, and we will get them in. Please let me know if you need electrical outlets.

4. A calendar of promotional events is enclosed to help you advertise Coke products.

I know this is "just one more thing from downtown," but the long-term benefits are worth it.

Thanks for your help.

John Bushey
The Coke Dude
(Bushey 1998)

With visionary leaders such as "The Coke Dude" to inspire them, students will be well prepared to perpetuate a world ruled by Salespeak. Of course, Pepsi (the girl), Mike (the actual student expelled for wearing a Pepsi T-shirt), and their fellow students did not begin encountering ads in high school. It begins much earlier.

Adopting Action Figures with Attitude

Advertisers aim at babies and small infants through their parents. For example, a California company sells milk bottles used for feeding babies that are designed to look like bottles of Pepsi, Diet Pepsi, 7 UP, Dr. Pepper, Mountain Dew, and Orange Slice ("Rock-A-Buy Baby" 1994). Salespeak begins in the crib. But it really cranks up for kids when they begin watching television and movies and playing with toys.

Very young children are not prone to remembering the name of a product. Nor are they inclined to memorize a list of reasons why a product might be a good one, or better than another one. Therefore, Salespeak aimed at the very young is drenched with "personality"—a clearly defined character with specific, easily identifiable qualities. In a word, "attitude." For example, Tony the Tiger growls benignly and roars, "G-r-r-e-a-t!" The personality can be linked directly to the product, as Tony the Tiger or Bullwinkle the moose are linked to cereal. Or the products can flow from a personality already entrenched, such as the dolls that streamed from Disney's *Little Mermaid* movie character Ariel, or the *Little Mermaid* sheets that adorned Pepsi's bed. In the larger context, most toys are essentially ads that kids can play with—Salespeak for other toys, films, and assorted items. Like the larger information environment, the world of children's toys is highly *intertextual*: one toy or message carries "traces" of additional toys and messages.

Stephen Kline (1993) describes how such "character marketing" influences kids' behavior when playing. For example, when kids play with a G. I. Joe or Hulk Hogan doll (the Salespeak term is "action figure" because it's aimed squarely at boys), they get much more than the toy itself and even more than all the "accessories" and other toys connected to it. They also get all the background material from the media attached to the toy—all the rules, rituals, manners of speaking, attitudes, lifestyles, and values created for the toy. Kline's research concludes that kids playing with such toys obeyed the rules of right and wrong communicated by the toys and their histories from previous TV programs.

Kline also concludes that kids do not "mix" or integrate the world view of one set of toys, such as G.I. Joe, with another set, such as Ninja Turtles. Because the Salespeak for toys clearly segments the market between boys and girls, and hence delivers a different set of rules carried by the toys and media back stories, kids often don't play with members of the opposite sex. Carrie McLaren (1997b) observes that kids would "find it easier playing together with a large cardboard box than with action figures." She's right: a large box is much more open-ended. But discarded boxes don't make money.

As a college freshman, I once attended a lecture given by Art Linkletter, who starred in the old, popular TV series "Art Linkletter's House Party" and authored the bestselling book *Kids Say the Darndest Things*. (I had time to kill between classes.) He told his small audience how a group of California businessmen had recently asked him to run for governor of California. Linkletter said the group told him he wouldn't have to do much—they'd do all the work for him, they just wanted him to run. Linkletter, of course, asked them, "Why me?" The men responded in words to this effect: "Art, everybody knows your face; everybody loves you. Everybody trusts you." Linkletter declined, and the group then paid a visit to Ronald Reagan.

Early on, we learn that personality and character, largely communicated from television, are all-important and all-powerful. The generation that elected Reagan president grew up on movies and television. The people who elected former professional wrestler Jesse Ventura to the governorship of Minnesota also grew up on movies and television—and Hulk Hogan action figures.

The National Truth Channel

Many other details of Pepsi's day are anchored in fact, not fiction. In Pepsi's not-too-distant world, Channel One television has become the

"National Truth Channel." Today Channel One, owned by a private corporation, beams daily commercials to more than 8 million American kids attending middle schools and high schools. It therefore imposes more uniformity on public school kids and their curriculum than the federal government ever has. For all practical purposes, it has indeed been our "national" channel for several years.

Although I made up the "Truth" part of "The National Truth Channel," I want to note that it serves as Doublespeak nested within Salespeak—a common occurrence in real life. For example, the term "corporate communication" (used in Pepsi's world, above, to refer to commercials) is a euphemism that the Benetton company actually used to refer to its ads. And although laser ads have yet to appear on the ceilings of classrooms, as they do in Pepsi's world, it is true that a few years ago, a company wanted to launch into geosynchronous orbit a massive panel that could be emblazoned with a gigantic corporate logo, visible for periods of time, over certain cities (Doheny-Farina 1999). Here, the promise of reality far exceeds what happened in Pepsi's fictional classroom.

Also, remember that "news story" about Zestra, a star of "corporate communication" spots that Pepsi watched on Channel One? More truth than fiction here, too. Since 1989, Channel One has sometimes blurred the lines between news, commercials, and public service announcements. In one study (Fox 1996), many students mistook commercials for news programs or public service announcements, such as those that warn viewers about drunk driving. The result was that students knew the product being advertised and regarded it warmly because, as one student told me, "They [the manufacturers and advertisers] are trying to do good. They care about us."

In the worst case of such blurring that I observed during the two-year period of this study, the students could hardly be faulted. Instead, the Salespeak was highly deceptive (merging with Doublespeak). That is, Pepsico's series of ads called "It's Like This" were designed to look very much like documentary news footage and public service announcements. The actors spoke directly into the swinging, handheld camera, as if they were being interviewed; the ads were filmed in black and white, and the product's name was never spoken by any of the people in the commercial, although the rapid-fire editing included brief shots of the Pepsi logo, in color, on signs and on merchandise.

Just as in Pepsi's world, described earlier in this chapter, real-life ads are often embedded within programs, as well as other commercials, products, instructions, and even "transitional spaces" between one media message and another. For example, when the girl Pepsi took a break from her "learning," she went to the school's Commoditarium, or mini-mall, to shop for items that had been advertised at school. Again, there is truth here. Although schools do not yet contain mini-malls, they do contain stores and increasing numbers of strategically placed vending machines. A ninth-grade girl told me that after students viewed Channel One in the morning and watched commercials for M&Ms candies, her teacher allowed them to take a break. The student said she'd often walk down the hall and purchase M&Ms from the vending machine. In such schools, operant conditioning is alive and well. This is not the only way in which many schools are emulating shopping malls. My daughter's high school cafeteria is a "food court," complete with McDonald's and Pizza Hut.

By establishing itself in public schools, Channel One automatically "delivers" a captive, well-defined audience to its advertisers, more than was ever possible before. "Know thy audience"—as specifically as possible—is the name of the advertising game. Marketers have become increasingly effective at obtaining all kinds of demographic and psychographic information on consumers. Channel One increasingly hones its messages based on the constant flow of demographic information it extracts from viewers, often under the guise of "clubs" and contests, which seek information on individuals, teams, classes, and entire schools ("Be a Channel One School"). Channel One's printed viewing and "curriculum" guides for teachers, as well as its Web site for students, also constantly solicit marketing information.

It's a Wonderful Day in the "Branded, Private Electronic Neighborhood"

Pepsi went to her computer lab to work and quickly drifted into an ethereal world of good-vibes Salespeak, which "interacted" with her in informal and personal ways. She was electronically massaged and called by name. Consumers interacting with advertisers, one-on-one, is the marketer's nirvana. This, too, already happens. Like the Salespeakers who use television, cyber-entrepreneurs are eager to use computers to spread Salespeak. They are equally excited about using computers to "track" consumers for collecting ever more specific and detailed psychographics—who we are, what we fantasize, what we do—for purposes of selling. One computer company plans to give away approximately 1 million computers in exchange for users who would be "willing to disclose their interests, income, and on-line browsing habits" ("Free Computers Offered by Fledgling Company," *Columbia* [Missouri] *Daily Tribune*, February 9, 1999, 7B). The company monitors the sites that users visit and the ads they click on (from a screen never devoid of ads). If users don't dial up to the Internet often enough, new ads are sent automatically to the computer terminal.

Although today's schools aren't yet as high-tech as Pepsi's school (which used "ConsumaScans" and "forehead prints" to analyze her responses to media), such approaches are not far-fetched. For example, market researchers now work directly in some schools, to determine "what sparks kids." One marketing company conducts focus groups in schools on behalf of Kentucky Fried Chicken, McDonald's, and Mattel Toys—all to improve advertising to kids (Labi 1999). To date, the most ambitious marketing venture is ZapMe! Corporation's offer of entire computer labs, fast servers with satellite connection, teacher training, and other lollipops to public and private schools, all for "free." The only price for this feast is that the systems will contain advertising and market research technology, in all its interactive and multimedia glory. However, the ZapMe! Corporation folks don't dare call it advertising. Instead they call it "brand imaging spots" and "dedicated branding spaces." Ah, Salespeak.

To date, 9,000 schools have signed up for this scheme, which is being piloted in several California schools. The ZapMe! approach is strikingly similar to Channel One television. In exchange for delivering this massive audience, schools receive some equipment from Channel One— monitors, a satellite dish (capable of picking up only Channel One's signal) and other equipment amounting to a total of about $50,000. Hence, it's hardly a shock that Channel One is found most often in low-income communities (McCarthy 1993, 4A).

ZapMe! President Frank Vigil tried to distinguish his company from Channel One: "Channel One is television. What we are is really an interactive learning tool, so we've very, very different" (Chmielewski 1998). Of course the Internet differs from TV. We've long known that when people interact with texts, they improve their retention and learning, internalizing those messages more quickly and deeply. ZapMe! wants to use this power to sell stuff. In addition to the constantly moving billboard on the screen, and in addition to the tracking of students for market research purposes, students are further immersed in ad culture when they collect "ZapPoints," which they can spend at an e-commerce mall.

Billions and Billions of Buyers and Bucks. You might think that the $50,000 worth of video equipment that schools receive from Channel One in exchange for their delivering audiences seems almost a decent trade-off, especially to poorer schools—but only until you consider that Channel One can charge advertisers as much as $200,000 for one 30-second ad (Hoynes 1997). Such sales pile up to an estimated $600,000 per day for Channel One (New York State Department of Education memo, May 23, 1995). The Internet ZapMe! Corporation, however, wants more than this. Much more. According to its Web site, ZapMe! will reach "a potential audience exceeding 50 million students in the United States and over a billion students worldwide." Sherman's march on Atlanta, the Allied landing in Normandy, and ZapMe!'s ad blitz into the world's classrooms. Ah, what progress democracy maketh.

The other "benefit" of beaming Channel One television into the schools is supposed to be its news program. However, research has concluded that Channel One news contains precious little news. The bulk of each broadcast (80 percent according to one study) is devoted to "advertising, sports, weather and natural disasters, features and profiles, and self-promotion of Channel One" (Honan 1997). Nobody in the schools can preview these daily broadcasts, because the signals are received inside of a locked metal box. And nobody at the schools has a key to open this box. Similarly, according to a press release from Commercial Alert (October 29, 1998), ZapMe! computers will contain "banner ads built into the browser interface" of their Internet access. Hence, nobody in the school can tamper with it. This is the state of democratic education.

Hitting Heads with Two-by-Four Billboards. Students using ZapMe! computers must view advertising on their computer screens. One direct use of ads is ZapMe!'s "dynamic billboard," a two-by-four-inch rectangle in the screen's lower left corner. Ad logos and messages now rotate, but these "dynamic" appeals will likely escalate to video, audio, and other whiz-bangs because, well, ads try to attract attention. Schools will be required to have students use ZapMe! computer labs at least four hours per day.

This is similar to Channel One's requirement, that schools must submit attendance records to guarantee that the program is aired during 90 percent of the school days, in at least 80 percent of the classrooms. Don't forget that every state has compulsory school attendance laws, which literally force kids to receive such messages. Also, Channel One costs taxpayers an estimated $1.8 billion annually in lost instructional time—$300 million of this to ads (Center for Commercial-Free Education, November 16, 1998). In short, taxpayers have already paid for this time that's being sold to advertisers. Channel One has convinced me that beaming glitzy ads to captive kids is highly effective. When kids see a specific item on TV at school, they often assume that the school itself endorses the product. Channel One has also broadcast commercials that closely resemble documentaries, causing kids (and adults) to blur ads with more nonbiased messages. Not only are many of the same commercials repeated endlessly, but kids also "replay" commercials themselves in a variety of ways—from singing the jingles, to repeating dialogue, to creating art projects that mirror products and product messages. Some kids even dream about commercials. In short, schools become echo chambers for ad messages. We should not be surprised, then, that such environments affect kids' behavior, including their consumer behavior (Fox 1996).

$pinning $ales in "Uncluttered Environments." Like Channel One, ZapMe! is motivated by what it calls an "open" or "uncluttered" market, one free of the usual teen "distractions" of family, music, television, jobs, and cars. An "uncluttered" environment also means little or no resistance

to the values and ideologies (e.g., materialism, competition) contained in most ads. If you have doubts about these corporations' intentions, linger a little while over their lingo. For example, in a press release, Martin Grant, Channel One's president of sales and marketing, said, "Channel One is a marketer's secret weapon. When used creatively by today's innovative marketers, it is an unparalleled way to reach a massive teen audience in a highly relevant, important, and uncluttered environment" (August 9, 1995). Another marketer once referred to in-school ads as "brand and product loyalties through classroom-centered, peer-powered lifestyle patterning." Translation: get 'em while they're young, captive, and have disposable income.

And consider this excerpt from the ZapMe! Web site: "Using fast and reliable satellite communications, we can create new methods of training, education, *sales* and even the *buying and selling of services and products*. Distance training, software distribution and high bandwidth data distribution are some of the exciting applications unfolding in the *global services market*. Join us in our pursuit of *expanding the market* by creating *complete application solutions*" (ZapMe! Web site n.d., italics added).

In the eyes (and prose) of this writer, dollar signs spin like wheels of fire on the Fourth of July. Just within the first sentence, sales are mentioned twice, and sales is what the sentence ends with, thereby emphasizing it most. And although "complete application solutions" includes more than sales, it certainly implies that sales will always be there (if not, entrepreneurs would not consider it "complete").

Living and Learning in the "Branded, Private Electronic Neighborhood"

Other, less visible problems occur when Salespeak invades schools. For instance, these two corporations "standardize" public education in ways that most of us never intended. Today, our most common or core curriculum in American education is the television commercial. More students watch ads for Bubblicious Bubble Gum than read Dickens's *A Tale of Two Cities*.

And now, ZapMe! executives promise Internet and cultural homogeneity for the thousands of schools that sign on with them. "Reduce Undesirable Websites!" they proclaim, because "in the ZapMe! Intranet environment, students [sic] access to undesirable websites is virtually eliminated." ZapMe! further assures us that "customized browser with search functions and other navigation tools guides us through the system." A "customized browser" is potentially the perfect tool for selecting, editing, packaging, manipulating, and controlling students' information.

We next learn that "ZapMe! editors search the Internet to collect and index information specifically focused for K–12 schools" (ZapMe! Web site n.d.). ZapMe! also tells us that they will be responsible for indexing and correlating this material to "a unified (National) curricular scope and sequence." They inform readers that they have "developed a proprietary-indexing scheme, which formats the content specifically for the K–12 market." Sorry, but who is supposed to choose and craft which information is best for students? ZapMe's executives? Not even close. And when they say they're going to "format" the content, I take it to mean they will cut it, slant it, shave it, dice it, tilt it, slice it, and wrap it all in glitzy technoid color, animation, video, and graphics—and ads. Too, "customized browsers" can short-circuit students' own discovery and thinking processes by directing them toward the ideas they are allowed to access—all the while leading them down endless electronic pathways strewn with ads. Finally, this ZapMe! quote refers to the "K–12 market." That's right; they define students as a "market." However, kids in schools were never, ever intended to be a "market." They are human beings who are required by law to be in school, which is supposed to be a marketplace of ideas, not a marketplace of Snickers, M&Ms, and Skittles. Students are learners, not merchandise to be hawked to advertisers in units-per-thousand.

ZapMe!'s Web site refers to its hardware and software as a "branded private electronic neighborhood." However, Mr. Rogers doesn't live there. Most residents in this neck of the woods will be surrounded by brands, if they are not walking brands themselves. Brands on every street corner, brands on every lawn, brands in every mailbox, brands lining every space down every winding boulevard to nowhere. These electronic messages will likely grow and change as marketers track the on-line movements of its young "visitors." Some current and new forms of Cyber-Salespeak (Robischon 1999) only suggest the possibilities. For instance, "interstitial ads" take shape on the screen, just slowly enough that, intrigued, you watch them materialize to see what they are. This, in essence, is a mini-commercial, which has a beginning, middle, and end. Watching this ad unfold allows you to participate in the message. This ad will disappear if you click to another page (where another one might be materializing).

"Pop-out ads" that appear in a smaller window next to the original Web page may be clicked on for an entire new venture into an infinite series of additional ads, some with video and audio features. "Banner ads" and "extramercials" wrap around the top of a screen and can even trail down the right-hand side, covering up the site's noncommercial content or information. Here again, *the act of moving this commercial* so you can read the actual content forces you to interact with the ad message and hence recall it better. Traditionally, a text's "editorial turf" or "message area" was sacred. Not anymore. It's like slapping a peel-off ad for Krazy Kola across a newspaper article reporting an airplane crash.

Another Cyber-Salespeak strategy is what I call "background tricks." For example, to focus attention on a new line of color printers, one Web site, known for its neon colors, turned its home page black and white. Increasingly, backgrounds (and many elements of foregrounds) will be composed of Salespeak. Finally, "animated ads" really capture attention. Most recently, to promote the Intel Corporation, the Web site for *USA Today* included an animated Homer Simpson scampering out of an advertisement and across the *USA Today* nameplate.

The leader in finding new ways to saturate the Web with Salespeak is Procter & Gamble. The firm's vice president, Denis Beausejour, stated that his company has "a vested interest in making the Web the most effective marketing medium in history" (Greenstein 1999). Beausejour would like to see "bigger, more complicated ads that appear automatically in a separate window on the screen when you go to a website or that allow you to send e-mail from within the ad" (Greenstein 1999, 105). Sending e-mail from within an ad means that we'll be more internally active within the ad, which deepens Salespeak's effects on consumer attitudes and behaviors. Beausejour is also "experimenting with technology that automatically downloads an ad in the background" (Greenstein 1999, 105).

Salespeak will likely take up more and more space on television, film, and computer screens, for more and more time, until they become a kind of wallpaper or permanent background. We will come to accept Salespeak as normal background, in addition to its increasing roles within various foregrounds (e.g., product placement ads). Especially in media, background serves as our anchor or base-point for "what is normal." When background and foreground are similar, they merge, just as for earlier generations, John Wayne, as actor and film character, became much the same as the open western landscape that so often spread out behind him. When Salespeak comes to dominate both background and foreground, our abilities to distinguish between the two will shrink and then disappear.

PRESS HERE TO FIND THE LOVE OF YOUR LIFE

To get a crude idea of what Cyber-Salespeak offers targeted and captive students, consider what happened to me as I was writing this chapter. Searching with the phrase "Internet advertising," the first search engine I tried yielded about 50,000 hits. Next, I randomly selected a site that sells Internet advertising services. I read about this company for a couple of screens, and then a large box caught my eye. The left side of the box contained a photo of a couple kissing, with a setting sun in the background. The right side of the box contained a large red heart and this message in a cursive style: "Press Here to Find the Love of Your Life." Who could resist such Salespeak?

I then got the same screen of the kissing couple, only much enlarged, with this message: "Welcome to Soul Mates" and "Press *HERE* to enter the site." Who could resist? Once in, I learned that this was a dating service. "New ladies just in from Thailand," it beckoned. While reading general information about this company, I learned that it was also seeking investors. I then randomly clicked on one of the men who had registered with Soul Mates, complete with photos, biographies, and descriptions of the women they were seeking.

The first person included was Paul, from Australia. The third line of text about Paul said he owns a boating business. The phrase "boating business" was a link to his company's Web site, so I clicked on it. Complete with color photos, descriptions of tours, and prices, this electronic brochure made me want to join a group of execs for an excursion around Sydney Harbor. But then I caught myself. "Whoa," I thought. "I've got to get back to my original purpose here!" So I returned to Soul Mates and checked out the women.

I found women from twenty-two countries and scanned their photos and written descriptions. There were thirteen groups of Japanese women. Alas, I didn't have time to "visit" women from Moldovia, Sevastopol, Hong Kong, Estonia, Minsk, or Olongapo City. Here is what I learned about "ordering" such women: "Write down the code number of the lady that you would like to write to and if there is a price write it down. If there is no price listed that means she belongs to the Bulk Order group whereby you can choose up to 6 ladies such as her for only US$25 or 14 ladies for US$50. Remember, minimum order is US$25. You can click the small picture to see the larger picture."

I then found out about "Special Priced Ladies": "Ladies that have a price tag near their bio-datas are called Special Priced Ladies. GOOD NEWS FOR ANYONE ORDERING 10 OR MORE ADDRESSES! YOU CAN INCLUDE ANY SPECIAL PRICE LADY AS A REGULAR ADDRESS—NO EXTRA CHARGE. BIG SAVINGS!"

At this point, I became a little dizzy. So many choices, so little money. I managed to stabilize myself (and sought refuge) by clicking on the "Soul Mates Gift Shop" icon. A worse mistake. Here I found photos of stuffed animals, along with their names, stats, and bios—just like the people at this Web site. These gift ads were aimed at the men visiting the Soul Mate Web site, and featured easy gifts to send to the women whose photos they fancied. Here's a sample entry:

Danny Dalmatian
Age—3 weeks, Height—9" (22cm), slim, very light, single

A spotty complexion makes Danny stand out in a crowd. Young, and keen to impress, this loving animal is simply seeking a permanent kennel in a special ladies bedroom (aren't we all!). If you think you can help put Danny to bed with your favorite lady then order him today. You know she will love you for it! Comfortably tucked up in his own quality box he is ready to board a plane and meet his new mistress and all for US$25. She will be sure to write to you to say thank you because she is provided with your address as well! (PS You will receive her address as well.)

In addition to Danny, I could have ordered Ken Koala, Ted Bear, or Roo (from Australia). There seemed to be a toy to represent the main nationalities of the men listed at Soul Mates. Then I spotted this instruction at the top of the screen: "Simply click on the photos below if you want to see an even CUTER picture." As overdosed as I was on these gimmicks, I clicked on it. (Could *you* resist?) For each one, I found a much larger color photo of the same stuffed animal. But right next to those cute critters—which I was guaranteed would impress the bejesus out of any of these women—lay a twenty-dollar bill (evidently, the price of the toy when the photos were taken).

No contest. Take that twenty and bring on the love of my life. Right from this site, I could use a credit card, Western Union, Thomas Cook, or other means. I could even use their "currency converter." Such a deal. However, the bucks didn't stop here. If you clicked on the "Success Stories" icon, you would find photos and glowing thank-yous to Soul Mates from men around the globe, gushingly grateful for making their dreams come true. I now felt deflated, hollow. Finally, I remembered I had some other purpose. But I couldn't remember what it was.

Such is life in a virtual world of Salespeak. If adults get sucked in, so do fourteen-year-olds. And ads carry explicit and implicit values and ideologies. The Soul Mates site assumes that women are merchandise, to be sold in bulk orders. Television—and especially the Internet—help us wander from one ad to another ad—which lead to other ads, ad nauseam. And when we encounter some ads as surprises—as when I discovered this one—we often follow them because it becomes an interactive game for us. When we interact with messages, we remember them better, raising the possibility that we will act upon them. But such links or ads are not placed haphazardly. They are planted there. Commercials can be embedded within other ads, as well as within "straight" information, each ad cloaked in varying degrees of disguise.

Channel One television entices many students to its Web site, which in turn leads them to United States Army recruitment ads and "reviews" of current R-rated movies. According to *Newsweek*, another corporation now provides free Web sites for school newspapers and, of course, weaves in ads, including some for the United States Navy, whereas another firm installs screen savers with rotating ads that include such imperatives as, "Pepsi: Develop a Thirst for Knowledge" (Stone 1998).

When captive students meander through virtual pathways—each paved with ads crafted for specific sites—marketers reach the brink of sales heaven, because they have nearly attained their eternal life: a one-to-one relationship between advertiser and "consumer." And once samples of this target audience are tracked and analyzed, the ads will be continually revised for even greater impact. The ZapMe! Corporation promises to employ ever-advancing technology to sell a "global market" of captive kids to advertisers. Schools, though, were originally set up to ensure democracy, to resist the propaganda that now resides at the head of the class and in the minds and hearts of the students. At this point, only one question remains: Which is worse: bleeding captive kids for profit, or passively watching it happen?

NOTES FROM THE WORLD OF SALESPEAK

More than anything else, dominant voices may be shaped by their environment. Consider the following facts about the environment that generates Salespeak:

- *$150 billion*: Amount spent by American advertisers each year, a cost that is passed on to consumers in higher prices. Landay (1998) summarizes our relationship with advertisers: "We pay their ad bills, we provide their profits, and we pay for their total tax write-off on the ads they place."
- *12 billion and 3 million*: The number of display ads and broadcast ads that Americans are collectively exposed to each day (Landay 1998).
- *2*: The number of times that we pay for advertising. First, advertising costs are built into the product. We pay again in terms of the time, money, and attention spent when processing an ad message.
- *1,000*: The number of chocolate chips in each bag of Chips Ahoy! cookies. The cookie company sponsored a "contest" in which students tried to confirm this claim (Labi 1999, 44).
- *$11 billion*: The amount of money dedicated to market research throughout the world (*World Opinion* Web site, November 11, 1998).
- *"Gosh, I don't understand—there are so many brands"*: This is what one marketing firm has its researchers say, after they go into stores and place themselves next to real shoppers, in an effort to elicit what consumers are thinking in an authentic context (from the May 30, 1997, issue of the *Wall Street Journal* [McLaren 1998]).
- *$66 billion*: The amount of money spent by kids and young adults (ages 4–19) in 1992 (Bowen 1995).
- *$16 billion*: Approximate number of American children who use the Internet (*Brill's Content*, December 1998, 140).

- *115.95*: The number of banner ads viewed per week by the average Web user (*World Opinion* Web site, November 11, 1998).
- *"Save water. It's precious"*: Message on a Coca-Cola billboard in Zimbabwe, where, according to the August 25, 1997, issue of the *Wall Street Journal*, the soft drink has become the drink of choice (necessity?) because of a water shortage (McLaren 1998).
- *$204 billion*: The estimated amount of Web-based transactions in 2001, up from $10.4 billion in 1997 (Zona Research 1999 on the *World Opinion* Web site).
- *89*: Percentage of children's Web sites that collect users' personal information (*Brill's Content*, December 1998, 140).
- *23*: Percentage of children's Web sites that tell kids to ask their parents for permission before sending personal information. (*Brill's Content*, December 1998, 140).
- *$29 million*: Net income for Nielsen Media Research during the first six months of 1998. (*Brill's Content*, December 1998, 140).
- *$36 billion*: The amount of money spent by kids and young adults in 1992 (ages 4–19) that belonged to their parents (Bowen 1995).
- *$3.4 million*: The amount of money received by the Grapevine-Colleyville Texas School District for displaying a huge Dr. Pepper logo atop the school roof. This school is in the flight path of Dallas-Fort Worth International Airport (Perrin 1997).
- *$8 million*: The amount of money received by the Colorado Springs School District in Colorado from Coca-Cola for an exclusive ten-year service agreement (Perrin 1997).
- *"A tight, enduring connection to teens"*: What Larry Jabbonsky, a spokesman at Pepsi headquarters, said his company seeks (Perrin 1997).
- *9,000*: The number of items stocked in grocery stores in the 1970s (Will 1997).
- *30,000*: The number of items now stocked in grocery stores (Will 1997).
- *99*: The percentage of teens surveyed (N=534 in four cities) who correctly identified the croaking frogs from a Budweiser television commercial (Horovitz and Wells 1997, 1A).
- *93*: The percentage of teens who reported that they liked the Budweiser frogs "very much" or "somewhat" (Horovitz and Wells 1997, 1A).
- *95 and 94*: The percentages of teens who know the Marlboro man and Joe Camel (Wells 1997, 1A).
- *Great Britain's white cliffs of Dover*: The backdrop for a laser-projected Adidas ad (Liu 1999).
- *$200 million*: The amount of money Miller Beer spends on advertising each year.
- *Time Warner*: A corporate empire that controls news and information in America. (There are fewer than twelve.) Time Warner owns large book publishers, cable TV franchises, home video firms, CNN and other large cable channels, and magazines such as *Time, Life, People, Sports Illustrated, Money, Fortune*, and *Entertainment Weekly* (Solomon 1999b).

- *$650 billion*: Annual sales of approximately 1,000 telemarketing companies, which employ 4 million Americans (Shenk 1999, 59).
- *350,000*: The number of classrooms that view two minutes of television commercials every day on Channel One ("Selling to School Kids" 1995).
- *154*: The number of Coca-Cola cans that students must find on a book cover and then color in, to reveal a hidden message ("Selling to School Kids" 1995).
- *50*: The percentage of increase in advertising expenditures during the past fifteen years (Bowen 1995).
- *560*: The daily number of ads targeted at the average American in 1971 (Shenk 1999, 59).
- *3,000*: The daily number of ads targeted at the average American in 1991 (Shenk 1999, 59).
- *Business Update*: An hourly segment broadcast on National Public Radio. Even though NPR is supposed to focus on "public broadcasting," it does not offer a *Labor Update*.
- *3.4 trillion*: The number of e-mail messages that crossed the Internet in the United States in 1998—a number expected to double by 2001 (McCafferty 1999).
- *80 percent*: The percentage of America's e-mail messages in 1998 that were mass-produced e-mailings, "most from corporations with something to sell" (McCafferty 1998).

It's hardly unusual for a free enterprise system to employ Salespeak. Advertising is a necessary ingredient for informing consumers about the goods and services they need. This is true for much of America's history. A sign hung in a trading post at the beginning of the Oregon Trail, 150 years ago, stating, "Sugar, 2 cents per lb.," contains necessary information for specific readers who had definite goals. Today, though, America is quite different.

First, unlike even forty years ago, most of today's advertising carries scant information about the product or service. Second, the more affluent America becomes, the fewer true "needs" we have. To make up for it, advertisers now focus not so much on what we truly need, but on what we may desire. Third, very few limits are placed upon advertising: we have little control over where it appears, who can see it (note how many of the previous items focus on young people), how often it appears, how messages are constructed, or how much money is budgeted for them (at the expense of, say, improving the product). The field of advertising itself is now a major industry. The Bureau of Labor Statistics reports that in 1995, more people died on the job in advertising than in car factories, electrical repair companies, and petroleum refining operations (*Advertising Age*, August 19, 1996). Because advertising has such free rein in America, it's become one of our most dominating voices, if not the most dominating voice.

ZEROING IN ON ZIPPIES: SALESPEAK AND
AUDIENCE ANALYSIS

> When you manipulate people—regardless of your motives—you
> take away their right to decide for themselves what they want to do
> and who they want to be.
> —Vance Packard, *The Hidden Persuaders*, 1959

The shape and delivery of Salespeak depends upon what information advertisers have about consumers—the marketer's audience analysis. In the old days, the Nielsen ratings measured the size of a TV program's audience on a program-by-program basis. However, since 1973, a new technology has been used, the Storage Instantaneous Audimenter, which measures the number of people watching minute-by-minute (Gleick 1997). Often with some inducements, today's sample audiences provide demographic information (e.g., age and income level), as well as "psychographic" data, an approach pioneered by Arnold Mitchell (1983).

Mitchell's "VALS" system focuses on values, attitudes, and lifestyles. "More than anything else," he says, "we are what we believe, what we dream, what we value" (Mitchell 1983, 3). Mitchell articulates subtle differences among nine interlocked lifestyles. For example, the "Need-Driven" groups include illiterate, older, and poor Americans, who live on the fringes of society. The "Outer-Directed" groups are externally motivated people who look outside of themselves, to others, for authority and standards. They look to the church, school, work, government, and other institutions. On the other hand, the "Inner-Directed" groups are internally motivated. They look inward, to themselves, for authority and standards, not to external authority figures and institutions.

Given marketers' knowledge of "what we believe, what we dream, what we value," it makes sense for Salespeak to tap into our emotions and our nonlogical feelings. In fact, emotion is probably the main ingredient of most Salespeak (unlike the old days, when verbal claims, logic, and argument dominated Salespeak). Many years ago, advertisers learned that emotion, based in physiological arousal, often motivates and sustains activity. And images, more than language, are the most effective vehicle for accomplishing this. Because we perceive images in an all-at-once fashion, we can hardly help but respond in an all-at-once manner, which, of course, is usually emotional in nature. When we look at Edward Hopper's painting *Nighthawks*, we might feel alone, quiet, or isolated. If we look at Leonardo da Vinci's Mona Lisa, we might feel wistful. Overall, images elicit undiluted emotional responses, usually unfettered by words and numbers and qualifications. That's the essence of pictures, the heart of electronic media.

For these reasons and more, Salespeak often relies on emotion—not logic, proof, argument, numbers, or words. One advertising researcher even states that emotions are "the basis for most decisions" (Edell 1990); that they are the reasons we make decisions in the first place. Also, emotions can distract us from logic, thereby reducing the number of rational options we might consider when responding to a message. Modern advertising, then, evokes internal experiences within us—feelings that we have moved from one point to another, from one emotion to another, from tension to calm, from imbalance to equanimity. Advertising research has greatly reduced its focus on consumer responses to logical claims. Instead, it focuses on the effects of not just general emotions, but specific emotions, such as warmth:

Aaker and Stayman (1990) define warmth as a "positive, mild, volatile emotion involving physiological arousal and precipitated by experiencing directly or vicariously a love, family, or friendship relationship" (54). Using a "warmth monitor," these researches concluded that warmth correlated at .67 with their subjects' galvanic skin responses while watching four warm commercials. In an earlier study, Aaker, Stayman, and Hagerty, 1986, found significant changes in "felt warmth" within seven to fifteen seconds, concluding that *feelings can be generated and changed within a single commercial*, even a 30-second commercial and probably within a 15-second commercial." (Fox 1994, 78, italics added)

A few examples of how such data and strategies translate into the messages aimed at specific audiences and contexts may help you understand how and why certain kinds of Salespeak take shape. For instance, the low-tar brands of cigarettes that now dominate the U.S. market are the result of psychological research conducted by the British affiliate of the Brown and Williamson Tobacco Company in the 1970s and 1980s as consumers were becoming aware of the dangers of smoking ("Tobacco Firms Studied Smokers' Reasons" 1998). Researchers working on Project Libra used a psychological tool called "consonance/dissonance" to examine smokers' internal conflicts about whether to keep smoking. This company even studied the unconscious needs of smokers who bought brands that offered coupons. According to a 1983 Brown and Williamson memo, "Raleigh and Belair smokers are addicted to smoking. They smoke primarily to reduce negative feeling states, rather than for pleasure. Given their low income, smoking represents a financial drain on family resources. Saving coupons for household items helps reduce the guilt associated with smoking" (1998, 5B).

This report concludes that these smokers are "very repressed people," lack self-confidence, and are not "totally rational" about how they choose cigarette brands. Brown and Williamson's latest venture is Circuit Breaker, a Web site (possibly the first for a cigarette brand) with Internet games and listings for nightclubs, music, and books. However, the site never mentions tobacco. Nor does it mention the sponsoring brand of cigarettes, Lucky Strike. According to a company official, this site is "a lifestyle site." Nonetheless, it collects marketing information from every visitor (*Advertising Age*, February 24, 1997).

One Canadian marketing firm focuses on " 'the non-conscious level' by observing play, fantasy, children's drawings and associations," accomplished by observing kids making consumer decisions in corner stores and malls, as well as talking with their peers in school playgrounds. This corporation also conducts focus groups. One approach involves seating ten-year-old girls with their best friends, face-to-face. The girls are encouraged to tell each other "the worst thing about getting your period" (Robertson 1999). Such psychological exploitation for profit flagrantly violates the American Psychological Association's founding principles: to "work to mitigate the causes of human suffering," to "improve the condition of both the individual and society," and to "help the public in developing informed judgments."

These APA principles seem downright quaint when you consider a recent trend in marketing research employed by mainstream conglomerates such as Shell Oil, Kraft, Starbucks Coffee, Coca-Cola, Daimler-Chrysler, and Procter & Gamble. These marketers, bearing names that reek of Sigmund Freud and Carl Jung, such as Archetype Discoveries, PsychoLogics, and Semiotic Solutions (Shalit 1999) hypnotize individuals and focus groups. Steeping themselves in "object-relations theory," these companies focus on how one's self relates to the physical world of objects. One eyewitness describes a session led by Hal Goldberg, a consumer researcher who specializes in focus groups conducted under hypnosis:

Goldberg . . . took them back, back—back to the last time they purchased gasoline. "What were you thinking?" Goldberg didn't stop, Oschle recalls, until the participants had regressed to a state of mewling infancy. "He just kept taking them back and back," he says. "Until 40 minutes later, he's saying, 'Tell me about your first experience in a gas station.' And people were actually having memory flashbacks. I mean, they were saying, 'I was three-and-a-half years old. I was in the back of my dad's brand new Chevy.' It was like it was yesterday to them. I was stunned." (Shalit 1999)

As a result of such research, Shell Oil refocused its advertising away from people who were at least 16 years old (the age at which consumers begin purchasing gas)—and toward children. In a speech, this hypnotist/marketer explained his approach: "When respondents are awake, they're reluctant to be frank and to tell you what they really feel. You'll find that respondents are much more willing to talk when hypnotized" (Shalit 1999, 15).

Another corporation studied a different group of consumers—young people who attend annual Lollapalooza festivals, an "alternative rock" and cultural festival that tours America each summer. The Interval Research Corporation focused only on those people who might attend the festival's Electric Carnival, a tent exhibit in which participants could play with video and computer technology (e.g., electronically altering their own voices and images). They defined this audience as 16–24 years old and referred to them as "zippies," "cyberpunks," "head-bangers," and "wannabees." ("Targeting the Stoned Cyberpunk" 1994). Interval Corporation further describes this "target" audience and how it might influence the product's design:

1. Their common preoccupation is the question of personal identity. They are largely self-absorbed and extremely focused on personal appearance. But they are vaguely aware that identity is primarily a construct of culture and family conditioning, variables over which they have little control. This leaves them feeling personally anxious and socially powerless (the Slacker angst). They are likely to be interested in exhibits that allow them to control the various elements of personal identity.

2. They feel marginal to mainstream society (although they are overwhelmingly white and . . . [can] afford the $30 festival admission fee). Thus the Electric Carnival needs to look and feel very different from school- or office-based experiences. The tent and all the elements in it should reflect a counter cultural aesthetic.

3. Shocking parents, family, friends, and community is often part of this group's self-definition process. They will want a record of the most socially unacceptable image of themselves to freak out their parents. We need to provide at least one printout of their self-creation. Ideally, this would be tied to completion and return of a survey after leaving the tent.

4. They don't want to fail, especially in public. Thus we need to set them up for success. Exhibits must be designed and tested to limit the frustration factor.

5. The majority of them will be drunk, stoned, tripping, or otherwise chemically altered. They are likely to have:

   • short attention spans

   • poor hand-eye coordination

   • impaired judgment

   • an altered sense of time

   Depending on the drug, they may be more aggressive (alcohol), more passive (marijuana), more impatient (speed), or more paranoid under usual circumstances. Thus:

   • they need the Electric Carnival to keep track of time for them

- they need brief, self-contained experiences
- interface images need to be larger and clearer than normal
- they need clear signs
- they need help understanding and making choices—facilitators
- they need a constructive outlet for expression of emotion, especially rage and grief
- we need to avoid heavy-handedness in controlling crowd. Humor? Costumes? ("Targeting the Stoned Cyberpunk" 1994)

Such characterizations contain much to complain about. I should also note that this focus on identity and high sensation is quite similar to the approach used by MTV, or Music Television, which also relies upon "mood and emotion" (Solomon and Quigg 1999). However, I include them only as glimpses of the massive forces marshaled in the pursuit of Salespeak—messages that, at bottom, always have something to sell. And even if we wanted to use such market research for more altruistic purposes, we could not, because it's usually secret information. Speaking as a teacher and researcher, Kline bemoans the loss of the data gathered from studying children for market purposes:

Nintendo U.S. has a fantastic research center which runs about 1,500 kids through a week. How am I to compete with them in understanding kids' fascinations with Doom and Mortal Kombat? Fisher-Price/Mattel undertook a global cultural research project . . . but try and get hold of world sales of Lego sets by theme or some of the evidence about cultural differences in play or attitudes of parents . . . well, you can't, because it's private data. (McLaren 1997b)

Finally, a recent trend in marketing itself—specifically, in how some market researchers are defining and rationalizing their work—promises even more effective Salespeak, but wrapped in humanistic rationales. Some marketing professionals now refer to themselves as "account planners" (Frank 1999), and their task is to *be* the consumer—to understand a brand's myth because, as one account planner states, "if you can understand experience, you can own it" (77). This requires public relations campaigns to change certain behaviors of people before an ad campaign is even created to increase sales. These marketers try to lay groundwork so that an ad campaign flourishes, when before, it did not.

For example, when Nike's researchers concluded that skateboarders were hostile to their brand, they developed a plan to "liquidate" this hostility, "to acknowledge and harness all those feelings of persecution" that the planners discovered skateboarders felt (Frank 1999, 78). The resultant ads asked, humorously, "what it would look like if other athletes were harassed and fined the way skaters so routinely are" (Frank 1999,

78). Skateboarders loved it. They even requested copies of these commercials to take with them when they were arrested and had to appear in court. All of this marketing is cloaked in the academic language and methodologies of the social sciences, especially anthropology. Why? Because it allows advertising to peddle its wares in the "democratic language of sensitivity and empowerment" (78). Such account planners believe themselves to be in the business of "raising consciousness": the Nike marketers who studied high school girls' basketball so that it could sell them shoes stated that they worked "to build role models for young girls." Indeed, some marketers view their job as socially altruistic, akin to running an orphanage or administering to the needs of a leper colony: "We are not at all about creating needs that people don't have. We are about meeting wants that people *do* have. If we can understand the way people want to live their lives—the way they want to see themselves— and then put brands to work in the service of that, I think that's a beautiful thing" (Shalit 1999, 12).

More effective marketing is one thing, but cloaking it in Doublespeak ultimately can only breed cynicism. Overall, understanding better how Salespeak is crafted can help us more critically interpret these messages. It can also help us remember Salespeak's sole, ultimate purpose—to sell. Keeping this simple notion constantly alive in our heads, every day, can even contribute to our health.

SALESPEAK AND HEALTH

Consumption—and the Salespeak that drives it—is now a way of life. It is our most powerful cultural force, helping to shape our attitudes, beliefs, values, and lifestyles. This voice is so pervasive and powerful that it affects four types of "health." First, Salespeak can affect our physical health. We may learn about a healthful practice or vitamin, but we may also be prone to engaging in unhealthful activities, lulled by media depictions of smokers and drinkers, as well as by direct ads for tobacco and alcohol. Second, Salespeak can affect our emotional health by delivering attractive, media-imposed definitions of beauty, sexuality, maturity, and problem-solving. Salespeak plays an influential role in other emotional health issues, such as instant gratification.

Third, Salespeak can affect our social health, since advertising can communicate attitudes, values, beliefs, and ideologies, including those of consumption, competition, and materialism. Finally, Salespeak can affect our cultural health, when we observe how, when, and if certain groups of people are represented in advertising messages. Advertising can promote and refute stereotypes of race, gender, age, and class status. In short, we must gain control over Salespeak so that it does not control us. Therefore, the following sections examine in more detail the ways in which Salespeak can affect young people.

Background

In the 1960s, marketers began to define children as a separate demographic category. By the late 1970s, research indicated that children had trouble distinguishing between television programs and commercials; that most children had little or no understanding of commercials' persuasive intentions, making them, "highly vulnerable to commercial claims and appeals" (Kunkel and Roberts 1991). In 1978, such research prompted the Federal Trade Commission to attempt to ban television commercials aimed at young children.

Ironically, the trend of marketing to children gained momentum, culminating in the establishment of Channel One in 1989, which now beams television commercials to a captive audience of more than eight million students in 40 percent of America's schools (Kozol 1992). Students attending Channel One schools have been found to reconstruct or "replay" the ads many times in many ways; they demonstrate little critical reading of ads, and they purchase the items advertised, sometimes for sale right there in the viewers's school (Fox 1996). One advertising executive said, "[Y]ou've got to reach kids throughout the day—in school, as they're shopping in the mall . . . or at the movies. You've got to become part of the fabric of their lives" (Report to the Legislature 1991, 16). Unfortunately, this trend will gain more momentum as technology, marketing research, and electronic media fuse and become more sophisticated and pervasive in students' lives—at home, at work, at play, or at school.

Salespeak and Physical Health

Ads for non-nutritious food, tobacco, and liquor encourage unhealthful choices. A study of eighty children found that TV commercials lowered children's ability to resist the temptation for low-nutrition food (Dawson, Balfour, and Walsh 1988). Blum (1983) examined the use of sports celebrities in TV commercials and magazine ads to promote the use of snuff and chewing tobacco, and points to the resultant increase in the number of young people using these smokeless tobacco products. Another study concluded that ads for alcohol became "increasingly salient and attractive [to kids] between the ages of 10 and 14 years" (Aitken, Leather, and Scott 1988).

In 1994, The American Academy of Pediatrics adopted strong policies opposing advertising to children. The academy estimates that, each year, children are exposed to 2,000 television ads for beer and wine. The academy believes that this may explain the increase in kids' liquor consumption. The academy also contends that the increase in children's obesity correlates with children watching more TV commercials touting foods high in salt, sugar, and fat (Schwed 1995). Combined, poor nutritional choices, liquor, and tobacco can wreak havoc on one's physical health, often for decades. This becomes more likely when Salespeak gains a foothold in promoting these choices during adolescence.

Salespeak and Emotional Health

Advertising has long appealed to young adults' acute awareness of physical appearance and sexuality. Surrounded by media images of sleek beauty, kids can develop emotional problems, ranging from feelings of inferiority, to eating disorders, to suicide (Pipher 1994). Appeals to sexuality have long been used to sell shampoo, deodorant, cigarettes, cosmetics, television programs, films, designer clothing, liquor, soft drinks, and even cars (Hayakawa 1962).

About half of the values identified in a study of Channel One's commercials are related to sexuality and appearance, including youthfulness/cleanliness, leisure/pleasure, status/self-esteem, and love/affection (Mueller and Wulfemeyer 1991). DeVaney (1994) agrees that Channel One's commercials emphasize sexuality and appearance; she even describes them as "Bacchanalian" (150). Her following description of a potato chips commercial shown on Channel One ("Cavorting on the Farm") illustrates the extent to which ads aimed at teens can employ erotic metaphors:

Scenario. In this thirty-second spot for Pringles corn chips, six teens (four girls and two boys) dance and play in a corn field. As the scene opens, one boy, standing in the middle of the corn field, is slowly detasseling an ear of very yellow corn. The other is standing on a ladder propped against a silo. He has a paint roller in his hand, but is facing away from the silo and into the camera. Four girls, waving yellow cans of Pringles at the boys, arrive in a speeding yellow jeep. Girls and boys come together. They dance and feed one another corn chips. Magically, the silo turns into a yellow can of Pringles. A large banner appears across the screen in block letters, "FEVER RELIEVER."

Audio. A musical jingle runs throughout this ad. The jingle compares corn chips to fresh corn and tells the students, "You have the fever of a fresh corn flavor." The rhythm and volume of the jingle gradually increase until they reach a "fever pitch." After the jingle ends, a rich deep male voice-over says slowly, "The fresh corn fever-reliever."

Video. The video track is in the form of a music video. Although a story is told, dramatic narrative codes are abandoned in favor of MTV codes. Approximately seventy shots occupy the thirty-second slot. Very fast-paced cuts articulate the shots, half of which are not matched, but are jump cuts. The boys are dressed in jeans and T-shirts, but the four girls are dressed in tight, bright clothes that call attention to their bodies. The two girls whose images occupy most of the music video are blond. Each wears an off-the-shoulder top. Their shoulders are bare. The pacing of the cuts increases as the rhythm of the music increases, until it reaches a fast-cut culminating scene. This scene is a very tight shot of a boy's lap. He is supposed to be seated in the corn field. His face is not shown. With one hand he holds a detassled ear of yellow corn erect in his lap. A female hand (no face) reaches for the corn. Magically, the corn turns into a stack of corn chips about the size of an ear of corn. The female hand plucks a corn chip, and the stack turns back into an erect ear of corn. By repeatedly intercuting the ear of corn held by the boy's hand and the female hand reaching for the corn/chip stack, the producer shows the stack of chips gradually diminishing. The scene closes with a close-up of the girl's ecstatic face. The scene switches to the closing series of shots next to the silo where the "fever reliever" banner is rolled. (DeVaney 1994, 146–147)

In such commercials, Salespeak blends with Sensationspeak (see Chapter 5 to create a powerful voice for young audiences. In this ad, potato chips become the same thing as an ear of corn—and both of these become the same thing as a penis. The primary way that the message maker constructs this meaning is by simple placement or proximity and some fancy camera work. Otherwise, there's very little connection among these things. This commercial illustrates immature and trivialized relationships between men and women, which, according to Moog (1994) contributes to kids' "stunted" perceptions of sexuality and gender identity. This prevents both men and women, Moog maintains, from developing humane and mature gender identities and relationships with other people.

If eroticism is used in this commercial to sell corn chips, you might reason, it can be used to sell anything, especially tobacco and alcohol. Advertisers have now begun to link sexuality with alcoholic products in ways that attract younger children: fifth-and sixth-graders not only remember TV commercials for beer (Schwed 1995), but they (and younger kids) also link the drinking of beer to "romance, sociability and relaxation" ("Flashy Beer Commercials Draw Children, Study Finds," *Columbia* [Missouri] *Daily Tribune*, February 12, 1994: A12).

Salespeak and Social Health

Advertisers bombard us with powerful messages reflecting values, attitudes, and ideologies that are not always conducive to social and environmental health. These include, but are not limited to (1) valuing appearance over substance; (2) valuing instant gratification over delayed gratification; (3) valuing action over reflection; (4) valuing consumption over frugality and recycling; (5) valuing competition over cooperation, and (6) valuing materialism over spirituality.

Greenfield (1984) reminds us that, in the 1950s, British children who watched television—the BBC, which contained no commercials—developed more materialistic attitudes than those who did not watch television: "Adolescent boys who watched television . . . were more focused on what they would *have* in the future; adolescent boys without television were more focused on what they would be *doing*. The longer the child's experience with television, the more this materialistic outlook increased" (Greenfield 1984, 51). This problem seems more severe with low-income, African American children. African American children view "significantly more TV than whites . . . an average of 6.85 hours of TV each day and 40,000 TV commercials each year." The result is that "Black families overspend in the attempt to be like the persons depicted in TV commercials" (Greenberg and Brand 1993).

It's important to note here that materialism involves more than just a belief in objects for objects' sake or "keeping up with the Jones's." It also involves the explicit or implicit view that intangible qualities, such as youth or popularity, can be obtained by purchasing some product, such as a soft drink. Greenberg and Brand (1993) concluded that Channel One viewers held "more materialistic attitudes" than nonviewers (150). Hite and Eck (1987) found that ads not only encouraged kids to adopt materialistic attitudes, but also generated friction between parents and children, limiting the development of kids' "moral and ethical values."

The ad in Figure 4.1 below seems to "limit" moral and ethical values by mocking and trivializing the traditional source of these values, the place of worship. When viewed in color, this ad's yellows, reds, blues, greens, and purples add considerable realism to the stained glass windows of each praying sports star. The balls of each sport serve as fitting halos around each sports god. Although somewhat low key, the line of small print that states, "Hours of worship Mon-Sat 10–7 pm Thurs 10–8 pm Sun 11–6 pm" clinches the message: that sports are holy, that Nike is sports, so Nike must be holy. Other, "larger" messages evolve from this ad: that what is holier than sports and even holier than Nike is spending money; that no entity outside of ourselves is bigger than Michael Jordan; that those who adopt the stance of prayer—the most private and vulnerable of human acts—are fair game for exploitation.

Salespeak and Cultural Health

How media portrays or "re-presents" gender, race, age, and social class can affect viewers' attitudes and actions toward that group. In 1933, Peterson and Thurstone found that a single viewing of D. W. Griffith's *Birth of a Nation* correlated with a negative shift in adolescents' attitudes toward African Americans. Other groups of people can also be affected.

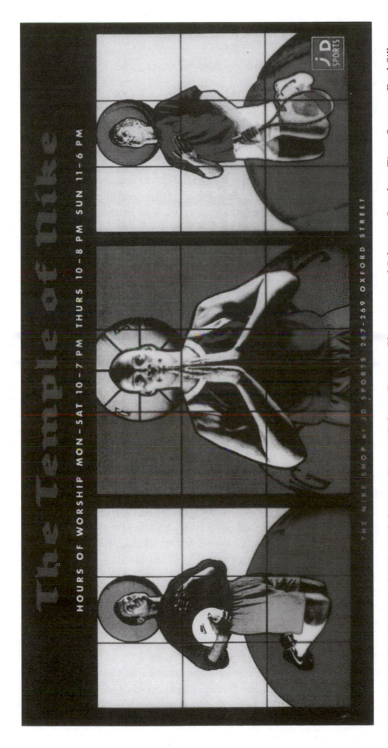

Figure 4.1. "The Temple of Nike" ad. Source: Simons Palmer Denton Clemmow and Johnson, London; Tiger Savage, Paul Silburn, Seamus Ryan.

The United Nations Commission on the Status of Women summarized three ways in which women in ads suffer from stereotyping: (1) women are usually portrayed as unable to think for themselves, deferring to men to make decisions; (2) loss of male approval is viewed as a threat, since the advertised products are used to gain approval from men; (3) women seem obsessed with cleanliness, expressing a "gamut of emotions" in embracing whiteness, brightness, and freshness (Report to the Legislature on Commercialism in Schools 1991, 91).

This report also concluded that almost all commercials with voice-overs are spoken by men, that men appear more frequently and in more roles than women, and that women are most frequently shown in family roles. When commercials show women in the home, they are doing things for men. Women are usually shown inside the house and men are shown outside the house. During children's programming, women and girls appear in commercials less often than men and boys (Report to the Legislature on Commercialism in Schools 1991, 92). Greenfield (1984) had earlier described TV commercials as "outstanding culprits" in stereotyping females:

One group of high school girls was shown fifteen commercials emphasizing the importance of physical beauty, while another group was not shown the commercials. The girls who watched the commercials were more likely than the others to agree with the statements 'beauty is personally desirable for me' and 'beauty is important to be popular with me.' However . . . television, even without commercials (for example, in Britain twenty-five years ago and in Sweden today) influences children to attach more importance to appearance in general and clothes in particular. (Greenfield 1984, 38)

Most adolescent females have watched commercials since they were young children—the formative years for developing their gender roles. Even three-year-old children who watch a lot of television demonstrated more rigid attitudes about what jobs men and women should have, as opposed to their light-viewing counterparts (Greenberg 1982). Young children can learn such rigid expectations from all types of characters in TV commercials. That is, human, nonhuman, and cartoon characters help kids form stereotypes of people's race, gender, occupation, and social behavior (Rossiter 1980).

Another study examined TV commercials for toys in an attempt to identify which of its features were associated with girls and which ones with boys (Ross et al., n.d.). The characteristics of commercials for male toys were loud music, rapid camera cuts, and sound effects. Conversely, ads for female toys used more background music and gentler camera shots, such as fades and dissolves. Most of the children who viewed mock commercials (using shapes instead of real toys) identified them in the same way—an identification that became more intense as kids grew older. Such filming techniques, then, can direct male children one way and females another.

The health issues explored so far have not included those "illnesses" created by advertisers themselves. For instance, "pronation" is an affliction corrected by buying Muscle Builder Shoes, whereas "bone hunger" can be fixed with a purchase of Scott's Emulsion; "smoker's fag" is remedied with Phillip's Milk of Magnesia, and "morning acidity" can be cured with a can of Libby's pineapple; "collapsed capillaries" can be strengthened with Ipana Toothpaste, and "perspiration aura" is healed with Mum Deodorant (McLaren 1999, 36). "Psoriasis" may be terminal. Finally, these types of health—physical, emotional, social, and cultural—may seem more difficult to maintain when you consider how ingrained Salespeak is in our social and cultural history, explored in the following section.

SALESPEAK IN THE AMERICAN GRAIN

Much of Salespeak flows from what the American Realist painter Thomas Hart Benton (1983) called the "parvenu" spirit, which runs deep in the grain of American values. Coming of age in the Midwest at the turn of the century, Benton continually fought hard to be an artist "in a world of 'practical' men," people who were products of the 1880s and 1890s, the period Twain called the Gilded Age, when Americans worshiped "Gold and Greenbacks and Stock—father, son, and the ghost of same" (Kaplan 1980). Today's dominant values are not very different. Benton's rendering of this period also rings true, for then and now:

There was . . . from the eighteen-eighties up through the Great War, the most complete denial of aesthetic sensibility that has probably ever been known. The natural human interest in the simple nature of things which is possessed to some degree by all men, was crushed almost utterly in favor of a short-range philosophy of action. This is recognized by all commentators on our civilization and is attributed, as a rule, to the exigencies of pioneer needs, where the mind was supposedly grooved to action alone. The claim is generally made that the hardships of pioneer life made the cultivation of aesthetic sensibilities impossible and that the pioneer psychology once established remained in the habits and ways of people, keeping them on a level of low sensibility. It is forgotten, however, that our aboriginal tribes, living under equal hardships, were able to cultivate aesthetic attitudes and practices to a very high degree. It is also forgotten that up to the time of the Civil War our pioneers themselves cultivated quite a number of arts. . . . No, it was not pioneer hardship that crushed aesthetic interest . . . and made the eighties and nineties so sterile in feeling and sympathy.

What really crushed it was the rise of the parvenu spirit during the great exploitative period following the Civil War, and the enthronement then of the ideals and practices of the go-getter above all other human interests. The psychology of the parvenu is destructive of the appreciation of the qualities of things. His is a quantitative mind. He is intent on expansion rather than on the cultivation and preservation of value in things. Things—all things—are, for his kind, merely instruments extending areas of control and promoting his wealth and power. Aesthetic values cannot survive when the particular pragmatism of the parvenu is socially dominant. . . . Where such values are denied in a society, as they must be when the go-getter's strictly material interests in economic expansion dominate the pattern of life, they become an oddity. (Benton 1983, 26–27)

Today, "strictly material interests in economic expansion" continues to dominate our lives probably more so than in the past. Salespeak and the forces that drive it help minimize true aesthetic values for authentic art, that which is generated by individuals who are not beholden to commercial interests. The "art" that dominates American life today often passes itself off as art, but it's often only Salespeak, however artfully executed. Regardless of how beautiful or glitzy the text, if its main or ultimate purpose is to sell something, it cannot be art (at least, not until its advertising power expires, after several years have passed). And without true art, human feeling is ignored and debased. However, if we accept commercially driven art as true art, then we have to view it in that way—as an indicator of who we are and what we value. And if we do this, what we find is that selling resides as the soul of our civilization.

Salespeak is born of many other historical and cultural forces: freedom of speech; westward expansion; a free-market economy; a body of literature, art, and music that privileges individualism; and discoveries in the sciences and social sciences. Today, much of art, music, philosophy, and architecture are collectively referred to as postmodernism. Or maybe postmodernism is the result of such forces. Regardless, postmodernism is a world view that rejects traditional ways of constructing meaning out of human experience. Instead, it often relies on recycling or repeating already-existing symbols and imagery. An oft-cited example of postmodern art is Andy Warhol's painting of many identical Campbell's soup cans. In terms of Salespeak, TV commercials, for example, often "recycle" or refer to other current or previous messages. Therefore, one message must be read in terms of another (this is also called "intertextuality"). For example, TV commercials for the Yellow Pages telephone directory included images of former Chinese Premier Mao Tse Tung, along with an abundant use of the color red, which elicited other messages related to the Chinese form of government.

In addition to intertextuality, postmodernism is often characterized by fragmentation, confusion, ambiguity, contradiction, and a lack of logical or chronological sequence. Videos produced for Music Television (MTV), for example, often appear to be directed in a postmodern style. Too, the worlds of Joseph Heller's *Catch-22*, Ken Kesey's *One Flew Over the Cuckoo's Nest*, and Kurt Vonnegut's *Slaughterhouse Five* are universes that reflect a postmodern view of life. For younger audiences in particular, Salespeak is often molded to fit within this paradigm.

In many respects, the grandfathers of modern Salespeak are Sigmund Freud and Carl Jung. They established the legitimacy of internal and unconscious meanings, which heavily depend upon emotions and visual thinking. Jung insisted that our communicating with internal and dream images is a normal thing to do—that there's nothing darkly voodoo or mystical about it. Freud's and Jung's theories of the unconscious were probably better understood by marketers than anyone else. Why? Because they applied their understandings of dreams and irrational desires to the modern marketing strategies needed for defining and targeting a growing number of different types of consumers.

At about the same time that Salespeakers were toying with Freud and Jung, two other schools of thought, general semantics and Gestalt psychology, were developing our understanding of Salespeak. Alfred Korzybski, Benjamin Whorf, and others were exploring the interactions between people, language, and reality. At roughly the same time, Gestalt psychologists such as Kurt Lewin, Max Wertheimer, and Wolfgang Kohler were establishing basic visual principles, such as "contiguity" and "proximity," which remain as staples of Salespeak. For example, in what is now called "association" or "transfer," simply positioning items next to each other more easily allows viewers to shift the qualities of one item to the other, even though they may be quite different. The presidential candidate who is filmed visiting a battleship knows that many viewers will transfer the militaristic values of the cannons to the candidate.

Another major source of Salespeak resides in America's history of fighting wars, from World War I to the Persian Gulf War. Especially during the two world wars, the government required massive amounts of propaganda to mobilize citizens—from Hollywood stars holding rallies to sell war bonds, to the thousands of huge posters produced by such artists as Norman Rockwell. Beginning in the early 1950s, the popularity of the war posters—with their dramatic, bold images and slogans—conditioned Americans to more easily accept TV sound bites as legitimate political discourse (Robertson 1994).

By 1992, even the mass publication *TV Guide* proclaimed that "some portions of the Persian Gulf war effort were stage-managed in an effort to rally public opinion for military action against Iraq" (Strong 1992, 11). This article details how the public relations firm of Hill and Knowlton helped to "package and rehearse" several incidents, including an emotional appeal by a young woman before a Congressional caucus hearing. This girl, identified as Nayirah, a Kuwaiti refugee, described how Iraqi soldiers stormed hospitals and tore newborn babies away from their incubators, leaving them to die. The girl's testimony received much media attention and was cited by then President George Bush. In reality, however, this girl was the daughter of Kuwaiti's ambassador to the United States. She had been rehearsed before video cameras by the Hill and Knowlton firm, which, by the way, was at that time headed by Craig Fuller, the former chief of staff to George Bush when he was vice president.

We increasingly rely upon staged TV events and sound bites. According to Solomon (1999a), between the Nixon-Humphrey race of 1968 and the Bush-Dukakis contest of 1988, "the average length of a sound bite on network TV news dropped from 43 seconds to nine seconds." Politics and show business now blur into a single ongoing spectacle, where voters (and the larger group of nonvoters) are mere spectators, not participants in shaping policy. All of these developments and more have nurtured the flowering of Salespeak.

Another change affecting Salespeak is that qualitative research has replaced much of quantitative research. That is, even hard science has shifted toward conducting research in ways that account for subjective reality and socially constructed truth, including the importance of context. Within this qualitative approach, the ancient study of semiotics, or the study of signs, has gained new life. Consumer research now focuses more heavily on consumers' psychological profiles, especially their emotions. By the late 1980s, the *Journal of Consumer Research* began publishing qualitative, ethnographic research on consumers' motivation and behavior (Holbrook and Stern 1997). Maddock and Fulton (1996) describe such marketing:

Marketing to the mind refers to the unconscious mind. This is the side of the brain that has been explored by few, and misunderstood by many. Yet, it is the motivating side. It is the emotional side. It is the visual side. It is the passionate side. In consumer behavior, it is the side that makes the initial ("gut") and final ("spend money") decision. The Silent Side is, or should be, to the advertising executive, the "sell to" side. Also, for the advertising person and the marketer, access to the unconscious will address and answer the question of *why* consumers do what they do. It explains, rather than just describes. (Maddock and Fulton 1996, 10)

On the other hand, we often ignore the fact that American culture has indeed valued the inner, emotional, intuitive side of life, and did so long before Freud and Jung arrived on the scene. Thomas Jefferson's "Dialogue with My Heart and My Head" vividly illustrates Jefferson's conflicting thoughts and feelings about a woman. Walt Whitman's life and work, celebrating the natural, the intuitive, heavily influenced American culture. Also, as noted in the previous chapter, American pioneers who settled the West were motivated just as much by "the romance of going" as they were by practical matters. They were "nomadic and romantic rather than economic minded" (Benton 1983). The most influential work of American literature, Mark Twain's *Adventures of Huckleberry Finn*, is not so much a story about a boy's trip down the river, as it is a boy's struggle with his conscience, his intuition. In recent times, the Vietnam War Memorial in Washington, D.C., with its downward-sloping walls, allows visitors to face the tragedies of war by looking into their own reflections in the shiny black marble. It is a monument dedicated not just to the people killed in war, but also to our internal lives. Even the idea of selling to children is not new (though selling to a mass audience of captive school students is). Consider the following excerpt from "Dealing in Futures: Insuring Sales for the Years to Come . . ." first published in 1919:

Some advertisers see little sense in spending money advertising "grown-up goods" to children; many, however, have found out the wisdom and profit in doing it.

Make a child think of "automobile" in the term of "Packard," keep that idea before it until it becomes an ideal, and when that child can afford it (and granted that Packards keep their relative position among automobiles), the man or woman the child has become will have the strongest incentive for buying a Packard. True, circumstances may compel the purchase of a Ford, but lurking in the mind will be the thought, "until I can buy a Packard." In any event, the Packard advertiser would have done everything he could and used his entire influence at the right time; but if he waited until the child had grown old enough to have absorbed from general sources the names of a dozen cars into its mind, he would have missed a wonderful opportunity. The waxlike mind would have been crisscrossed by the other names; the soil would have other seeds besides his and it would be a continual struggle for supremacy. First impressions are strong—which is particularly true of advertised goods. (see McLaren 1997b)

Several years after the above article appeared, Salespeak again lurched forward to gain "supremacy" over our "waxlike" minds, when the Procter & Gamble Company needed some type of radio segment to hawk its detergents and soaps. Hence, the company devised a fifteen-minute serial melodrama. These became known as soap operas and motivated millions of women to listen to their radios. Twenty years later, P & G identified, again ahead of the pack, the potential for mass audiences in the new technology of television. The company sidled its soap operas over to TV and the rest is history. But not quite. Greenstein reports that P & G is on the brink of committing advertising dollars whole hog to the Internet, since it believes that cyberspace has "the potential to dwarf television as a way of bonding with consumers" (1999, 104).

Jefferson? Huck Finn? Packards? Wars? Soap operas? What could be more American? Only one thing: Salespeak, the glue that holds it all together.

SALESPEAK AND TRADITIONAL AMERICAN MYTHS

It's hard to imagine a capitalist society without communication dedicated to glorifying consumption. In "The Strange Disappearance of Civic America," Putnam (1996) traces the evidence that points toward television (and its accompanying spread of Salespeak) as the main cause for the decline in Americans' involvement in active citizenship. Our traditional values of "democracy in action" are going dormant, because we increasingly choose not to participate in civic life. Americans continue to avoid voting, as well as joining organizations such as bowling leagues, labor unions, professional associations, literary discussion groups, Kiwanis Clubs, the Red Cross, and many others.

Over the decades, television's growth has paralleled this lack of involvement in civic life, this decline in "social connectedness." Putnam systematically rules out other competing causes for these declines, including the "usual suspects" of busy-ness and time pressures, economic downswings, economic affluence, suburbanization, mobility, the changing role of women, and others. The major culprit remaining is television. In addition to affecting the traditional American theme of democracy in action, Salespeak is an integral part of the following traditional American myths or sets of beliefs and values.

Happily Ever After

One persistent American characteristic is sheer optimism, especially "the happy ending"—the unshakable belief that "everything turns out okay in the end." If anything, Americans have always prided themselves on optimism, on fixing problems. We have traditionally insisted that novels, stories, folktales, movies, and TV offerings wrap up all loose ends in a positive way to ensure a happy ending. When critic I. A. Richards (1921) studied this phenomenon in his college freshmen, he labeled it "happiness binding." Our acceptance of Realism, in which not every piece of bad luck, problem, character flaw, or natural disaster is resolved for the best, is a relatively recent genre in literature and film. Nonetheless, texts intended for mass audiences still end happily ever after. Today, we continue to possess little tolerance for unhappy endings and maybe even less patience for unresolved, ambiguous endings. Salespeak texts capitalize on this seemingly innate desire. Whatever tension, conflict, or problem has been established in the narrative is resolved by a product or service—by purchasing something. With the arrival of Mr.

Clean or the shiny new Ford, everyone is smiling. Not only is the commercial's plot resolved happily, but the people involved are also intrinsically transformed into more positive beings. If the problem of our dull kitchen floor is solved by a can of Johnson's Wax, then the people in the kitchen also become happy. Investing tangible goods and services with intangible values boosts sales because we want to acquire those values— but we also want that happy ending, no matter what.

Individualism and Independence

When Salespeak warns us about the dangers of ring around the collar, B. O., fly-away hair, foot odor, cellulite, halitosis, and dull teeth, it's telling us that something's wrong. When Salespeak implores us to buy the latest model of car, it often suggests that doing so will make us more popular with the opposite sex—that we're not already popular enough. When Salespeak parades images of beautiful people wearing a certain brand of clothes or perfume or shoes, it often implies that these items will make us somehow better than we currently are. Most of the time, Salespeak's dominant message is, "You're not good enough the way you are." This is the sole, most powerful message of Salespeak. So how does this message, repeated over and over, in so many different ways, relate to the strong American traditions of individualism and independence? It does it in more ways (and in more complexity) than I can provide here, but let me summarize three important ways that Salespeak interacts with the American theme of individualism and independence.

First, our powerful streak of individualism and independence has not been durable enough to shield our psyches from allowing messages intended for a mass audience to affect us. Although consumers generally know that Salespeak is aimed at huge numbers of people, the intimacy achieved by television and other media, combined with the large budgets that pay for highly effective messages, often override our sense of independence. Doubt seeps in and we begin to compare ourselves with the ideal images of mass media, and think, "Well, maybe *my* teeth *do* need to be whiter."

When mass technology displaces our sense of individuality, something else occurs at the same time: our belief that the things advertised can deliver the intangible qualities promised by the Salespeak—that Gap trousers will somehow generate sex appeal, that Lunt sterling silverware will somehow beknight us with class. What happens when these products do not supply us with the intangible values, attitudes, and other qualities promised? There are three main results. First, when disappointed, we might buy more things. Second, we might cast about, buying different things. Third, we may become frustrated and eventually disillusioned. Why? Because we've been conditioned to believe that we're individuals who have the power and freedom to improve ourselves, yet we can never seem to overcome the daily deficits fed to us by Salespeak.

Second, the ever-present message of "You're not good enough" preys directly upon our traditional sense of individualism and independence. That is, if we become convinced that we're not good enough, we can merely change our brand of toothpaste or shampoo because we're individuals who have the power to change ourselves for the better. It is our constitutional right to improve ourselves. The American creed "Pull yourself up by your own bootstraps" used to mean that we were independently responsible for learning English, getting a decent job, and becoming financially independent. However, since our economy and standard of life have developed and since the advent of Salespeak through mass media, it now more often means that we're independently responsible for having whiter teeth or greater sex appeal. We now pull ourselves up by our bootstraps not by doing things, but by purchasing things—even if it means acquiring things we don't need, or consuming more than we produce.

Third, because of the prevalence and intensity of Salespeak, and because an information society can provide few active ways for us to exercise our sense of individuality, we do it vicariously via the media—through engaging with the technology itself (e.g., playing video games, surfing the Web), or through interacting with media representations. For example, McLaren (1999) interviewed self-described "Arielholics"—adults who are engrossed in any object, clothing, toy, film, or print message that involves Ariel, the lead character in the Disney film *The Little Mermaid*. (Such immersion in the personalities of media stars is studied by academics, who call it "fandom.")

After finding about fifteen Web sites that focused just on Ariel, McLaren interviewed Doug, who has watched *The Little Mermaid* "about 150" times, maintains a Web site focused on Ariel, spent six years' worth of weekends pursuing Ariel-related merchandise, and stopped eating seafood, which he describes as "a personal act of devotion because [he] loves seafood." In short, Doug and other "fans" vigorously participate in the lives of media stars and media representations as a way to individuate themselves, to find a unique identity. They accomplish this mainly through consumption. And in a world of media "tie-ins," where one product or message leads to many other products and messages, fans such as Doug follow rich chains of Salespeak. In essence, Salespeak can provide one's identity, or displace it, or replace it, depending upon your point of view.

Hero Worship

Doug's passion for all-things Ariel might also be defined as hero worship, another traditional American theme. Our penchant for finding heros has certainly intensified since the advent of media and information technology. We do, though, own a long history of hero worship. From George Washington to Colin Powell, many ballyhooed military leaders have become president or run for public office. Salespeak is fundamental to hero worship, ranging from the sloganeering of "Tippecanoe and Tyler Too," to the camera positions that filmed Dwight Eisenhower making America's first political TV commercial in the early 1950s. (The "average citizens" asking questions of Eisenhower in the series of ads "America Asks Eisenhower" were filmed looking up at Ike, as if he were majestically above them; in reality, the questioners and Eisenhower were taped in different locations at different times.)

Electronic media, especially film and television, has replaced the military as a dominant structure in American life. Therefore, most of the heros and antiheros now worshiped come from the screen: Charlie Chaplin, Greta Garbo, John Wayne, Paul Newman, Marilyn Monroe, Archie Bunker, Luke Skywalker, Madonna, Oprah, Homer Simpson. A film or TV show is a product, which is sold to advertisers in units of viewers-per-thousand. Unlike the military, the media industry depends heavily on profit, which means Salespeak. You may be well familiar with the extent that sales determine the creation of media texts—who makes them, what message they bear, how the text is crafted and delivered, how it is advertised, and so forth. The point is that Salespeak is intricately and thoroughly woven into media texts. For instance, in the horror flick *The Faculty*, Tommy Hilfiger clothing makes up 90 percent of the wardrobe worn by the stars (Gerbner and Cones 1998). This approach, however, is far more than mere product placement, in which a commercial item appears in obvious view for a few seconds in exchange for a fee or some trade-off. In this film, this brand of clothing "stars" for an hour or more. Also, Hilfiger provided half of the film's ad campaign funding about $15 million.

Most interesting, though, is that this film's stars appeared in television and magazine ads as the characters they play in the film. During these ads, they of course wore the same Hilfiger clothes. In the past, plugs for movies were done by the actors appearing as themselves—not in their fictional roles. Other ad campaigns (e.g., those for Anheuser-Busch, BMW, and Smirnoff) have also employed actors to engage in Salespeak as their fictional characters, as people who step out of their film setting to hawk real-life vodka or cars. Because of this thorough marketing approach, *The Faculty* becomes little more than a long, more complex commercial, which audiences pay to see. (The idea of consumers paying for advertising is not new: it occurs when we wear clothing that bears brand names and symbols.) Gerbner and Cones (1998) question the reasoning behind using films for advertising:

The film industry commercial zealots appear to be completely oblivious to the fact that if it is worth $15 million dollars to the Tommy Hilfiger clothing line to give prolonged exposure to the clothes in a film, presumably because that will influence the thinking and behavior of many of the young people who see this film (i.e., encourage them to go out and buy Tommy Hilfiger clothes) then it is also very likely that exposure to the violent acts included in this horror film may also be emulated by some of the moviegoers who witness those acts as portrayed through this most powerful communications medium of the 20th century. Duh! (Gerbner and Cones 1998)

This blurring between marketing and entertainment means that the only heroes we are given by the media are those who have been judged to be potentially profitable. The insane randomness of war, which used to produce our heroes, has given way to the microcalculations of profiteers. Heroes manufactured only by those with something to sell promise only to deliver more Salespeak, in turn supplying new heroes for consumption, as the cycle continues.

SALESPEAK AND EMERGING AMERICAN MYTHS

Although we are rank with emerging myths that involve Salespeak, only a few important ones are included here—ones that seem to be huge unquestioned assumptions of the American mediascape.

Fantasy Is as Good as Reality (Maybe Better)

New technology multiplies itself. The massive Unix computer gives way to the desktop machine, which spawns the laptop, which spawns the palm-held computer. In turn, each generation of hardware spawns other items that "enhance" them—from the mouse, to the joy stick, to the latest upgraded software. With new technology comes new media, which also replicates itself: from the traditional movie screen to the IMAX; from the poster, to the one-second TV commercial, to the ad messages on beepers, to the DVD. New media and genres, as well as the old ones, depend upon a large measure of induced fantasy as we immerse ourselves in entertainment of all types, including serious forms such as war or national issues.

For example, the Gulf War was a serious, deadly experience, but it was nonetheless wrapped in media messages akin to a TV mini-series, complete with titles, logos, musical sound tracks, computer graphics, controlled press conferences, and star reporters wearing field jackets. Operation Desert Storm and Operation Desert Shield could have been the titles of Errol Flynn, John Wayne, or Sylvester Stallone movies. The reasons for such packaging have more to do with persuasion, with selling a war to the public, than with entertainment for its own sake. The point is that both—selling or persuading through entertainment, as well as entertainment for its own sake—are rampant, causing them to blur in the public's eye, a natural response when each takes on qualities of the other.

It is only normal that generations that grow up with media entertainment increasingly accept it as the norm, as the universal background for their lives. In short, we increasingly prefer fantasy to reality, privileging the enhanced, dramatized, and fictionalized over the unadorned facts of existence. One problem with this is that a national issue such as a war should be examined as foreground. However, when it's packaged as entertainment, it begins to recede into the background. In effect, it becomes another video rental off the shelf, something we approach not as an issue to debate and judge, but as a performance to engage us, uncritically, during down time.

All Salespeak, All the Time

This emerging myth states that it's manifest destiny that technology spread Salespeak everywhere, every day, around the clock. A willing citizenry and rapidly developing technology ensure that Salespeak will reside everywhere. One recent example is digitally adding product placements to TV programs ("TV Show Uses Technology to Insert Product," *Columbia* [Missouri] *Daily Tribune*, March 30, 1999: 15A). A can of Coca-Cola was placed onto a desk and a Wells Fargo billboard was inserted into the background of scenes from the drama *Seven Days*. These items were not there when the scenes were filmed. Such product placements occur in addition to regular commercials. It's only a matter of time until the regular commercials become somehow integrated or subtly linked to the product placements, making the bleeding of ads into TV content more "natural."

The only places left untouched by Salespeak are churches and other places of worship. These, too, will fall once cyber-church replaces actually going there, and parishioners get zapped by ads for Smirnoff vodka as they wend their way to and from virtual confession booths. The other "empty" space awaiting advertising is the sky above. However, as noted earlier, at least one corporation has already considered launching satellites to install massive corporate logos over city skies at night. About the only thing we can be sure of is that Salespeak will take new forms and appear even more frequently. Technology will enable Salespeak to become the new American background—the new electronic baseline of universal normalcy.

Such normalcy necessarily includes conflict, to varying degrees, between corporations, a kind of consumer and brand factionalism—not the "cultural cleansing" as we see today, for example, in the Balkans, but "consumer cleansing" or "product cleansing." Today, we can see the beginnings of such conflict, where the battles have remained on the playing field—the American psyche. Witness the competition between Pepsi and Coke, Nike and Reebok, a currently mild form of media-induced consumer factionalism. The increasing spread and intensity of Salespeak will likely escalate.

This seems inevitable when a culture elevates product and brand loyalty to human, cult, and icon status, such as Mickey Mouse, Joe Camel, and the Budweiser frogs. It used to be that only famous people were asked to press their hands into Mann's Chinese Theater in Hollywood. But recently, Gerry Thomas, the inventor of Swanson's TV dinner, pressed a replica of the original TV dinner aluminum tray into that theater's cement sidewalk ("Swanson Reheats TV Dinner on Anniversary to Boost Sales," *Columbia* [Missouri] *Daily Tribune*, March 30, 1999: 15A). Murray Kessler, president of the Swanson frozen foods division, said, "It's part of American culture." The report matter-of-factly concludes, "TV dinners have become an American icon since they were unveiled in 1954." Such worship of products, as well as the messages that promote them (witness, for instance, the Clio Awards for TV commercials), necessarily includes intense feelings of devotion and loyalty, beginning, as we have seen, in childhood. Such "product ethnocentrism" has already generated real conflict, as kids have been killed for their name-brand clothing and running shoes.

Salespeak messages competing within the American psyche create reality, not just reflect it. Salespeak affects the tenor of our culture, distorting and fragmenting reality, debasing authentic art, and desensitizing human feelings. This is not the type of conflict that is ever likely to become direct, clear, organized, physical, and real. Rather, it is likely to cut even more deeply into our collective psyche, which, as we have seen time and again, does indeed translate into definite actions and behaviors.

CONCLUSIONS

This chapter has merely glanced at (or ignored altogether) many hazards of Salespeak. Therefore, the following "conclusions" are based upon this chapter's implicit, as well as explicit, information.

Salespeak and the Commodification of E-v-e-r-y-t-h-i-n-g

Increasingly, we are paying for commercials—to wear them, to see them in films. We are beginning to view ads as "not ads" and as "more than ads." Another growing trend is the embedding of ads within ads. As an MTV segment plays (an ad for a CD or tape), a window in the lower left corner airs "testimonials" from consumers about the song or artist that fills the rest of the screen. Or, a line of text runs across the bottom of the screen, again advertising the ad. In short, these segments consist of ads as foreground *and* as background. We may focus on Mariah Carey singing and dancing (foreground) and then redirect our primary attention to the fan from New Jersey, amidst a screaming crowd, extolling Carey's many artistic and personal virtues, hence placing Carey in the background, as the testimonial becomes our new foreground. Here, background and foreground alternate with each other. Either way, we're still watching a commercial, as one commercial becomes a kind of "break" from another ad.

Although this book often focuses on individual media messages, they hardly constitute the larger picture, which is the point of this chapter— that through Salespeak (and often because of it), we think of nearly everything as something we can purchase: ideology, personality, integrity, lawn chairs, companionship, history, refrigerators, learning, whatever. We believe that intangible qualities and values can be plucked off a shelf and paid for, that we can obtain that quality instantly. In many ways this is a logical response, because technology's speed has reduced our awareness, knowledge, and value of processes—those actions, thoughts, conversations, and periods of time for work that are necessary to accomplish any worthwhile task. And an awareness of processes is crucial for comprehending the abstract but very meaningful qualities of human life. For example, the marriage vow, "for richer, for poorer," is most meaningful for those couples who have experienced the processes of daily life when finances were good and bad. A person about to enter a long-term relationship may harbor the illusion that he understands this concept because one afternoon he visited a large number of Web sites focused on family finance. Finally, technology has made advertising and consumption the single most ubiquitous element of daily life. So it's somewhat natural that whatever we want, we want to buy it, right now.

Salespeak and McCulture

The social and cultural homogeneity created by technology's ability to spread Salespeak threatens the survival of specific cultures, creating a single "McCulture," in which Salespeak is the dominant discourse. Most of the world's media is owned by a handful of corporations (Miller 1996). According to McChesney (1997), there are "nine firms which dominate the world": Time Warner, Disney, Bertelsmann, Viacom, Rupert Murdoch's News Corporation, Sony, TCI, Universal (Seagram), and NBC. Most of these are U.S. based, translational media corporations, which form a system to "advance the cause of the global market and promote commercial values, while denigrating journalism and culture not conducive to the immediate bottom line or long-run corporate interests" (McChesney 1997, 11). When most of us talk about technology "shrinking the world," we think about the great speed of communication. This speed, however, ultimately leads to sameness.

Salespeak and Environmental Destruction

McKibben (1990) and others have detailed the ways in which Salespeak leads to environmental destruction. We cannot escape paying the price for large vehicles contaminating the air as millions of people perpetually wait in line in traffic jams, fast-food restaurants, and drive-in banks. We can't forever ignore the massive amounts of paper, plastic, petroleum, and other resources that fuel a society submerged in consumption. Among other values and practices, those of competition, materialism, consumption, freedom of choice, and the individualized mobility afforded by automobiles are all part of America's dominant ideology, all mainly fueled by Salespeak.

Salespeak and Mental Health

Salespeak chips away at our mental well-being by telling us that we have problems that can mainly be fixed with money. When appearance and style are most valued, our ability to think, not just solve problems, withers. When we're quagmired in sorting out the differences in the quality, quantity, and prices of seventy-nine types of salad dressing, it's much harder to imagine an alternative world. And when our perceptions are based almost exclusively on appearances, on the assumption that everything is for sale, that all things, people, beliefs, and values are mere commodities, then the only golden rule to guide us becomes a price tag. Of course, consumption can have a placating effect, appearing to address a perceived deficit. But with time, a gnawing feeling may return, whispering that "the product wasn't that great, anyway." And when consumption doesn't work, our habit is to spend more money, or to spend it differently. And when that doesn't work, Salespeak provides no answers—only confusion or frustration, which often turn to cynicism.

Also, Salespeak can influence our mental health because marketing has become so "experiential." Having so many brands competing within such an affluent society has elevated them to the point where they no function as surrogate human processes. That is, brands can now operate not just as mere representations of products, but as processes that link with consumers. The chairman of a Manhattan ad agency concludes that brands have become so anthropomorphized, that they "enter our lives as relationships—in order to either enhance or dissolve other relationships" (Shalit 1999, 27). And such relationships can include those with other people. The young viewer of the Gap TV commercial for khaki pants may develop a "relationship" with this series of ads, which focuses his attention not just on the product itself, but also on the models and their actions and what they might suggest to him.

For example, these commercials may hint to him that his own girlfriend may be less seductive than the girls he watches, that the crowd of dancing teens in the commercial may somehow reduce his own feelings of social isolation. Robert Deutsch, a cognitive anthropologist who works in advertising, defines brand in encompassing terms: "Brand is when a person creates—the word I like to use is designs—a metonymic link between their own self-story and the story of a product, such that to be loyal to the product is a misnomer. It's loyalty to the self" (Shalit 1999, 30). In this view, brand and self not only communicate with each other, they are one and the same. Brands R Us. In short, our mental health is hard enough to negotiate when just human beings are involved. But when you throw in relationships with brands as if they were people, things can really get screwy.

We know little about how Salespeak may affect other types of behavior, but the issue is at least beginning to be explored in literary fiction, film, and video. Documentary videos such as *The Ad and the Ego* (Boihem and Emmanouilides 1997) and *Affluenza* (de Graaf and Boe 1997) are creatively examining the psychological and social ills generated by our culture's overemphasis on materialism and consumption. After reading Bret Easton Ellis's *American Psycho*, a book that Canadian serial killer Paul Bernardo considered bedside reading, Dyson noted, "The cultural environment where such a book comes from is fascinating. . . . The parts with the description of consumer goods are boring. It makes you look forward to the killing, actually. Because of that it was kind of an eyeopener to me. I never thought of the causal relationship of mindless consumption and the lack of real human interaction, eventually leading to violence" (Dyson 1999a).

Salespeak and Free Speech

Despite the personal, social, and cultural damage wrought by Salespeak, and despite the fact that Salespeak is so prevalent that it crowds out other types of messages that are not motivated by a desire to sell something, the free speech issue is always raised in defense: "Doesn't free speech guarantee the right of anyone to say anything?" I strongly believe in free speech, but when I consider the enormous power of Salespeak and the problems it generates, free speech becomes a lame excuse. How, given our current state, can we continue to treat large corporations as if they were individuals? Today, it's absurd to think about mega-businesses in the same ways we think about individuals, yet we to do this. Corporations, the main source of unified, multichanneled Salespeak campaigns are special interests. Therefore, they are bound to place the public welfare second to their own interests. In very basic terms, democracy conflicts with capitalism. Democracy is based upon inclusion, whereas capitalism is based upon exclusion.

At the same time, media organizations' own checks against what they broadcast, their standards and practices departments, have become marginalized. At least since the mid-80s, corporate downsizing—and the corporate culture that assumed leadership during this period—have helped ensure that consumers are treated as "targets" and that bottom lines always win. Also, government deregulation of broadcasting has encouraged further disregard for anything except profit. Not all media makers, of course, are consciously conspiring to manipulate us for profit, although this occurs far too often, as in the cases of Channel One television and the ZapMe! Corporation, examined earlier in this chapter.

Finally, those who maintain that corporations should have the same rights of free speech as individuals often assert that "the marketplace of ideas" is the best determinant of which ideas rise or fall. However, in practice, this means that only those who can afford to mass-market their ideas—that is, media conglomerates such as Time Warner and Disney—will have a stall (and a bullhorn) in the marketplace. And the corporations that can afford these places often rely upon violence and sensationalism because they sell well around the globe, because they translate easily into all languages. Explosions, gunshots, and sex require no subtitles. The free speech of far poorer independent media and individuals has scant opportunity to be heard. If something doesn't make a certain profit, it's gone. This is how free speech is most often snuffed.

RECOMMENDATIONS

Most old solutions have long been pre-empted by whiz-bang technology and the consumption mania it spreads. I recently received a long letter from a high school junior in Iowa, who explained that he'd read some of my writings. This student debater was researching ways in which the federal government could oppose advertising in public schools. One of his ideas was somehow to declare consumerism a religion, and then remove advertising from schools under the existing law separating church and state. Although this idea may appear outlandish, it nonetheless represents the type of thinking that the overpowering world of Salespeak now demands.

On the other hand, when we take actions in response to Salespeak, we can end up fueling its flames. For example, when beer advertisers became aware of their target audience's growing cynicism about advertising, they countered with the "nod and wink" strategy, designed to tap into this very cynicism. That is, advertisers created ads that poked fun at advertising, such as Sprite's campaign, "Image Is Nothing, Thirst Is Everything." When advertising enjoys free rein in a free-market economy, it can neuter any consumer criticism by incorporating these opposing viewpoints into their ad messages. In a way, consumer awareness often spurs Salespeak to new heights. Despite these challenges, I offer the following recommendations.

Pursue the Personal Video Recorder

Despite the fact that this recommendation may well result in a game of technological one-upmanship, we should pursue the development of the personal video recorder, a new machine with a computerlike hard drive enabling it to "pause or rewind a live program, record while you play back, and compile any kind of programs you like." Most importantly, the PVR can also skip commercials. As you might expect, such a machine has so frightened some media conglomerates that they are threatening to file a lawsuit to stop it from being sold (Solomon 1998b). Skipping TV commercials before they begin (instead of muting them) would be a considerable step forward. However, if such technology becomes common, advertisers may, in turn, create even more attractive enticements. For example, some commercials would likely begin to look more like regular programs. Even though the PVR may provide only a temporary respite from Salespeak, it's worth a try.

Ban Professionals from Exploiting Young People for Commercial Purposes

Professional associations, especially groups such as the American Psychological Association and the National Education Association, were founded for humane purposes—to help people, to heal them, understand them, and teach them. These original principles were intended to apply to individuals as well as to the whole of society. However, too many professionals have drifted away from these humane aims and values. Instead, some psychologists, for example, use their knowledge and skills to exploit and manipulate children. More than ever before, psychologists use their understanding of human behavior to design more effective advertising campaigns aimed at children. In addition, methods of psychological research—especially focus groups crafted to lay bare children's fears, dreams, and desires—are employed to develop more effective advertising. These young research subjects are often unaware that they are even being manipulated. Even though other countries have laws protecting children from advertising (e.g., Canada, Greece, Sweden, Norway), the APA's Ethical Principles of Psychologists and Code of Conduct, for example, does not even address this issue. Groups such as the APA, NEA, and others should make public statements reaffirming their helping and healing missions and monitor professionals who abuse and disregard them. In a September 30, 1999, letter to Richard Suinn, president of the APA, sixty psychologists urged that organization to "amend the APA's Ethics Code to establish limit for psychologists regarding the use of psychological knowledge or techniques to observe, study, manipulate, harm, exploit, mislead, trick or deceive children for commercial purposes" (American Psychological Association 1999). If professionals cannot restrain their colleagues from exploiting children, then the government should.

Ban Advertising in Schools

If each school that requires students to watch commercials (e.g., Channel One schools, discussed earlier in this chapter) received the same amount of money spent to produce each commercial shown, then this gross imbalance would be somewhat fairer. Each school should also receive payment each time a commercial is repeated. Billions of dollars in additional revenue for each school would help the current playing field level out a bit. But these scenarios are sheer fantasy. Therefore, we need federal legislation to ban all forms of print and electronic advertising in schools. This ban would return the schools to what they once were—a marketplace of ideas, not a marketplace of products and packaged ideologies wrapped in the guise of entertaining TV ads and programs. America must officially define public school students as citizens and not as consumers.

Enact a Federal Law to Protect Young Consumers

Advertising at its best is making people feel that without their product, you're a loser. Kids are very sensitive to that. If you tell them to buy something, they are resistant. But if you tell them that they'll be a dork if they don't, you've got their attention. You open up emotional vulnerabilities and it's very easy to do with kids because they're the most emotionally vulnerable. (Written by Nancy Shalek, president, Shalek Advertising Agency, quoted in Nader and Ruskin 1999.)

The Federal Trade Commission (FTC) should be responsible, as it once was, for protecting children and young adults from exploitive advertising. Public Law 96–252, passed by Congress in 1980, actually prohibits the FTC from establishing rules to protect children from exploitive advertising. Because children at a very early age are heavily targeted by advertisers—at home, at school, at play, and everywhere else—this law should be repealed.

Tax Advertising

There is hardly a public space in America where advertising does not intrude. For this reason alone—because we have no "ad-free zones"—advertising in public spaces should be restricted, as well as heavily taxed. If advertising cannot be banned wholesale in schools (as it should be), then the second-best solution is to impose hefty taxes on advertising, especially in "sensitive" locations, such as near places of worship, schools, and other places of natural, architectural, historical, and cultural beauty and/or importance. Baker examines this recommendation's rationale and constitutionality. He declares that such laws are needed because "individual efforts . . . cannot succeed adequately given the existing economic and legal framework" (Baker 1994, 136). Such taxes should be used to educate and retrain teachers and others in media education, to purchase technology and training for schools, to fund graduate training and research in media literacy, and even to fund the removal of advertising from public places.

Stop Passing Advertising Costs to Consumers

Gerbner (1998) reminds us that the airways are public property, not private domain: "broadcasters operate by virtue of a license issued by the Federal Communications Commission (FCC), in exchange for their promise to provide 'public service.' " Gerbner laments the unfair way in which we pay for television. We pay for *Baywatch* when we buy shampoo at the supermarket. That is, the high costs of commercials are built into the price of the shampoo. What's more, much of the profits earned on products are plowed back into the company's advertising budget, not into improving the product. What's even more, this money can be written off at tax time, as business expenses. Hence, we pay more than once for advertising we may not like or want. Gerbner advocates that people insist that the FCC and Congress enforce the terms of the license. He also proposes that "all programming over the public airwaves be produced by a public corporation (as in all other democratic countries) accessible to citizens (which private corporations are not)." This would involve the public in subsidizing it, not corporate or advertising subsidy.

Pay for TV by the Program

Another partial solution is to institute a "pay by the program" TV system. McCannon summarizes the advantages of this plan:

- We could have *real news* without the ratings-induced tendency to give us sex, violence, and kitties in trees [see Chapter number 5, "Senationspeak"].

- If the system were national in scope, larger markets would provide *real variety*. We could have whole channels devoted to Hispanic women's interests, jazz, snowboarding, classical music, golf . . .

- Genuine variety might lead us out of the current tendency to dumb down and coarsen the national culture through the epidemic of sitcoms and action (violent) programs.

- There would be no 30-second political ads, so we would have to figure out a way to genuinely inform citizens about candidates' real positions. How democratic.

- If people paid by the program, they would consume television more carefully. TV would not just be "on" all day. People would consider the cost of the program versus, say, a walk in the park. . . . Families might spend more time watching together or even talking, reading and playing with one another. (McCannon 1999)

Much of this chapter boils down to Salespeak from the media on one hand, and education on the other. However, in most discussions of Salespeak, media, and the media literacy movement, we often overlook a basic issue—the intrinsic worth of education. Because of many of the forces mentioned in this chapter, we usually talk about education as a means for students to achieve material success. In a culture that sells and glorifies things, even elevating them to iconic and mythic status, it's little wonder that we forget that the chief value of education has always been intrinsic—that the only thing that matters, as Cookson (1998) reminds us, is "arousing to life the wonderful ideas that lay sleeping in the souls of children."

Finally, given its technological capabilities, its massive funding, and its popular appeal, Salespeak easily fills any social or cultural vacuum, as it does for Pepsi, the young woman described at this chapter's beginning. And most of the voids filled by Salespeak are large ones. For instance, Christianity has established most of our ethical codes for the past 2000 years, but for increasing numbers of people, it no longer motivates ethical behavior. In the West, at least, little or nothing else remains to fill this void, not even communism. Salespeak, then, fills each vacuum, floods quickly into each crevice. People unanchored to any kind of compelling moral guidelines tend to flounder when they search for meaning in their lives and try to establish their own identity. Unanchored people are good for business, good for Salespeak, as they continually try to purchase meaning and morality in the marketplace. As Lapham (1997) asks, "If I knew who I was, why would I keep buying new brands of aftershave lotion, and how then would I add to the sum of the gross domestic product?" In such a world, Pepsi's life will belong less to her and more to her namesake.

Learn about Salespeak

America's media literacy movement is growing and becoming better organized, especially through the efforts of such umbrella organizations as The Cultural Environment Movement, founded by George Gerbner, dean emeritus of the Annenberg School of Communication. The CEM is a nonprofit coalition of independent organizations and individuals from every state of the United States and fifty-seven countries on six continents. This coalition is "united in working for gender equity, general diversity, and democratic decision-making in media ownership, employment, and representation." From all indications, CEM is a dedicated, practical, imaginative, and humane organization.

A note of caution. Although it's great that the number of media literacy organizations in America is growing, some of them have become somewhat co-opted by corporate interests. One large clearinghouse of media literary information refuses to distribute materials which document Channel One's adverse effects on students. Similarly, I watched a video distributed by a large media literacy organization about "how to watch TV critically." I kept wondering when the video would stop the fluff and get down to answering the question. It never did. As I watched the credits roll at the film's end, I noticed that one of the sponsors was Whittle Communications, the corporation that established Channel One, which beams commercials to captive audiences of kids. Media literacy organizations and individuals who espouse media literacy should not be subsidized by the very people who profit from the exploitation of children.

Sensationspeak

The excellence of every art is its intensity, capable of making all disagreeables evaporate, from their being in close relationship with beauty and truth—Examine King Lear and you will find this exemplified throughout; but in this picture ["Death on a Pale Horse"] we have unpleasantness without any momentous depth . . . in which to bury its repulsiveness.

—John Keats, 1817

OKAY, THESE ARE YOUR OPTIONS . . .

If you don't want to learn how, when, where, and why sportscaster Marv Albert was indicted on charges of ripping a woman's flesh with his teeth, or how boxer Mike Tyson bit off a chunk of his opponent's ear, you can catch the program, "When Animals Attack," and "World's Most Dangerous Animals." If you have grown weary of the Bill Clinton and Monica Lewinsky sex scandal, you may view the program, "World's Scariest Police Chases."

And if you don't want to hear more about sportscaster Frank Gifford's extramarital affair, simply tune in to "Cheating Spouses: Caught on Tape" or "When Good Pets Go Bad." If you've already seen the film *Twister*, and if you're tired of "Alien Autopsy," and if you can't take any more media coverage of Princess Diana's deadly car accident, you might catch "World's Deadliest Storms Caught on Tape" or "World's Most Shocking Medical Videos." This is Sensationspeak: communication that madly strokes our senses, intense messages that are unconnected to truth, order, beauty—"unpleasantness without any depth."

These "options" constitute one small fragment of Sensationspeak. In *Busted on the Job*, a TV program airing on the Fox Network, food employees hack and blow their noses into tacos, and a secretary defecates on her boss's chair. One planned program, *Crash Test*, will feature several items being blown up, such as exploding 1,000 parking meters and throwing a Corvette off a building (Stein and McDowell 1999). Sensationspeak is also becoming more invasive as well as seeping into local media. The Fox Network's New York station, WNYW, became at least the twentieth station to air hidden-camera footage of gay men soliciting sex in bathrooms:

It all started during sweeps week in Seattle in February and spread to San Diego, San Antonio and cities across the country, resurfacing for sweeps week in May in New York. The Rupert Murdoch owned Fox . . . led with promo spots declaring: "You'll think twice" about allowing your kids to use a public restroom because "sexual deviants are roaming our stores and malls." . . . Richard Goldstein, Executive Editor of *The Village Voice*, said many of the reporters came soliciting sex. "They did the thing that caused the behavior, and then they filmed it. They're presenting it as a clear and present danger to children." ("Media Mash XIII" 1998)

Invasive and local Sensationspeak also occurs without the pretense of protecting children. A San Francisco radio station, KYLD, regularly ridiculed a retarded man called "Hammerin' Hank":

" 'They have him on the show to make fun of him, laugh at him, degrade him,' the source said. At a live party, the radio station sponsored some time back at the Sound Factory, tickets to a concert were offered to the first woman to get him sexually aroused. A striptease did the trick. At that moment, the Dog House Gang [the station's morning show DJs] tore down his jogging pants to expose his genitals, and the whole club started laughing." (*San Francisco Chronicle* 1998)

Why would local TV stations in large cities show footage from cameras hidden in restrooms during sweeps month? Why would listeners tolerate the degradation of a retarded man, or anyone? Why do major networks show programs such as "When Animals Attack" and "World's Worst Plane Crashes"? Why would a station broadcast a suicide on live TV? Why would CNN's coverage of the Oklahoma bombing disaster garner its highest TV ratings ever—even "eclipsing the record viewership of the O. J. Simpson trial" (*New York Times*, April 28, 1995, A10)? And why would the *New York Times* even report on such ratings? Because it's all shocking, which entertains us. We will accept anything if it's entertaining. And entertainment is ruled by profit.

OVERVIEW

In this chapter, you will find a brief history of modern Sensationspeak, "You Asked for It," which defines this voice in more detail. Then, after exploring how Sensationspeak relates to Salespeak, I focus on some common reactions to Sensationspeak, many of which hinder our relationships with this voice. Next, "Notes from the World of Sensationspeak" provides a series of facts that reveal the expanding boundaries of this voice. I then review three influential types of Sensationspeak: Celebspeak, Alienspeak, and Hatespeak. After this, I explore the question of whether Sensationspeak is linked to actual violence. Then, after investigating some examples of "hidden" Sensationspeak, I explore some of the roots of Sensationspeak in American history, including its role in our relationships with death. Next, "Sensationspeak and Traditional American Myths" examines such legends as "rags to riches" and "the happy ending." The next segment speculates about how Sensationspeak connects to a few emerging myths of technology. This chapter ends with a series of conclusions and recommendations, which include litigation, legislation, and education.

YOU ASKED FOR IT

When I was a kid there were kids who went home to empty houses, and they did what kids do, put on the TV. There were game shows, cartoons, some boring nature shows, an old movie, "The Ann Southern Show," Spanish lessons on educational TV, a soap opera.

Thin fare, boring stuff; kids daydreamed to it. But it was better to have this being pumped into everyone's living room than, say, the Ghetto Boys on channel 25, rapping about killing women, having sex with their dead bodies and cutting off their breasts.

Really, you have to be a moral retard not to know that this is harmful, that it damages the young, the unsteady, the unfinished. You have to not care about anyone to sing these words and to put this song on TV for money.

—Peggy Noonan (Minow and Lamay 1995, 8)

Today, our official landscape of reality—what's in the news—is much like our current entertainment: both focus on stimulating our senses. Each time the ante is upped in blood, gore, violence, and humans and animals in pain, higher doses of Sensationspeak are required to achieve the same effects in the audience. Sensationspeak has steadily escalated, from the days of circus man P. T. Barnum to Robert Ripley's syndicated column (and now, museums), "Believe It or Not!" In the 1950s, a popular television program, *You Asked for It*, starred Art Baker as host. Viewers wrote to Baker (a genial, fatherly, TV version of Ripley) requesting what they wanted to see on television. As a child, I lay on our living room floor and watched this program, transfixed by the young girl dancing atop an airplane wing as the craft flew across the black and white sky.

Two decades later, *That's Incredible!* appeared on TV—far glitzier, even shallower. By millennium's turn, Sensationspeak is the norm, not the exception that it was in the 1950s, when tabloid newspapers did not blare from grocery store checkout counters. The gentlemanly Art Baker has been replaced by the crude Howard Stern and a multitude of others. Kaul (1999) sums up the world of Sensationspeak this way: "Nothing, apparently, can gain attention in the chaotic atmosphere of our popular culture unless it is loud and shocking and, preferably, naked. Life increasingly has come to imitate professional wrestling. Literally."

WHAT IS SENSATIONSPEAK?

Sensationspeak is any print or electronic message in which the content and/or form stimulates the senses more than the mind. The term "Sensationspeak" also applies when nonstimulating messages occur rapidly, intensely, and in great volume. Although Sensationspeak can stimulate rational thought and motivate humane instincts, it often does not. Indeed, Sensationspeak is usually gratuitous—unhinged from larger concerns for order, beauty, truth, or a desire to change the world for the better. Sensationspeak often has little or no context. For example, a Benetton magazine focused an entire issue on images of dead and mutilated animals. These messages offered no information about how to stop animal abuse, nor did they include any information on animal rights. This company merely tried to sell clothes through pure Sensationspeak.

Sensationspeak is often driven by emotion. It relies upon verbal and visual imagery and surprise, as well as extremes in volume, tone, frequency, and speed. Sensationspeak carries many verbal, aural, and visual shocks (also known as JPMs or jolts per minute) ranging from loud noises and music, to explosions and collisions, to rapidly edited scenes. As a movie director said, "We are constantly accelerating the visual to keep the viewer in his seat" (Landay 1998). In addition to speed, sex is used to keep viewers in their seats—especially sex coupled with violence. Sex and violence can occur within the same scene, or they can be juxtaposed or alternated with each other in separate scenes. Either way, the frequent pairing of sex with violence has prompted some observers to use a single term, "sexandviolence."

Often designed for mass audiences, Sensationspeak "travels well" across the boundaries of age, race, class, gender, and culture. That is, the visceral shocks and jolts per minute of Sensationspeak require little explanation and few subtitles: a gunshot or a kick in the face makes equal sense, regardless of your age, gender, culture, language, socioeconomic status, or neck size. Because Sensationspeak is transient, designed to provide short-term solutions to fictional conflicts and is aimed at mainly young audiences, it is a slave to current style, especially other media messages. Therefore, it often strives to be witty, sexy, gimmicky, or glamorous. Consequently, Sensationspeak has a brief shelf life and is easily forgotten. However, its long-term effects tell a different story, a topic dealt with later in this chapter (see "Are Sensationspeak and Real Violence Linked?").

Finally, and maybe most important, Sensationspeak functions as an extensive set of stories—a body of narrative or myth that shows us and tells us how to live and how not to live, just as fairy tales and fables did for past generations. Like the tales of ancient times (e.g., myths involving wolves, witches, and natural disasters), Sensationspeak addresses our natural need to peek at the dark sides of life, just to see how dark it can get; to experience it vicariously rather than actually. However, when we're surrounded with too many stories of how *not* to live (e.g., the Andrew Cunanan murders; the Menendez brothers' murder of their parents; Jeffrey Dahmer's killing and cannibalism), it's possible that we can grow, over time, to accept them as the model of how to live, almost by default.

SENSATIONSPEAK AND SALESPEAK

Sensationspeak shares several characteristics with Salespeak (see Chapter 4). First, like Salespeak, Sensationspeak appropriates previous styles, elements, and images, blurring the boundaries between "high" and "low" modes of representation. The Benetton ads mentioned previously pretend to focus on animal rights (a "high" mode of representation), while using the images of dead and mutilated animals to shock us (a "low" mode of representation). A film such as *Starship Troopers* may glamorize Nazi-esque values, a "low" mode of representation, while at the same time, its creators claim that such Nazi references function to satirize or parody Nazi themes (a "high" mode of representation). Despite such claims of altruism or satire, it's hard for Sensationspeak to have it both ways, because whatever shock is generated can often distract us from anything else the message might have to offer.

Second, like Salespeak, Sensationspeak is self-reflexive: other media report on it. It becomes "news" to report that demonic possessions increased at the release of the film *The Exorcist*. It becomes "news" when *Time* magazine reviews how ABC covered the FBI's confrontation with Branch Davidians in Waco, Texas. Third, Sensationspeak overlaps with Salespeak in that it "sells" or persuades us that violence, sex, aggression, and instant gratification are acceptable, legitimate, optional behaviors.

Fourth, like Salespeak, Sensationspeak can distract us from larger social issues, such as corporate dominance and environmental deterioration— a phenomenon Postman (1985) refers to as "amusing ourselves to death."

Finally, if you follow the multiple threads of a specific case study of fictional or nonfictional Sensationspeak, such as the O. J. Simpson trials, you will likely find blurred boundaries, just as you would find in a specific case of Salespeak. For example, a newly released feature film, spin-off toys, fast-food products, other entertainment media, news-reporting media, and advertising might echo each other, reinforcing each other's products. Sensationspeak can be similarly resonant and recursive, some of which is calculated and some of which is due to business hopping the bandwagon.

COMMON RESPONSES TO SENSATIONSPEAK

Whenever Sensationspeak arises as a topic in public discourse and informal conversations, several knee-jerk responses surface, but I'll note only a few of them here. One of them is a red flag that, somehow, the "far right" or religious fanatics such as Jerry Falwell or Paul Weyrich have contaminated our thinking. This red flag quickly leads to the suspicion that whoever is talking about Sensationspeak "must favor censorship" or "must not believe in free speech." In reality, censorship is seldom an either/or issue. Nor does this argument often include any weighing of the differences between a megacorporation's right and an individual's rights. Although I personally don't believe that corporations pursing profits are entitled to the same free speech rights as individuals pursuing ideas, I do believe that such questions as, "Who is free speech for?" and "What is the purpose of free speech?" are, in many ways, useless questions. Why? Because there is no necessary *or* unequivocal connection between the symbol (First Amendment) and the thing symbolized (free speech). We can never agree on such questions. Additionally, when media organizations and advertisers claim "You're infringing on our freedom of speech!," we forget that profiteering is the greatest restriction on free speech. That is, anything that doesn't make a certain amount of money is instantly dropped.

A second automatic response is that whoever acknowledges Sensationspeak is engaging in a "recurring moral panic" over a new technology. Sorry again, but Sensationspeak has deep roots and transcends technology, though new technologies have certainly spread it. In addition, it's not the technology so much as how messages are selected and crafted. A third common response is to blame, wholesale, the makers of Sensationspeak—its directors, producers, and writers. Again, sorry, but it's more complicated than this. Although creators must bear responsibility, we must also remember that the deregulation of TV in 1984 led to increased product licensing. Within a year, most of the best-selling toys were related to TV shows, most of which were violent (Frank 1999).

Also, consumers must take some blame here. When cable TV spread during the 1980s, consumers rushed to it because of improved TV reception and its greater choice of channels. They did this without understanding that these channels and programs would be free of the same controls which apply to network television. As Considine observers, "Without FCC controls, explicit language and graphic images of both sex and violence began to find their way into American living rooms where they were often encountered by children and teens in the absence of parental supervision" (1993, 10). Although there is certainly truth in this, it also returns us to such questions as, "Who owns the airwaves?" and "Should the right to free speech be granted to large corporations in the same way as it is to individuals?"

A fourth response to Sensationspeak is that such material, in any form or medium, debases or trivializes other communication. The opposing view is that it does not, because we perceive that such information exists quite apart from other communication. Some people even talk about it as existing in a different "space." The truth likely resides somewhere between these polarities. However, as with all other averages or continuums, sometimes the extremes will dominate.

Missing from most of these common responses is a concern for the values that undergird Sensationspeak. For example, the heavy coverage of Donald and Ivana Trump's divorce seldom focused on anything other than the amount of money involved in their settlement. To be sure, we could have learned other lessons and meanings from the Trumps' situation, but the media messages mainly focused on money, thereby fixing consumers only on materialism.

NOTES FROM THE WORLD OF SENSATIONSPEAK

- 5 million: The number of hits per day averaged by *Playboy* magazine's Web site (Schlosser 1997).
- 109: The average number of "graphic and gruesome violent acts per hour," based upon ten movies starring Arnold Schwarzenegger (Gerbner 1994).
- 8 to 1: The ratio by which TV references to premarital sex during the family hour outnumber references to sex within marriage (Media Research Center Report on the Family Hour TV, 1996).
- 20–25: The average number of violent acts per hour in Saturday morning children's programming (American Psychological Association 1993).
- $750 million to $1 billion: The range of money spent by Americans in 1996 on telephone sex (Schlosser 1997).

- 12, 18, and 53: The number of killings (respectively) portrayed in these three films: *The Godfather, Godfather II*, and *Godfather III* (Gerbner 1994).

- $665 million: The amount of money Americans spent on hard-core pornographic video rentals in 1996—up from $490 million in 1992 and $75 million in 1985 (Schlosser 1997).

- Phoebe's boyfriend won't sleep with her. Since the guy "won't put out," the gang speculates he must be gay. Later, Phoebe barely contains her glee when she finally "makes it" with her boyfriend. She succeeded because she explained to him that she wasn't expecting a commitment just because they had sex: the plot of *Friends*, prime-time network TV program (aired in March 1996).

- 18 and 264: The number of killings (respectively) portrayed in the 1988 movie *Die Hard* and the 1990 movie *Die Hard 2* (Gerbner 1994).

- $175 million: The amount that Americans spent in 1996 on pornographic videos to watch in their rooms at major hotel chains, such as the Hilton, the Hyatt, and Holiday Inn (Schlosser 1997).

- *Crash*: The title of a 1997 film about people who are sexually aroused by automobile wrecks. In this film, a man "sexually penetrates a woman's wound." This movie was also "the subject of panting coverage on 'Entertainment Tonight' " (Grossman and Hewitt 1997).

- One-third to one-fifth: Estimated amount of hard-core pornographic videos being sold in America in 1997 that are made and filmed by amateurs (Schlosser 1997).

- 300,000 kilometers per second: The speed of electrons, the basic unit of Sensationspeak (Landay 1998).

- 150: The average number of pornographic videos produced in the United States each week (Schlosser 1997).

- February 1992: The date in which the NBC series *I Witness Video* showed a replay of murders taped by amateurs with video cameras. According to *TV Guide*, "For the first time in history, a major network started programming death as entertainment" ("What You Need to Know about Television Violence" 1998).

- A male character asks, "Does size matter?" A female character responds, "Give women some credit. Of course it doesn't matter. Unless you're having sex." (Penis size as running joke in episode of *Caroline in the City*, prime-time network TV program, March 1996).

- 500: The number of titles sold by Homegrown Videos of San Diego, California, that portray ordinary people engaged in sex (Schlosser 1997).

- $20: The amount of money paid by Homegrown Videos for every minute of pornographic videotape it accepts from the public for commercial distribution (Schlosser 1997).

- 2 times per minute: The average number of times viewers change channels using remote control devices (Landay 1998).

- 133: The number of "acts of mayhem per hour" in the film, *Teenage Mutant Ninja Turtles* (Gerbner 1994).

- A group of friends bemoan a shortage of contraceptive sponges. With supplies limited, Elaine interviews her date to determine if he is "sponge worthy." Plot to episode of *Seinfeld*, prime-time network TV program (March 1996).

- 500 percent: The amount of increase in the annual production of hard-core pornographic videos since 1991 (Schlosser 1997).

- 8,000: The number of murders seen on TV by the time an average child finishes sixth grade (TV-Free America Web site).

- 200,000: The number of violent acts seen on TV by the average 18-year-old American (Huston et al. 1992).

- Three to five: The average number of violent acts per hour on television; there has been no appreciable change in this number over the past two decades (American Psychological Association 1993).

- 1,000-plus: The number of studies that attest to a casual connection between media violence and aggressive behavior in some children (Gerbner 1999).

CELEBSPEAK: LIFESTYLES OF THE RICH AND FAMOUS AND INFAMOUS

Although there are many forms of Sensationspeak, the following sections focus on three major types: (1) Celebspeak—the communication we use in our obsession with celebrities, (2) Alienspeak—the communication about supposed beings from other planets, and (3) Hatespeak—the communication used to express negative attitudes and behaviors toward certain groups of people. Like the other voices explored in this book, the greater the spread of technology, the more ubiquitous Sensationspeak becomes.

Celebspeak includes the words and symbols surrounding our worship of celebrities, found in tabloid newspaper headlines; radio and TV interviews with "stars" of television, film, sports, high finance, music, and politics; fan club newsletters; TV docudramas; Web sites and chat rooms based on specific luminaries; celebrity endorsements in advertising, and so on. Celebspeak has many causes. For instance, a "brand-oriented" society is likely to think of people in the same ways it thinks of objects and commodities. That is, a celebrity, as a brand of person, does not differ terribly from name-brand clothing. Second, our obsession with celebrities helps fill the void created by America's great lack of authentic community in our daily lives. American life is often devoid of communal spaces and times for interacting with others outside of home and work. The celebrities we come to feel that we "know personally" can be considered as media replacements for friends, neighbors, and even extended family members from whom we are isolated.

When average people are surrounded by Celebspeak, the repercussions affect individuals as well as society. First, Celebspeak seems to make us want more—more details and images of Leonardo DiCaprio, more details about Madonna's bedroom. Celebspeak often takes two routes. The first one is to build the celebrity up, as audiences participate in discovering and following that person's career and personal life. The second one is following that same person's fall from grace. Celebrities who make this yo-yo trip several times (whether actual or hyped) become icons, such as Elizabeth Taylor and the late Frank Sinatra.

Another effect of Celebspeak is that it eventually makes many of us begin to crave media exposure for ourselves. You don't have to look very hard for evidence of the average person seeking notoriety with a larger audience: community TV channels; copycat crimes (see the later section on copy catviolence); audience participation in nearly any venue; celebrities, from sports stars to actors and professional wrestlers, being elected to public office; the rapid growth of personal Web sites, which are accessed by large audiences; and virtual reality software. This effect operates, of course, when audiences identify to a fairly high degree with what they behold in media.

One example of how to act out your own celebrity fantasies comes from a company in Anaheim, California, Tinseltown. For a price ($44.95), in addition to dinner, you get to become a celebrity for an evening, as you step onto a red carpet and are besieged by reporters, camera operators, and autograph hounds. An emcee describes your glittering life as you accept your Oggie Award, Tinseltown's version of the Oscar. You get to watch yourself on a large screen as you appear with Henry Fonda in *On Golden Pond*. Your photo is splashed on several large screens while your adoring fans scream and applaud. According to the senior vice president of this "fantasy adventure" company, "Everybody that sees themselves on that screen is imagining that millions of viewers are watching them" ("Dinner with Fame on the Side," *Columbia* [Missouri] *Daily Tribune*, January 3, 1999: 6C). We are no longer just a nation of watchers. Now we want to be watched, as well.

A third effect of Celebspeak is that overvaluing glamour and charisma distorts our notion of what fame really is. Many of us may regard fame as far more important than actual accomplishment and behavior. We may not perceive of fame as a burden, because we seldom get past the glamor and glittering surfaces. We tend to think of fame as a goal in and of itself—not as a by-product of real accomplishment. This perpetuates our pursuit of fame. If more people knew the downside of celebrityhood, I doubt we would pursue it so doggedly by consuming media. However, if our constructions of celebrityhood ever collapsed, so would much media, advertising, and sales—America's main floor.

A fourth effect of Celebspeak is that we fail to differentiate between fame, mere notoriety, and infamy. Mother Theresa was famous because of her long work with Calcutta's impoverished people, but an unknown scorned spouse on the *Jerry Springer Show* is notorious only during that episode's airing. (The unknown people who appear on the Springer show and others of its ilk are merely following in the footsteps of what they have witnessed throughout their lives—that "famous" people, such as Madonna and Ivana Trump, appear on TV to bear blame and spread it.) However, because both the scorned spouse and Mother Theresa appear on TV, it's easy to lump them together as both being famous. Mother Theresa may have appeared on the same channel as the embittered spouse—or on a different channel but at the same time, or on the same TV set—or they may have appeared nearly next to each other, as the viewer channel hopped with the remote control. The principle of proximity from gestalt psychology holds true here: the meanings associated with one thing can "rub off" onto a very different thing, merely because the two are near each other.

Fifth, we tend to accept celebrities, mainly actors, as legitimate embodiments of the roles they portray in fictional films and TV programs. After actor Robert Young began playing Dr. Marcus Welby in the popular TV series *Marcus Welby, M.D.*, he was forever regarded by the public as a kindly, real doctor. At century's turn, we are hardly questioning this blurring of reality and pure fiction. In 1999, the U.S. Senate Subcommittee on Public Health played to a full house of spectators who had come to listen to a visitor urging support for the Pediatric Autism Research Act. The person testifying was not a doctor, nurse, researcher, or academic expert. He was Anthony Edwards, the actor who plays Dr. Mark Greene on the popular TV drama *ER*. Approximately six Hollywood actors per month address congressional hearings ("Cause Celebs" 1999). When pressed, actors such as Edwards can point to other reasons that qualify them to provide expert testimony. For instance, they may be connected to the issue through friends, family, or interests outside of acting. Nonetheless, the fact that the actors are celebrities who are also superficially associated with the issue is the main reason for their appearance. You would think (or hope) that the people who are elected to Congress would know better. Instead, they officially certify that celebrities who have no experience with the issue are nonetheless experts. Here, Sensationspeak meets Doublespeak.

Sixth, the more awestruck we are with celebrities, the less likely we tend to value our own achievements and lives. If we submerge ourselves in Celebspeak, the relationship becomes one of spectator and participant. And scant few spectators would ever dare compete with their idols. We develop the mind-set that spectators should consume only the news and other texts created by the participant-celebrities. (However, as noted earlier, more noncelebrities are desiring to become participants and minicelebrities also, and technology is aiding this shift.) The more awestruck we are, the more passive we become. The National Commission on Civic

Renewal concluded that America is becoming a "nation of spectators" ("Report Says U.S. Is 'Nation of Spectators,' " 1998, 11A). Basing its claim on statistical and anecdotal evidence, the commission stated that Americans need to participate far more in school, church, and community organizations. The report also concluded that the entertainment industry should be held "as accountable for civic harm" as the tobacco industry is for physical harm. We've become so blinded by the klieg lights that we seldom recall the truth: throughout history, ordinary people have accomplished far more than those bathed in spotlights.

Seventh, our often frenzied worship of sports heroes, actors, and others can be viewed as displacing the worship of traditional symbols of organized religion. Images of Michael Jordan seem to outnumber images of crucifixes or Stars of David or any other religious symbol. What has long been called the "worship of false idols" has been spread by technology. It makes sense that the more we invest time, money, and psychic energy into celebrities, the less we'll have for religious symbols, which, of course, also lack the dizzying attraction of their competition.

Finally, Celebspeak is fueled by the natural frailty of our own psyches—our need for approval and validation. We tend to idealize famous people mainly by assuming that their public personas match their private selves. However, this can seldom be true. We also tend to believe that achieving success and fortune provides celebrities with a kind of internal security or peace, because they no longer have to gain the approval of others, as most of us mere mortals must do. But this can seldom be true, either.

Sue Erikson Bloland (1999) believes that adults idealize celebrities because it is "a way of sustaining the belief we held as children that we are protected by people more powerful and capable than ourselves in a world too frightening to endure without the comfort of this illusion" (62). She further reminds us that humans are the only animals who shoulder the knowledge of their own deaths, and that consequently, we invest our own energies and time into larger-than-life celebrities "to make us feel safe." As Erikson Bloland (1999), Korzybski (1933), Hayakawa (1991), and many others have observed, this idealization of others diminishes and denies our own lives. How can a lowly commoner see her own potential (and build on it through actions and changes), when she is focused on a superhuman other?

ALIENSPEAK: THE TRUTH IS OUT THERE (AND SO IS PASTRAMI ON RYE)

Alienspeak is any communication about beings from other planets, whether depicted as science fiction or reported as fact. Of course, Alienspeak is not concerned with whether such beings exist. The little gray people with almond-shaped heads and bug-eyes are now American icons, and the Roswell incident (the purported discovery in 1947 of a crashed alien spacecraft, along with dead aliens, in New Mexico's Area 51) approximates an ancient creation myth. In addition to an explosion in books and alien-oriented Internet sites, an entire cable TV network focuses only on science fiction. Indeed aliens have so thoroughly invaded the media that we no longer question whether they actually exist: a 1997 *Time*/Yanelovich opinion poll revealed that more than one-third of all Americans believe that intelligent beings from other worlds have visited Earth (Cabbage 1997, ID).

This lack of proof or certainty about the existence of aliens, this basic ambiguity or "unknowability," resides at the core of much Alienspeak, making it an open text—a kind of Rorschach ink blot onto which we project our own state of affairs or the state of our culture. Alienspeak probably reveals more about our collective psyche and social situation than it does about anything else. For example, America's climate in 1947, when the term "flying saucers" first entered our culture, fostered a fear of aliens. In June 1947, Kenneth Arnold, an Idaho businessman, reported seeing nine saucerlike crafts as he flew his private plane over the Cascade Mountains of Washington. A reporter later referred to such craft as "flying saucers." A mere two weeks later, the Roswell event supposedly occurred. Throughout that summer, roughly 800 sightings were reported from across the country (Cabbage 1997).

At this time, most Americans didn't think these were interplanetary visitors. Instead, we feared the visitors were Russian secret weapons. All of this occurred at the same time that the communist witch hunts were heating up in Washington, D.C., fueled by the House Committee on Un-American Activities and the late Senator Joseph McCarthy of Wisconsin. By 1956, the fears of aliens from outer space and aliens from Moscow sufficiently coalesced to produce the feature film *Invasion of the Body Snatchers*, in which beings from space snatch the minds of small-town Californians, robbing them of their individuality, creating uniform zombies who serve the state as good comrades were thought to do. The psychology and motivations of film and TV aliens seem to mirror our collective psyche. The fear and anxiety of the Cold War years' body- and mind-snatching alien portrayals gave way to the 1980s' film portrayal of the kindly and benign *E.T.*, a little lost guy who wanted only to "phone home."

Once the Red Scare ran out of steam, the Roswell incident also lost power, and we seemed to forget about both dramas for thirty-one years. Then in 1978, Jesse Marcel, the intelligence officer at the Roswell air base at the time of the reported crash, gave an interview to the *National Enquirer*, the tabloid that had established itself in supermarket chains a few years earlier (Fox 1989). Marcel claimed that the debris found in 1947 was indeed from an alien spacecraft. The Air Force investigated UFO sightings from 1948 until 1969, offering explanations for all but 5 percent of the 13,000 UFO sightings reported. In 1994, the federal government's General Accounting Office also investigated UFOs and claimed that the Roswell incident was part of Project Mogul, a secret program developing balloons that were used to spy on Russian nuclear tests (Cabbage 1997).

The sometimes forgotten parallels here are that, first, interest in UFOs took off at the same time that America was fearful of earthly alien invaders, the communists. Second, the growth of alien lore since 1978 also roughly parallels the boom of electronic media in America, especially television and computers. From 1965 to 1996, the average American's time spent watching television increased by about one-third, and by the late '80s, three-quarters of all households had more than one set (Putnam 1996). During the 1990s, talk radio and the Internet mushroomed. For instance, in 1999, Art Bell's radio program *Coast to Coast AM*, which often focuses on all things alien, boasted 9 million listeners per week, making him the fourth-highest-rated radio talk show host in America. Bell's Web site (www.artbell.com) reports 44 million hits between 1997 and 1999 (Corliss 1999). All of this means more Alienspeak than ever before. Alienspeak's growth over a mere twenty years must constitute some kind of record.

Despite these parallels, as well as evidence contrary to the existence of aliens, Alienspeak will likely continue its ascent. Alienspeak has grown rapidly through several media texts and genres. In addition to the wildly popular fictional films such as *E.T., The Extraterrestrial* and *Close Encounters of the Third Kind*, "abduction" stories have deepened our belief in aliens. These stories consist of people reporting "lost time"—a period for which they cannot account for their whereabouts. Later, under hypnosis, these people describe how aliens took them aboard a spacecraft and conducted medical-type experiments on them, often probing their genitalia. Another classic media text media text perpetuating our belief in aliens is the *Alien Autopsy* film, a TV "documentary" in which people in contamination suits examine a small alien body. Despite widespread claims of fraudulence, this film has aired in America, as well as in thirty-two countries (Corliss 1995).

The newer forms of Alienspeak represent hybrids of investigative journalism, technical information, science (including scientific speculation), conspiracy theory, comedy, fantasy, theology, poetry, and cinematic special effects. Alienspeak can even merge with Salespeak. A double-page ad in *Spin* magazine (vol. 15, no. 9, September 1999) depicts an enlarged, grainy, black and white photo of a flying saucer that fills the entire left-hand page. Filling the opposite page is this statement, surrounded by white space (line breaks noted): "If aliens are smart enough/to travel through space, / why do they keep abducting the / dumbest people on earth?" Below this message is a small pack of the cigarettes being advertised. This ad simultaneously captures the aura of aliens and makes fun of people who truly believe in them.

Although Alienspeak is an evolving and mixed genre, it nonetheless contains a few common qualities.

Characteristics of Alienspeak

Web sites and other media focused on aliens share the following features, several of them similar to another genre of Sensationspeak, tabloid newspapers: (1) their central premise—that aliens from space actually exist—is sometimes assumed for readers and viewers; (2) they often employ a civilized, cerebral tone; (3) they use incomplete, unclear sources of information; (4) they use one dubious piece of information to help substantiate another; (5) they "concretize" certain points with small details, imagistic language; and (6) they use suggestive, ambiguous imagery. Of course, the features below do not apply to all forms and examples of Alienspeak.

Alienspeak **Assumes** *the Existence of Beings from Other Planets.* Alienspeak texts often operate from a base assumption of reality—a stance or frame of reference that assumes *for* viewers and readers that the existence of aliens has long been established, and that therefore, it's pointless to even consider this "old-hat" question. Although many Alienspeak texts (e.g., reports of unidentified flying objects, feature magazine and newspaper articles) maintain the stance that "we don't yet know if aliens exist," and thereby remain "open," more recent examples of Alienspeak assume that we do. Unstated or implied assumptions are difficult for many readers and viewers to identify, and they are therefore hard to refute. Several teams of scientists are indeed searching for evidence of other civilizations in our galaxy, but it's not a done deal.

For example, a few years ago, a late-night TV program, loosely fashioned after the popular *Entertainment Tonight,* included a male and female anchor sitting at desks, reporting on various items related to UFOs and aliens. The anchors provided voice-over to film clips and spoke directly into the camera, a la *Sixty Minutes,* which specializes in investigative TV journalism. After a story about alien implants, one anchor reported the name and telephone number of a physician who would remove alien implants from people, free of charge. This material was reported in a matter-of-fact manner, emphasizing only the service and the fact that it was free. The doctor's name and number appeared on the screen, just as legitimate public service information might be provided about a natural disaster or food bank. What was not emphasized, what was not even acknowledged, was any doubt that aliens even exist in the first place. The doctor and his offer could well be authentic, but what they assumed for viewers to be truth remains, of course, a profound mystery.

This rhetorical stance of assumed reality also occurs on Internet sites focusing on aliens, hence making their existence more believable, especially for unsophisticated or inexperienced readers. One now defunct Web site, bearing a 1993 date, contains official-looking lists of UFO sightings by astronauts, including Gordon Cooper, Ed White, James McDivitt, James Lovell, Frank Borman, Neil Armstrong, Buzz Aldrin, and others. This site also claims that when Neil Armstrong and Edwin "Buzz" Aldrin landed on the moon in 1969, they witnessed several spacecraft lined up on the "far side of the crater edge," watching their every move. The site then quotes Maurice Chatelain of NASA as explaining that the phrase "Santa Clause" was first used by astronaut Walter Schirra, aboard *Mercury* 8, to indicate the presence of a UFO next to his space capsule. We then learn that James Lovell, aboard the *Apollo 8* command module on Christmas Day 1968, used the same code language, stating, "Please be informed that there is a Santa Claus." This reference to Schirra's earlier use of the phrase helps validate Lovell's later use of it, creating the appearance of precedence—and hence validity.

This stance is manifested in other genres of Alienspeak, including books. Sometimes, just the titles reveal unwarranted assumptions. Consider Harrison's (1997) book *After Contact: The Human Response to Extraterrestrial Life*. According to one reviewer, this book includes chapters on "various aspects of the postcontact situation, such as first impressions, initial impact, interacting with extraterrestrial intelligence, and the long-term consequences" (Tough 1998, 625). What's more, the reviewer tells us, "four disciplined but fascinating chapters speculate on the psychology and sociology of aliens themselves, as well as their culture, social organization, and supranational systems" (625). I'm not sure who is farther out on this deep-space limb—the book's author, the reviewer, the American Psychological Association for publishing this review, or me, for reading it.

Finally, Joseph P. Firmage, who quit his successful career in computers to study aliens and UFOs, makes available his entire book *The Truth* on the Internet. In his writing, Firmage clearly acknowledges that his topic has never been established in fact. He describes his book as a "hypothesis of the unity of science, faith, and history." However, similar to his book's title, his Web site address is http://www.thewordistruth.org. Even though Firmage offers clear disclaimers, his writings, read by more and more people, are unrestrained in what they assume.

Alienspeak Employs a Civilized, Cerebral Tone. Unlike most other forms of Sensationspeak, Alienspeak—especially science fiction print literature, television, and film—is characterized by a civilized, cerebral tone. Compare the lack of noise, gore, and violence, along with the quiet, genteel style of the *Star Trek* film and TV offerings, with other forms of Sensationspeak, such as Oliver Stone's film *Natural Born Killers* or any film with Arnold Schwarzenegger. In Alienspeak, you will typically find more dialogue (spoken with more inflection); longer scenes; more varied vocabulary; longer utterances or sentences; greater emphasis on ideas and concepts, that is, topics not visible on screen, and more frequent use of manners and formal address (e.g., "Mr. Spock, may I have a word with you?").

Although some of this civil tone is attributable to Alienspeak's unavoidable links with science and technology, part of it seems due to its creators acknowledging the uncertainty of alien existence, keeping this doubt "on the table" via a sort of distancing through tone, maintaining a respect for readers and viewers. The clearest example is the print text that explores the possibilities of alien existence without expressing belief one way or the other. A far more subtle example is *Star Trek*, in TV and film. In one way, it assumes the existence of alien life, given its futuristic setting in time and non-Earth locale. However, the extent to which its creators develop the show's internal logic and construct reasons for the show's plot developments reveals respect for viewers who know that we don't yet know about alien life, but want to pretend we do. The creators of this text enable viewers to achieve a more subtle suspension of disbelief than they are often given credit for.

Alienspeak Uses Unclear, Incomplete Sources of Information. Media, especially Internet sites, have notoriously lacked accurate and complete documentation for their sources' information. This is partly because no one monitors Web sites for such things. Web sites therefore often identify their sources of information in ways that are ambiguous and difficult to verify. For example, the 1993 site noted earlier mentions only names of speakers, with no affiliation or title identified. Gordon Cooper's testimony was labeled only as having been delivered to a "United Nations committee." Other quotes come from "a taped interview by J. L. Fernando." Other sources are identified ambiguously, such as, "unnamed radio hams [operators]" and a "certain professor who wished to remain anonymous."

This Web site lists four titles as sources. I assume this Web author synthesized information from these sources (whether they are books, reports, or something else is not made clear). However, in an Internet search in 1999, I could not find any of the titles or authors (which doesn't necessarily mean that they don't exist). Actually, I did find one title listed, *The UFO Encyclopedia* by Jerome Clark. However, the site lists John

Spencer as the author. What's more, Clark's book was published in 1998—five years after the date of this Web site's publication. Confusing, to say the least.

Alienspeak Concretizes Its Claims with Small Details and Imagistic Language. Also like tabloid journalism, this site uses small, concrete details and imagistic language to help persuade readers that the information is true. For example, if a tabloid headline claims that "Hitler is Alive!," he does not live in South America. Nor does he live in Buenos Aires. Rather, we're told that he lives in a *suburb* of Buenos Aires. Even a horoscope (traditionally the most general of messages) in tabloids can be very literal and concrete: "Attend an evening barbecue on July 24." Similarly, Web sites about aliens invariably contain vivid specifics—rhetorical devices intended to convince skeptics.

For instance, the astronaut Web site also contains a "List of UFO Bodies Allegedly in the Possession of the United States Government." This list names the day, month, and year the bodies were found, and their location (sometimes vaguely stated, such as South Africa; other times more specifically, such as Kingman, Arizona). The site also specifies the number of bodies recovered, which ranges from one to sixteen per location. This information is said to come from "The UFO Crash/Retrieval Syndrome (Status Report II: New Sources, New Data) by Leonard H. Stringfield, January 1980" and published by Mutual UFO Network Inc., in Sequin, Texas. Even more detailed is the following description (narrator not identified) of one of the alien bodies recovered. Note the use of imagistic language, such as adjectives, metaphors, and similes. This information came from Stringfield's report, which contains "interviews [with] several medical doctors who did autopsies on ET [extraterrestrial] bodies from UFO crash sites" (Stringfield n.d.).

ET had large heads and were around 4 ft. tall. They have small noses and mouths with no ears or hair . . . an eye diameter of about an inch. He has his left hand raised in a salute [in a photo]. That hand has 4 fingers on it with one finger twice as long as either outside finger. The photo was taken at a range of 3 ft. From the waist up. Brain capacity is 1800 cc versus 1300 cc for the average human. The skin is grey or ashen and under the microscope appears meshlike. This meshlike appearance gives it the reptilian texture of granular skin lizards like iguana or chameleon. There was a colorless liquid in the body without red cells, no lymphocytes, no hemoglobin. There was no digestive system, intestinal, alimentary canal, or rectal area in the ET autopsy. (Stringfield n.d.)

The purpose of concrete details and images in written prose is to provide verification, or to create the illusion of reality. Sprinkle in some terms from an eighth-grade science textbook and you have something convincing enough for many readers. But the power of such passages goes beyond this. Despite the rapid growth of cinematic production and other technologies that reproduce images, our culture remains fairly wedded to the notion that seeing is believing, whether the images are pictorial or verbal.

Alienspeak Uses Suggestive Imagery. Finally, both print and electronic media employ suggestive or ambiguous imagery to help generate interest and belief in the existence of aliens. Such open-ended imagery is another form of assuming reality, discussed earlier. One of the most popular current Web sites for UFO and alien buffs is The Black Vault (www.blackvault.com), created by John Greenwald Jr. when he was fourteen years old. Several years later, Greenwald continues to collect material once classified as Secret and Top Secret from the U.S. government via the Freedom of Information Act. Greenwald scans into his Web site the actual declassified documents he has received from the FBI, NASA, CIA, Department of Energy, the Defense Technical Information Center, and other agencies. Although this site is an archive of information, it nonetheless employs screens consisting of black skies full of stars as background and labels information with terms such as "sectors," "levels," and even "The Galactic Chamber," thus intensifying the reality of aliens.

Likewise, the initial screen on Joseph Firmage's Web site (thewordis truth.org, described earlier), is solid black with a few phrases in white. His organization's logo appears at the top, consisting of two smaller circles, one atop the other, within a larger circle; a vertical line divides the circles. Like most logos, it's ambiguous, but it suggests a figure eight, the yin and yang symbols, the male and female symbols, and other oppositions that might be encompassed or reconciled (via the logo's outer circle). The main entry screen, in black, blue, and white, shows the top half of an Earthlike sphere, which is covered by a meshlike grid. The figure eight shape begins within the sphere and rises up out of it into a black night sky filled with stars and nebula. Atop this sphere, one religious symbol blinks off, to be replaced by another: a Buddha turns into Christ on the cross, which turns into a Star of David, and so forth. Such "open texts" do not literally prescribe. Instead, they nod toward a belief in beings from other worlds and higher states of consciousness, by providing a visual, implied assumption of the authenticity of aliens.

Overall, Alienspeak does little to help us determine the truth or falseness of alien life, which is supposed to be its purpose. (In this way, Doublespeak is a foundation of Alienspeak, too.) Like the other voices in this book, Alienspeak presents us with mirrors, riddles, and other geegaws of entertainment and self-absorption. The fact that Alienspeak is Disneyfied may be irrelevant to the ultimate truth or falseness of its claims. That is, Alienspeak is the product of its culture, so we can't expect too much of it. It's especially unrealistic to expect it to shed any light on such a large and universal question as the existence of alien life.

However, another type of Alienspeak not explored here is the personal narrative—the stories of people who claim direct experience with aliens. These accounts contain sufficient detail, variety (in types of people, ages, occupations, backgrounds, etc.) and "honesty-through-naivete" in their reports, that many intelligent people have to acknowledge that something is going on. We don't seem to have the structures to understand clearly what this "something" is. Mass hysteria? An unknown plane of consciousness? A compelling need to rise above lives submerged in materialism? The truth really is out there, floating around with reality sandwiches.

HATESPEAK: WWW.GODHATESFAGS.COM

At the White Aryan Resistance (W.A.R.) Web site, the first menu category is called Racist Cartoons. Its subcategories are Nigger, Spic, Jew, Whigger, Anti-Government, and Heterophobe. This is Hatespeak. The Internet address for the Westboro Baptist Church in Topeka, Kansas, is www.godhatesfags.com. This site's opening screen defends its choice of addresses: " 'GOD HATES FAGS'—though elliptical—is a profound theological statement, which the world needs to hear more than it needs oxygen, water and bread." This is Hatespeak.

Like the other voices explored in this book, Hatespeak comes in many forms: graphics, visuals, font styles, animation, audio recordings, jewelry, and crossword puzzles, to note a few. The Westboro Baptist Church Web site contains a "Perpetual Gospel Memorial to Matthew Shepard," the University of Wyoming college student who was beaten and murdered in 1998 because he was gay. This section states, "Matthew Shepard has been in hell for 253 days. Eternity − 253 days = Eternity." What dominates this screen's black background is a photo of Shepard's face, which bobs up and down as flames shoot up around it. Below this graphic is a button to click, which plays a recording of what is supposed to be Shepard's voice as he burns in hell. It squeals, "Agghhh! For God's sake, listen to Phelps!" (Fred Phelps, pastor of Westboro Baptist Church, created this site.) This, too, is Hatespeak.

The introductory screen of the Stormfront Web site of the White Nationalist Party contains a large black, white, gray, and red Celtic cross. This group's slogan, "White Pride World Wide" appears within the cross. In the background is a gray, threatening sky. The word "Stormfront" appears in a red, German Gothic font; the letter "f" is shaped like a downward-pointing dagger. Along with Nazi and National Socialist

Figure 5.1. Symbols of Hatespeak: Nazi swastika (left) and White Nationalist symbol (right). Source: White Nationalist Web site: http://www.stormfront. org.

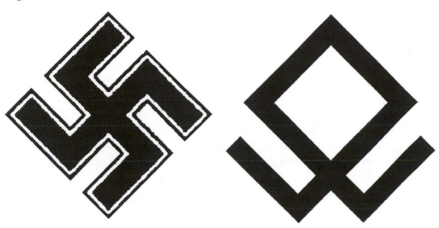

symbols (and a few Confederate flags thrown in), this site displays its own collection of symbols and graphics, all evoking Nazi World War II designs. Figure 5.1 shows the similarities between the Nazi and White Nationalist symbols.

Because of their similarities, many viewers will transfer or associate meanings of the Nazi symbol with the newer graphic. This site even offers Nazi jewelry—rings, pins, key chains, pendants, and earrings—all adorned with swastikas, iron crosses, and Celtic crosses. Other white supremacy Web sites (e.g., the World Church of the Creator) contain pages for children. These include games such as Sieg Heil!, which features Aryan heroes as well as crossword puzzles, one of which contains clues such as, "White children are _____" and "My _____ is dedicated to my race." All of this, too, is Hatespeak.

Hatespeak is communication that expresses negative and destructive attitudes and behaviors toward certain groups of people on the basis of their race, age, ethnicity, religion, sexual orientation, and other affiliations. Hatespeak can be direct or indirect. American Hatespeak is typically aimed at women, Jews, African Americans, Hispanics, immigrants, those in favor of abortion rights, gays, lesbians, bisexuals, and the federal government. A more recent group targeted by Hatespeak is Whiggers—white people who embrace African Americans or their culture. This relatively new term replaces the earlier "white nigger."

Although at century's end, Hatespeak is not uncommon in music lyrics, TV, radio talk shows, and film, it seems to reside mainly on Internet Web sites, which are replacing the printed pamphlets that used to be passed out on street corners. Therefore, unlike the pamphlets of old,

Hatespeak reaches not just a few hundred people at any one time, but hundreds of thousands of people on-line, including children. When I looked at the Westboro Baptist Church's site, on June 21, 1999, I was visitor number 871,466; this is only one site out of an estimated 250 Hatespeak sites (McCafferty 1999, 7). Let me point out one essential difference between these two communication settings. Just as some school-children believe that their school somehow sanctions or endorses the products of the commercials that air within classrooms (Fox 1996), the home setting can likewise legitimate the Hatespeak received in its safe surroundings. In other words, Hatespeak messages received along with non-Hatespeak messages takes some edge off of Hatespeak. The Internet dumps Hatespeak into the same pot of soup with everything else—right there beside the sports scores, weather forecasts, and e-mail from family members. Seeing a rotten apple on a shelf by itself is one thing, but receiving it mixed in with a bushel of good and average apples is quite another. In this way Hatespeak will likely become more valid, more mainstream.

Hatespeak often generates public discussion that invariably falls into two camps: those who believe Hatespeak represents free speech and those who believe it incites actual physical violence. This debate, though, usually ignores the issue of psychological violence altogether, which occurs when a viewer processes Hatespeak, as well as afterward. In addition, the evidence shows that Hatespeak does indeed lead to actual violence (see the following section, "Are Sensationspeak and Real Violence Linked?").

The Media Context of Hatespeak

First, Hatespeak represents a very limited choice that viewers have made, not the free and open choice typically claimed in defense of Hatespeak—the old, "We're just giving people what they want" argument. People sitting at home in front of a TV set do not choose from among programs that are *not* available. They choose from what *is* available. Neither does public Hatespeak (e.g., Springer's TV show, radio call-in shows) fully serve the "democratic" function claimed by proponents, who feel they are providing a voice for participants who are often denied media access. Although there is a bit of truth in this claim, the larger truth is that these participants are manipulated, trivialized, and exploited for profit—something more akin to a freak show than a legitimate opportunity for social or political representation. Nor do we know the complex web of participants' personal and work lives, and how these may have interacted with media to help motivate participants.

Third, Hatespeak (and other forms of Sensationspeak) are reported by other media and treated as news events. In 1998, both ABC's *20/20* and NBC's *Dateline* reported on the perversion of the Jerry Springer TV program. However, according to Solomon, "[B]oth networks chose to broadcast their in-depth Springer coverage in the midst of the ratings sweeps period. Nice to have it both ways" (Solomon 1998a, 1).

Finally, setting up a conflict situation and an either/or context for viewers places the media into the role of mediator. That is, the voice of the editor who monitors and comments on the anonymous telephone call transcripts printed in the daily newspaper becomes the arbitrator, the one who states foul or fair. Likewise, after people psychologically and physically abuse each other on the *Jerry Springer Show*, Springer himself enters in to arbitrate, to tell us what is right and wrong. These elevated roles help perpetuate Hatespeak because they communicate that a wiser parent figure will be there to settle things—that Hatespeak is, in effect, normal behavior.

Aside from the fact that media becomes invested with untoward influence here, the larger fact is that media sets up such conflicts in the first place, and then, even more media texts bemoan and moralize over what happens. A more subtle manipulation occurs on news programs, such as when anchors tell us, "This is a terrible shock. Here, let's take another look." I do not mean to place blame upon media emcees, who come and go. We should, though, question media owners, as well as the concentration of media ownership—the circumstances that enable a small group of people to control most of the media (McChesney 1997).

The Hatespeak mentioned so far seems harsher than the following example from syndicated radio host Bob Grant:

It wasn't too many years ago that most people could walk down the street and never have the pungent, sickening aroma of curry wafting up their nostrils. I don't mean to single out people who come from a country that eats curry, uses curry, bathes in curry, dives in curry, swims in curry, sleeps in curry, but it is true. As a matter of fact, there is a community not too far from where this great radio studio [WOR] I'm sitting in is located, called Iselin, New Jersey. For all practical purposes, ladies and gentlemen, when you enter Iselin, you have left the United States of America and are now in a modern version of a small city in India. (Naureckas 1997, 3)

The day after this broadcast, in Iselin, swastikas and ethnic slurs were spray painted on two Indian immigrants' businesses and one house; one business was hit with gunfire. Hatespeak should be viewed for what it is: psychological violence, an attack upon people's inner lives, a form of social betrayal that results in short-term and long-term effects on both its perpetrators and its victims. Even the "milder" forms of Hatespeak, such as that inflicted by this radio talk-show host, lead to actual, physical mayhem. With Hatespeak, it's not just a matter of messages leading to actions, because here, the messages *are* the actions, are the event itself, destroying without physical action.

ARE SENSATIONSPEAK AND VIOLENCE LINKED?

Yes. Although the number of Americans who understand this relationship is growing, no critical mass yet exists to effect substantial policy changes. The evidence for believing that Sensationspeak in the media can lead to violent behavior is scattered throughout many fields and disciplines; therefore, the following sections represent only a partial response. Before exploring how Sensationspeak and violence are connected, let me emphasize that nobody will ever determine a cause-effect relationship between Sensationspeak and violent behavior. Media and violence involve far too many variables for that to occur. Therefore, the question "Does media cause violence?" is the wrong question, an invalid one.

Second, the issue of media's link to violence should never displace or distract us from the equally important issue of the availability of guns in our culture. Gitlin (1994), for example, believes that the huge number of firearms ("some 200 million") in America and our easy access to them is a greater concern than crime induced by media. "Assume, for the sake of argument, that *every* copycat crime reported in the media can be plausibly traced to television and movies. Let us make an exceedingly high estimate that the resulting carnage results in 100 deaths per year that would not otherwise have taken place. These would amount to .028 percent of the total of 36,000 murders, accidents, and suicides committed by gunshot in the United States in 1992" (Gitlin 1994, 3).

I share this concern. Making guns much harder to obtain may save lives faster. However, the 100 deaths linked to media that Gitlin cites represent only those clear, obvious cases of definite media influence and harm (e.g., death). Of equal concern should be media's more subtle, corrosive, partial, recurring, or residual effects on everyone else—on media's indirect effects that harm people, physically and psychologically, without killing them. In short, we have to address the *culture* of violence.

Sensationspeak and Violence Are Linked Because Research Tells Us So

The statistics quoted in "Notes from the World of Sensationspeak" earlier in this chapter offer only glimpses of the large amount of research that has been accumulating on the effects of media since the Payne Fund Studies nearly seventy years ago (Peterson and Thurstone 1933). Although we still have much to learn, especially about media's subtle, long-term, effects, we know far more than most people realize. Such research includes content analyses, which monitor the types and amounts of violence in media texts; longitudinal correlational studies, which follow a specific group of children over several years or more; naturalistic studies, which explore how children respond to media as it is introduced into their culture; and case studies, which explore one person's responses to media. Media violence affects people of all ages, types, and backgrounds, often in different ways. Overall, a report of the The American Academy of Pediatrics concludes,

Over 1000 studies—including a Surgeon General's special report (1972) and a National Institute of Mental Health report 10 years later (1982)—attest to a causal connection between media violence and aggressive behavior in some children (Strasberger 1993; American Psychological Association 1993; Comstock and Strasberger 1993; Dietz and Strasberger 1991; Klein, et al. 1993). . . . The vast majority of studies conclude that [this] link is undeniable and uncontestable. (Gerbner 1999)

In addition to the American Academy of Pediatrics, many large organizations, including the Cultural Environment Movement, The Center for Parent and Youth Understanding, The Canadian Association for Media Literacy, and others, agree that media representations of violence may

- facilitate aggressive and antisocial behavior.
- desensitize viewers to future violence, actual and portrayed.
- provide viewers with models of behavior to imitate.
- increase viewers' perceptions that reality is meaner and more dangerous than it actually is.
- convince viewers that violence solves all types of problems.
- convince viewers that there are no options to violence.
- convince viewers that violent behavior can be fun, entertaining, and funny.
- convince viewers that criminals and police make up larger portions of the population than they really do.
- convince viewers that violence is practiced by heroes as well as by villains.
- convince viewers that violence occurs out of context, carrying no consequences of pain, fear, anxiety, alienation, loneliness, ruptured relationships, and so on.

More than a decade ago, one leading researcher proclaimed that the controversy over whether media violence affected behavior was finished ("What You Need to Know about TV Violence" 1988). Unfortunately, even with this amount of "hard" evidence, this seems far from the case.

Sensationspeak and Violence Are Linked Because Other Evidence Tells Us So

In addition to controlled studies using quantitative and qualitative research methods, a wealth of informal or "anecdotal" evidence demonstrates connections between media violence and violent behavior. Consider the media's influence on young people's actions during a mere two-month period in 1993 (Considine 1993). First, in Texas and Ohio, firefighters reported that young children started fires after watching TV's *Beavis and Butthead*, including a fire set by a five-year-old that killed his younger sister. Second, Touchstone Pictures (owned by Disney), changed its film *The Program* after one boy was killed and many others injured when they lay down in the center of a highway, imitating a scene in the film.

Young children are also imitating what they see pro wrestlers do on TV. In Winnipeg, Manitoba, for example, eight elementary schoolchildren were suspended for using an obscene gesture common to pro wrestling shows—pointing to genitalia and making an obscene comment. In a yearlong study, researchers at Indiana University found almost 1,700 instances of this gestures, or about thirty-three per two-hour show (Thomas 1999). People can even imitate sensationalized media texts in organized, systematic ways. American teens (typically ages 14–19) are increasingly imitating the jeering antics of TV's popular World Wrestling Federation (WWF) and World Championship Wrestling (WCF). Such cable and network programs consist of elaborate costumes and "behind the scenes" story lines, all played out with body slams, pile driving (dropping an opponent on his head), vulgar gestures, flamboyant entrances, and snarling tirades against foes.

Many teenagers across the country have formed their own amaterur WWF-type groups (called Backyard Wrestling or BYW). These local groups engage in matches, videotape them, and then sell the tapes or broadcast them over the Internet. Teens take on WWF-style nicknames (e.g., Mauler Mark and Kevin Perfection) and props as they engage in matches in members' backyards. Participants imitate various holds and moves seen on TV and cavort in rings made of old mattresses. Many of these organizations promote themselves through Web sites, which feature biographies, photographs, interviews with wrestlers, message boards, and teasers about upcoming bouts.

After browsing through several Backyard Wrestling sites, I found lots of black screens with macho graphics and font styles. I also found a kind of mocking tone, as well as plenty of blurry photos taken in the backyard (and misspellings in the sites' text). It mostly adds up to nothing very unusual—teenage boys messing around, having fun, fantasizing about a glitzy TV show-biz "sport." However, two sites out of ten were not so normal. One site included photos of participants' bloodied faces. Another site was more disturbing.

I randomly came across a screen titled "This is Some of the BCW Stars Attacking a Teacher at School, Whatch [sic] Him Get a Stone Cold Surprise!!!!!!!!!!" Note the imitation in that Stone Cold Steve Austin is a popular mainstream wrestler. The next title read, "Beating of High School Gym Teacher." As I scrolled down this page, several photos, one by one (as if taken from a video), reveal a group of teenaged boys facing a male teacher, striking him, and surrounding his motionless figure on the floor. The teacher is black, and all of the boys are white (one of whom has a shaved head). The camera operator is positioned behind the teacher and facing the boys. On this page is a button to click if you want to "hear it!" In this garbled audio recording, we first hear a student say, "We're making a film here." Then the teacher says, "You're not supposed to be in gym class." Next we hear the jumble of voices and scuffling noises before another adult evidently interferes at the end and says, "Break it up!"

The audiotape and photos seem to be authentic, though I don't know for sure. Regardless, this site promotes racial violence almost as much as Backyard Wrestling. The content of some Web sites can harbor very different messages than what they present themselves to be. We have to wonder, in this site's blur of media, prejudice, and violent actions, what led to what? How? And how much did the boys' desire to shoot a film and show it to large Internet audiences fuel their willingness to intrude inappropriately into a setting and, worst of all, inflict violence on a teacher? I cannot answer these questions. But on this Web site, the creators seem proud of this taped beating. They seem to regard it as a kind of trophy or prize pelt for their group. Like most Backyard Wrestling sites, this one is enamored with drama, action, and violence. In addition, an opening screen on this site boasts how visitors are increasing by "100s and 100s every day." Growing numbers of people, consciously or not, blur the differences between reality and representations of reality.

At the end of the 1990s, a series of murders at public schools focused attention on media and violence. The school-yard killings of five people in Jonesboro, Arkansas, in March 1998, appear to have spawned a spate of copycat crimes including school shootings in Springfield, Oregon; Fayetteville, Tennessee; Los Angeles, California; Houston, Texas, and the mass murder at Columbine High School in Littleton, Colorado. Like the Backyard Wrestling clubs, many of these crimes were more planned than spontaneous. Of course, they generated much Sensationspeak. Consider the following newspaper report, describing how one student gunman entered his school's cafeteria:

He was wearing a trench coat, toting three weapons, like some character in an Arnold Schwarzenegger or Clint Eastwood movie. He was arrested with a .22 caliber rifle and a 9 mm Glock pistol. The Jonesboro boys, who allegedly shot from a nearby hillside, resembled young Rambos, dressed in camouflage and toting rifles with scopes. . . . Witnesses said Kinkel put a foot on one kid's neck and shot four times, that he approached an older, bigger boy and just shot him in the head. (Lokeman 1998)

Also, *Time* magazine (May 3, 1999) employed its classic Sensationspeak formula in its coverage of the multiple killings at Columbine High School in Littleton, Colorado. The cover sports two large color photos of Eric Harris and Dylan Klebold. Each is clean-cut and smiling, looking very suburban-normal. Their photos are surrounded by smaller black-and-white photos of the twelve students and one teacher they killed. The large headline blares, "The Monsters Next Door," the word "Monsters" appearing in red, the others in white.

Inside, the report begins with a cropped group photo of the shooters' class, which consumes most of the two-page spread. Eight students openly smile into the camera, their heads positioned straight ahead. However, in the upper left corner of the photo, Harris and Klebold— "the boys in black," as the caption tells us—have their heads tilting down, with their eyes narrowed, staring upward, affecting a kind of sneer. The large reverse type across the double page states, "On March 4, Eric Harris and Dylan Klebold sat for this class picture. On April 17, they both went to the prom. What they did next left their school . . ." With this titillating lead for readers to turn the page, we see another huge, double-page photo of a girl's face wreathed in agony: her head is titled back in disbelief, hands grasping either side of her forehead, mouth agape in shock. These words run across both pages, in even larger reverse print and all-caps: ". . . IN SORROW AND DISBELIEF" ("The Monsters Next Door" 1999).

The revulsion of this crime may deserve such intensified reporting. But such treatment goes for the gut, creating the brightest, biggest spotlight possible to draw readers, like moths, to its dazzle—readers who can be enamored of fame or infamy, in very different ways. As long as we define ourselves by media ("I am reproduced electronically, therefore I am"), whether its fame or infamy often doesn't matter. A teenager who mimicks the showy pro wrestlers of cable TV was asked what he thought the life of a megastar TV wrestler would be like (Thomas 1999). The boy replied that it would be "like a million people cheering and loving you. And if they hate you, it's the same feeling." Love and hate become the same thing, as long as klieg lights glow.

Harris and Klebold, who committed the Columbine shootings before taking their own lives, lived within a world of media violence. They followed shock rocker Marilyn Manson and were devoted to the brutal computer game Doom. Klebold named his sawed-off shotgun Arlene after one of his favorite characters in Doom. Harris even said, "That f— ing shotgun is straight out of Doom." In Harris's last videotaped suicide message, he identified a compact disc that he liked so much, that he willed it to a friend. Its title is "Bombthreat Before She Blows." Harris and Klebold viewed such violent films as *Reservoir Dogs* and *Natural Born Killers* multiple times (Gibbs and Roche 1999).

It's important to note that Harris and Klebold were not enamored just with violence, but with media itself. They created a video about their guns for a film production class, a kind of postmodern "rehearsal," blurring simulation and reality. In their last videotapes before the murders, Klebold said about their planned assault, "Directors will be fighting over this story." The two boys then discussed which director would be most appropriate, Steven Spielberg or Quentin Tarantino. As FBI agent Mark Holstlaw concluded, "They wanted to be famous" (Gibbs and Roche 1999, 44).

In their cover story on "The Columbine Tapes" (December 20, 1999), *Time* magazine adds fuel to the glorification of media, even while reporting on the boys who sought media fame by murdering their peers. Aside from the large photos of a Columbine survivor in agony, and aside from the huge blood-red print, the lead story begins by merging the killers with one of their favorite gory films: "THE NATURAL BORN KILLERS WAITED until the parents were asleep upstairs before heading down to the basement to put on their show" (Gibbs and Roche 1999, 40). Similarly, in the *Time* issue discussed earlier ("The Monsters Next Door"), the contents page states, "Two young men stage a fire storm at their high school." Stage? Stage, indeed. The students in trench coats (the "young Rambos" described earlier), the newspaper reporter who made the film comparisons, Klebold and Harris as consumers of violent media, as well as creators of it, and the editors of *Time* who refer to the Columbine murders as a "staged" crime, committed by "natural born killers"—all of us are enmeshed in this nightmarish confusion.

Clear, simple answers as to why these boys committed this crime do not exist. We all want straight, crisp explanations, and quick resolutions. But they don't exist. These would only be more sound bites, which can never address this hugely complex event. These boys were not "monsters" as *Time* pronounced. That's far too simple, a Sensationspeak sound bite. Carl Jung and others would agree that the monster inside one of us also exists within the rest of us, but that we succeed in keeping it subdued. A myriad of factors contributed to this crime, including family life, the school's culture, the availability of weapons, police response, and each boy's idiosyncratic personality and behaviors, their relationship with their parents, each other, and their previous experiences with media. Nonetheless, it's clear that Sensationspeak (and the culture it helps create) likely played a significant role in the development of Harris's and Klebold's identities. And this is possibly an easier issue to address than most of the other factors influencing the crime. Why we fail to do so may be the greatest mystery of all.

But hope flickers. In fact, we have actually reached a milestone in our collective understanding of Sensationspeak (though the event made scant little news, of course). On March 8, 1999, the U.S. Supreme Court refused to free filmmaker Oliver Stone from a lawsuit that says his movie *Natural Born Killers* led a couple to shoot a woman during a robbery. The court agreed with a lawsuit alleging that Stone intended to incite viewers to commit similar crimes. This film "has been implicated in fifteen copycat murders from Nebraska to Paris" (Dyson 1999b). To my knowledge, this Supreme Court action is the first significant public and official acknowledgment that Sensationspeak and violence are linked.

Sensationspeak and Violence Are Linked Because, Well, . . . It's Natural

The large truth of the previous arguments is that Sensationspeak is an artificial construct that should not have to affect our actual behavior. However, it's also true that it's natural for Sensationspeak to influence our actions, in at least two main ways. First, Sensationspeak and the larger media culture now constitute a significant part of our daily environment, regardless of our age, gender, culture, and socioeconomic status. And, like other forms of life, humans tend to adapt to their environment: to survive, we try to blend in with our surroundings. Although I don't want to devalue other theories of intelligence, psychologists, anthropologists, and others largely agree on "the importance of adaptation to the environment as the key to understanding both what intelligence is and what it does" (*Encyclopedia Britannica* 1994–1999). We usually adapat to our environment by changing ourselves, by changing our environment, or by finding a new environment altogether. Also, psychologists generally agree that effective adaptation draws upon many cognitive processes, including perception, reasoning, memory, learning, and problem solving. We can adapt to our media environment in an infinite number of ways, ranging from those that are healthy and productive, to those that are unhealthy and destructive.

For instance, when possible, we can reject our environment and find an alternative, or we can accept some of it, or we can interpret it and modify its meaning so as to fit into our own context. Or, we can adapt by emulating it, as the Littleton, Colorado, student gunmen and others described in this section seemed to have done. It stands to reason that the deeper and more varied our media environment, the more likely it will spawn casualties—those who, like Harris and Klebold, cannot adapt to it in positive ways. By the same token, our media environment will spawn successes—those who adapt successfully, those who, for example, choose to emulate the honesty they perceive in *Forrest Gump* or the integrity they discover in *Saving Private Ryan*.

Second, it's natural for Sensationspeak to influence our actions, because throughout recorded history, we have looked to representations of reality to discover possibility. We have always turned to art, sculpture, literature, music, dance, film, television, and the Internet to find what we cannot see near us, in each other. We use our eyes and intuition to fathom those bits of hope or despair or fear that artists catch first and then translate into concrete terms we can understand. What is faith and organized religion without religious icons? What is mystery or wistfulness or knowledge without da Vinci's Mona Lisa? What is isolation and alienation in modern America without the paintings of Edward Hopper?

Throughout history, our gaze has invariably turned toward images and icons to show us what we are, where we've been, and what we might become. We instinctually look beyond ourselves, to representations, for solace, guidance, inspiration, distraction, fantasy, and fear. And today's representations of reality occur upon ubiquitous screens. In this way, our turn toward media is traditional, natural. The fact that we often fail to acknowledge such natural connections between Sensationspeak and our actual behavior often creates obstacles in our humanely processing Sensationspeak.

"GOOD TEENAGERS, TAKE OFF YOUR CLOTHES!"
HIDDEN SENSATIONSPEAK

The visceral, in-your-face qualities of Sensationspeak help it sell itself. In this sense, Sensationspeak can be thought of as a very pure form of Salespeak, since that's mainly why it's sensationalized—to sell. One Sensationspeak phenomenon involves somehow "hiding" or embedding sensationalized words and images into a media text, often into "family fare," such as the Disney films *Aladdin, The Little Mermaid*, and *The Lion King*. These films and others have been reported to contain hidden messages, what some might refer to as "subliminal" messages, because of their subtlety. Such messages are supposed to occur just below the threshold of consciousness, where our conscious defense mechanisms cannot process them (Key 1976).

In the past, whenever I read about hidden messages in media, I reacted like most other people probably do: "Those religious fanatics are at it again!" I shook my head and turned the page. Several years ago, I read that the American Life League, a "Christian anti-abortion group," claimed that Disney films contained risque messages ("Group Culls Disney Films, Finds More Scenes Offensive" 1995, 8A, and " 'Lion King' Sex Scene Has Christian Group Seeing Red" 1995, 14A). I kept some articles for four years before I decided to see for myself. I rented the videos and scanned for the spots in question. One article directed me to a scene in *Aladdin* that supposedly contained the audible line, "Good teenagers, take off your clothes." I found the scene (when Prince Ababwa visits Princess Jasmine in her castle room, just before they ride the magic carpet) and cranked up the volume. I watched and listened four times. Nothing there.

Feeling a little sheepish, I tried it one last time, with my eyes closed and head turned, so I could focus just on the soundtrack. Then I heard it quite clearly. I tried it several times again, just for verification. It's there, all right—a voice whispers just as Jasmine, facing the audience (and the Prince), pulls some curtains back. The first two words, "good teenagers," are a little hard to hear, but "take off your clothes" is quite plain.

Just then, my 16-year-old daughter entered the room. She knew nothing about such messages. I said nothing to her, because I wanted to verify what I'd just heard. Telling her to listen closely, I replayed the same scene, stopped the video, and waited for her response. She said, " 'Take off your clothes'?" She then told me that when this whispering voice interjects into the scene, Princess Jasmine's eyes become very wide. We watched it again, and she was right. I reasoned that I didn't catch it the first four times because I was too distracted by the visual elements. Of course, I now had to check out *The Little Mermaid* and *The Lion King*.

In *The Little Mermaid*, the scene in question is the wedding, when the suitor is about to marry the maniacal sea witch, who is disguised as a beautiful young woman. The couple walks down a large ship toward an old man who will perform the ceremony. Once again, it took me four times to spot the Sensationspeak. Just as the couple steps up to the official (an old, short man who appears to be standing on a box), we see his entire body in profile. At that moment, if you look below his waist, you will see his white pants poke straight out as he becomes sexually stimulated. (This time, I asked my wife to verify what I am reporting, which she did.) *The Lion King* also came through. I found the spot where Simba, the lion hero of the film, walks to a cliff's edge by himself and plops down on the ground. An overemphasized cloud of dust swirls above him into the air on the left side of the screen, forming the letters, S-E-X.

Embedding faces and other messages into art has long been practiced, at least since the eighteenth century, when artists embedded faces and other messages into tapestry, flowers, landscapes, and buildings (Zakia 1976). When my son was 9, we visited an art gallery, and he pointed out to me how Paul Gauguin's face was blended into one of his paintings. Such deceptions were often intended to poke fun or somehow comment on current events. However, the messages about such hidden Sensationspeak may be more potent than the Sensationspeak itself. Stories about these verbal and visual subtleties are nearly the stuff of urban folklore. We usually hear about them in undocumented, fragmented, confusing ways, such as the old late '60s legend in which listeners supposedly hear a voice say "Paul is dead," over and over, if they play a certain Beatles song backward.

Similarly, when the film *The Exorcist* appeared, newspapers were full of brief accounts of people "possessed" by Satan, of crucifix-bearing priests summoned to dark bedrooms, of viewers fainting while watching this flick. Such stories usually spread informally, orally, and in print. Regardless of their truth, these tales create extensive webs of people thinking and talking about a commercial product—people actively participating in the life of a product (just as we are doing right now). The main result is that sales go up. Here, Sensationspeak functions as a type of Salespeak.

Participating in such activities allows us to engage in a type of one-upmanship with others. She who passes on the vulgar morsel buried in *Aladdin* is somehow privileged over her listeners; after all, in an age of massive public information, she seems privy to exotic "insider" information. Such messages create interest in audiences who wouldn't ordinarily rent the *Aladdin* video (though who knows how much, if any, extra revenue this might have generated for Disney). Also, these hidden messages create a sense of indignation and even paranoia in those who are especially offended by them.

Overall, in addition to their shock value for some audiences, these messages likely amount to a little Salespeak and a smattering of amusement for a handful of bored technologists in the editing room (playing their own version of one-upmanship). However, the main effect of hidden Sensationspeak may well reside in baiting and discrediting the conservative groups that bring them to the public's attention—another skirmish in the culture wars. Although my own beliefs differ considerably from those of the American Life League, those folks are correct about what's hidden in the Disney films.

SENSATIONSPEAK IN THE AMERICAN GRAIN

Like the other voices in this book, Sensationspeak is entwined with American history and values. Like most cultures, our history is notched with one group of people displacing another. This usually involves physical violence, which often became sensationalized by storytellers, yellow journalism newspapers, and dime novels. Beginning with the American Revolutionary War, Sensationspeak was often blended with the persuasion of Salespeak and a dose of Doublespeak to produce the most effective hybrid messages for mobilizing support among the colonists against

British rule (see Chapter 3, "Doublespeak"). Each major war after that served as a kind of incubator for developing new hybrid messages, from Thomas Hart Benton's highly sensationalized paintings depicting monstrous, bloodthirsty Nazis during World War II, to the video-game versions of sanitized-but-real warfare projected on TV screens during the Persian Gulf War (Robertson 1994; Gerbner 1994).

Along with official conflicts, Sensationspeak (where fact and fiction often blurred, just as it can in today's Web sites) was further advanced by oral and printed tales of a variety of early American action figures such as Daniel Boone, Davy Crockett, Jim Bridger, Sam Houston, Buffalo Bill Cody, Wild Bill Hickock, General George Custer, and Jesse James. In addition, early posters and print accounts portrayed captured slaves as animalistic wild men. From about 1850 until 1900, the enormously popular dime novels featured the sensationalized thrills and melodramas of western frontiersmen such as Deadwood Dick and Diamond Dick. The price of these pulps was dropped from a dime to a nickel so that young readers could afford them (Sensationspeak has long focused on the young). The most popular of the early books was *Seth Jones: or, The Captives of the Frontier* (1860), which sold 60,000 copies the first day, later achieving the 500,000 mark and translation into ten languages (Donelson and Nilsen 1997, 417).

Death and American Sensationspeak

Although sensationalized print messages have long relied on the painting of vivid pictures with words, the invention of the camera reigns as the supreme tool of Sensationspeak. From still photographs, to movies and television, to digitization, pictorial images can zip past the slower, more reflective verbal processing required by print. Pictures are tailor-made for Sensationspeak.

In the last 100 years, we have increasingly used photographs to reflect death and the grotesque. By their very nature, of course, deathly images constitute the dark side of Sensationspeak, from accounts of grisly murders on the frontier, to today's lyrics and theatrics of musical groups such as The Insane Clown Posse and Marilyn Manson. Throughout history, such images have allowed us to ponder what death is, to wonder about our own mortality. In addition to this primary function, deathly images can serve other purposes.

Soon after photography became available, and up into the 1930s, people commonly photographed their recently deceased loved ones, dressed up, lying in caskets, or sometimes propped up in favorite chairs. Photos were rare, and it made sense to have a memorial photo made before burial. During the Civil War, photographs of dead infantrymen, stretched out on stubbled battlefields, mouths agape, helped to document the horror of Americans killing each other, as well as to enlist support from the home front. Especially from the 1870s through the 1890s, desperados of the frontier, such as the Dalton Gang and Ned Christie, were photographed in death, heads propped up, bodies stretched across plank sidewalks—trophies for law enforcement, sensational "crime doesn't pay" messages for young people, and curios for everyone else.

In the past fifty years, we have continued to be entranced with images of death and the grotesque. Proulx (1997) summarizes how, since the 1970s, our interest has exploded, with,

scores of books and exhibitions of work in the so-called post-mortem genre, which embraces the morgue photography of Jeffrey Silverthorne and Rudolf Schaefer, police shots of crime victims from early in the century, Rosamond Purcell's exquisite prints of dead animals, skeletons, and preserved mutations, Akin and Ludwig's photographs of body parts preserved in museum formaldehyde, Olivia Parker's mementos of death, and the stunning assemblages of Joel-Peter Witkin that combine dead human and animal parts with still-living dwarves, hermaphrodites, homosexuals, and transexuals in complex scenes that make ironic comment on Western aesthetics and culture. (Proulx 1997, 31)

From the 1950s through the 1970s, one of the most well-known photographers of death and especially taboo subjects, such as living abnormalities and oddities (i.e. Sensationspeak), was Diane Arbus. Arbus and Michael Lesy—whose *Wisconsin Death Trip*, chronicled death, disease, murder, suicide, madness, and disaster during the 1890s by juxtaposing old photos and newspaper clippings—helped us accept death and disfigurement as legitimate subjects for photography. Proulx sees this "growing photographic frankness about death" as paving the way for our acceptance of the powerful photos and video that came out of the Vietnam War and later, the AIDS crisis. Also during this period (and continuing to the present) America has been awash in sensationalized images of serial murder and street killings, in entertainment as well as in the "reporting" of these crimes. A *Newsweek* cover (August 15, 1994) depicts a large black-and-white photo of a young black person sprawled upon a tile floor, legs and arms outstretched, blood pooled near the head. On a nearby wall, two thin lines of blood drip down to form a puddle near the baseboard. Today, in addition to the news and feature film offerings, family-hour TV shows such as *World's Scariest Videos* and *When Animals Attack* keep death and the grotesque within easy reach, around the clock.

We continue to stare into images of death and the grotesque for the same reasons we always have—to try to comprehend our own mortality, to contemplate the whole of life. However, our increased interest in such images has also coincided with our transformation from an industrial society to one based on information and technology. It may be that our gazing upon death has an upside. If we are not too distracted by the mere sensationalism, these messages can function as "open texts"—as unrestricted and uninhibited in the meaning we create when interacting with them. In other words, in a world that bombards us with information—most of which carries specific content and agendas, especially Salespeak—we may have increasingly turned toward the blank texts of death and the grotesque as a kind of relief or refuge. Wandering here, free and unencumbered, may somehow help restore us, so that we can return to the avalanche of facts, figures, details, and yes, sales pitches of our daily lives.

SENSATIONSPEAK AND TRADITIONAL AMERICAN MYTHS

A concern for Sensationspeak is nothing new. More than 100 years ago, Henry David Thoreau cautioned readers that "the mind can be permanently profaned by the habit of attending to trivial things, so that all of our thoughts will be tinged with triviality." Although Sensationspeak is embedded within many American myths and values, I will focus only on the following: rags to riches; competition and individualism; "happiness-binding," or the insistence that texts end on a positive note; and equality and virtue in action.

Rags to Riches

We activate the American myth of the Horatio Alger rags-to-riches story by watching others, such as entertainment celebrities, politicians, and sports stars, move from anonymity and/or poverty to fame and riches. The operant cliché here is "meteoric rise," usually followed by "tragic downfall." These figures accomplish this in many ways: in their real lives, in print and on screen, in the public personas they assume, and in the fictional characters they portray in TV, film, and advertising. Real or fictional, each role reinforces the others, thereby more deeply imprinting the rags-to-riches value on us. Whether viewing the film *Annie* or following the career of the budding Hollywood starlet, the roller coaster trajectory of such stories constitutes a distinct form of Sensationspeak. By feeling childlike in comparison with such blinding myths, we disempower ourselves.

Competition and Individualism

Sensationspeak thrives within the traditional American myth of competition and one-upmanship. If you weren't sufficiently grossed out by last week's *Guinness Book of World Records* TV episode of self-inflicted torture, then try this week's masochism. Engaging in the extremes of life—the longest kiss, the most hot dogs consumed—remains a way for us to assert our individuality, another revered American value. However, we assert this largely by watching others do it.

The Happy Ending

The American value of sheer optimism, especially our desire that all texts "turn out okay in the end," is linked to Sensationspeak, just as it is to Salespeak (see Chapter 4). Texts intended for mass audiences still end happily ever after. We continue to insist on happy endings, and we have little patience for unresolved, ambiguous endings. In texts dominated by Sensationspeak, when humans suffer through great harm and mayhem, this return to happy endings is unhealthy, because viewers seldom see the consequences of violence and other forms of Sensationspeak. The characters in, say, a TV drama, after suffering the murder of a family member, the loss of their home, and the psychological breakdown of another family member, pop up in the last scene, sitting around the dinner table, smiling and chatting—all of this within minutes of experiencing life-changing traumas. In reality, such major traumas often ravage human beings. When people in real life experience the same traumas, they may well spend months or years in recovery. They may also be plagued with a series of new problems brought about by the experiences, such as nightmares, insecurities, ulcers, divorce, depression, alienation, insomnia, and nervous conditions, to name a few. This ingrained pattern of glossing over the consequences of Sensationspeak prohibits our achieving even a rudimentary understanding of the effects of physical and psychological violence.

Overall, we become desensitized to violence, however it manifests itself. A recent Associated Press poll ("Poll Shows Tolerance for Violence in Films" 1999, 2A) reveals that 40 percent of adults would be less likely to see a film if they knew it contained violence—20 points *lower* than what people said to the same question a decade earlier. Further, those people most concerned about violence and sex in media are also those who attend movies less frequently. Together, these results point toward our increasing desensitization toward the Sensationspeak of sexandviolence.

Finally, Fiske (1993) and others clarify that media teaches us "what's normal." That is, after watching a media text, where the plot and action occur as forms of "disruptions" or as elements positioned in the foreground, we return to normal life—to the background. McLuhan (1964) and others maintain that the message of any media text is the background, not the foreground. Hence, when we return to the calm and happy ending, we learn that we can recover instantly from the trauma, that it leaves no trace.

Equality and the Virtue of Action

Computer and video games, which have been America's best-selling toys for the past several years, are tailormade for people who no longer have to till the soil by hand, build fences, hunt food, or tame the frontier. By circumstances as well as by their own choosing, many people have few significantly physical demands left in their daily lives. The scant tactile involvement with video games is enough to inflate the illusion of actually *doing* something—and usually not *for* people and other creatures on the screen, but *to* them. The video games that hit the shelves in 1996 are typical. "I counted 52 different games in all. Twenty-three were racing videos, 13 were weapons centered, another 13 were one-on-one fighting games, and 3 were other sports. Just over 50% of the games were centered on violence" (Smith n.d.)

This Sensationspeak is part of the American value of trying to achieve equality—at thumbing our nose at those whom we perceive to exercise power over us, just as the game Crime Patrol does. This game is played on a large screen TV. Like most video games, the player is made to appear as if she is holding a gun, pointing at the screen, to kill as many criminals as possible. It has long been virtuous for Americans to take action, to remedy that which isn't right.

Unlike many games, this one uses realistic looking people—gangsters and drug dealers—instead of monsters or aliens. According to Smith (n.d.) "these characters taunt you while they commit crimes and surround themselves with material goods and women in bikinis." In the late 1700s, we may have thumbed our noses at King George. Today, we resist assorted terrorists, aliens, or drug dealers on screen. Today, pointing and clicking a computer's mouse to accomplish something seems to be a more deeply ingrained pattern than, say, loading a musket was for American colonists. In a sense, we can speculate that a society steeped in technology and media may have an even greater need to take action than previous generations. And our needs to take action are often realized by consuming more media and technology—a self-perpetuating cycle.

SENSATIONSPEAK AND EMERGING MYTHS OF TECHNOLOGY

The rise of technology—and its attendant myths and values—is also having profound effects on Sensationspeak, just as it has on Doublespeak and Salespeak. The following sections try to describe some of these changes.

Not Being There

Technology has made sex and violence more accessible than ever before. Witness the rise in the number of homes with TV sets, as well as the number of sets per household (three is the norm). Witness the increase in cable channels and Web sites focused in some way on sex and violence, such as the racist attack displayed on the Backyard Wrestling site described earlier. Witness also the rise of "adult" videos available in hotels, the increased production and rise in profits made from pornography, the increase in cellular phones and phone sex.

The ubiquity of sex and violence has many implications for us, but so does the anonymity of it all. By this, I don't mean that our electronic trails can always be covered. I do mean, though, that our electronic engagements with sex and violence are generally ones that require little or no commitment to our being there in any way, shape, or form. When we call, or watch, or listen, nobody has to know our name, face, behaviors, attitudes, values, or histories. Instead, we can exist in a kind of technological shadow. We are similarly removed during routine daily transactions. This anonymity or isolation may eventually result in profound changes in individuals' lives, as well as in our culture. For instance, such anonymity may help us desire more Sensationspeak, not just in quantity, but in quality, too.

This technological shadow also helps deflect America's best minds from solving problems. For instance, once people communicate or pontificate on the Internet, they can become convinced that they've actually addressed the problems in real ways. Similarly, the Internet's linking of like-minded people can create insular nests for hiding, for intellectual escapism. Franck (1998) speculates what it might have been like if the Internet had existed in Germany in 1939: "A lot of sincere, concerned Germans spent their brilliance discussing how terrible it was that their neighbors were being carted off to slaughter in trains." Many linkages and "communities" formed on the Internet could also be described as gripe sessions, which mainly create an illusion of activity, thereby defusing whatever steam might be gathering.

Aim & Shoot, Point & Click

At this writing, the in-school mass murder in Littleton, Colorado (following shootings at schools in Arkansas, Texas, California, Canada, and other places) dominates the news. Legislation is being introduced in Congress to make it legal to charge 14-year-olds as adults. The explicit violence and cold attitudes (i.e., tone) that dominate America's popular music, film, television, and computer/video games speak for themselves. In 1996, the majority of video games on the market were based upon violence, such as Brutal, Lethal Enforcers, Killer Instincts, Mega Bomberman, Weapon Lord, Power Monger, Third World War, and Surgical Strike (Smith n.d.).

However, the spirit, attitude, and point of view that reside behind these images of mayhem are likely more damaging than the physical violence itself. For instance, every computer and video game I've looked at (including the innocuous *Star Wars* games) has one feature in common: when players look at the screen, they are looking down the barrel of some weapon, which the viewer is ostensibly holding. The player's focus changes only when the gun is pointed at some other target. Throughout the game, players seldom view anything except what they're aiming at with a gun. The question, then, is never, "Should I shoot?" but "Who or what do I shoot?"

When looking at life down the barrel of a gun becomes the standard, universal point of view, of course young people will assimilate this pattern of behavior—especially when it's reinforced constantly, in varied ways. This aiming and shooting that serves as the modus operandi for so many games is, in many respects, a variation of what we do with computers all the time—point and click. We point and click—or aim and shoot—and instantly, something changes. I have no doubt that pointing and clicking is the most common, most repeated pattern of American life. It's what we do if we want something (on the screen) to change. When we are raised in a culture that employs pointing and clicking and aiming and shooting all the time, side by side, for purposes of altering our environment, then we should expect violent crimes.

CONCLUSIONS

After encountering some instance of Sensationspeak, you may wonder, "What could possibly be next? What stroking of the senses could top this?" I don't know, either. However, if Sensationspeak continues to sprawl, it may generate a conservative backlash. If it's regulated (as Denmark did in 1969, when it legalized pornography), it could turn into a black market taboo and become even more appealing. The concerns about media in the wake of the Littleton, Colorado, school murders (and, to a much lesser extent, the lawsuit against Oliver Stone's *Natural Born Killers* noted earlier in this chapter) indicate growing public awareness.

However, at the same time, Sensationspeak, information overload, and technological whiz-bang combine forces to stunt public memory and action. Already the horror of Littleton has nearly faded from public consciousness. We are naturally appalled at certain episodes of real and media violence, but then we become too distracted with the next eruption—a Washington sideshow here, an overdosed celebrity there—and we forget everything, until the next terror erupts and the hellish cycle repeats itself. It's difficult to determine just what the greatest crime is: (1) the instigators of the violence, (2) the Sensationspeak surrounding it and hence perpetuating it, or (3) whatever subsequent media distractions deflect our attention from saving children's lives.

Another factor driving Sensationspeak is profiteering. Media violence will run hog-wild as long as it reaps profits. Television networks, for example, pursue huge profits from mass audiences. The Telecommunications Act of 1996 provided for considerable commercial control of the U.S. airwaves (e.g., Fenton 1998). As noted earlier, we have accumulated solid research (to say nothing of common sense) that tells us that media violence helps destroy life. The public has long been preoccupied with this question, to which we have long had the answer. It seems no accident that a media that makes massive profits on violence would rather focus attention on its consumers' motivation than on its own. We should stop debating whether media violence influences behavior and begin debating whether corporations should make profits from such violence. In America today, there are three types of violence: actual, documented violence; media and print representations of violence; and the business of those who traffick in it. It's hard to view one of these as worse or better than the others. With this partial background, then, I offer the following conclusions.

Sensationspeak Polarizes Us

A natural, inevitable effect of Sensationspeak is that it often positions people at opposite ends of any ideological spectrum. From either position, any shades of gray that reside between these extremes, where truth often resides, seemingly disappear. It is true that certain issues, such as abortion, seem not to have any middle ground. But it is not just the intensity of our passion that keeps us from viewing the middle ground; it is also the inflammatory messages from both ends of the debate.

For example, the Web site of the Child-Care Action Project, a group that focuses on the "Christian analysis of American culture," reviewed the film *South Park: Bigger, Longer, and Uncut*. First, many adults would likely agree that this film is indeed a stellar example of Sensationspeak (as they would likely also label the *South Park* TV series). After all, this site lists the number of times the characters uttered the word "fuck" (131 times) and other conventionally obscene words (119 times). This site further notes that in the film, "Body parts dripping with blood were ripped from a child by a surgeon" and the dead child "was then seen with an exploded chest," and that the character of Saddam Hussein "waves his disembodied male member around—and it was not a cardboard drawing like most other images in the movie; it was of photographic resolution ("Movie Most Foul" 1999, 28).

Few would likely argue that this film is not a clear example of Sensationspeak, one that, given its "target" audience, clearly resides at the extreme end of the spectrum. However, residing at the *opposite* end of this spectrum is the language used by this Christian organization to judge the film: "the most foul of the foul words" and "*South Park* is another movie straight from the smoking pits of hell: . . . an incredibly dangerous movie" ("Movie Most Foul" 1999, 28). Such fire and brimstone may motivate a *South Park* sequel, so the cycle can begin again.

Sensationspeak May Affect Us in Subtle Ways

Although thrills, chills, and even copycat crimes are direct effects of Sensationspeak, many of us may be influenced in far subtler ways, over a longer time period. For example, the symptoms of ADD, or Attention Deficit Disorder, are restlessness, boredom, distraction, and difficulty focusing on any one thing longer than a few minutes. Some experts now wonder about "culturally induced ADD," possibly caused by Sensationspeak—not just in the content and intensity of messages, but also in their frequency and volume (Shenk 1999). Other states associated with Sensationspeak include atrophy of physical and mental abilities, isolation, delusion, voyeurism, desensitization, cynicism, and narcissism. Take voyeurism, for instance. If we are a culture that prefers to watch from the sidelines, what happens to our ability to act? And to act authentically? Increasingly, we can engage in voyeurism anonymously, yet we have no idea how this circumstance influences our identity, our relationships with others, or anything else. If we attend only to shock, who and what gets left behind in the calmer dust? We know very little about the long-term, residual effects of Sensationspeak.

Sensationspeak Is America's Blind Spot that Bleeds

Our collective refusal or inability to acknowledge the links between media violence and actual violence (including more subtle, slowly activated violence) is our greatest blind spot, our supreme act of denial. This is not like other blind spots; it's not something that might happen or is about to happen unless we see it. Rather, it's happening all the time, a kind of constant bleeding. Again, the continued prevalence of Sensationspeak over time has desensitized us to it, even though good minds in America fret about it on the Internet, believing they have accomplished something.

Sensationspeak Fills Any Vacuum

Like Salespeak, Sensationspeak fills any vacuum, drowning out alternative voices in the process. Here are a few of the many reasons for this.

First, Sensationspeak, by its very nature, is so loud and distracting, it's very difficult even to hear alternative voices. Second, packaging and selling scandals, violence, and freak shows allows us to easily find every value we want in messages—from the far right of the political spectrum to the far left. I believe this is easy because people appear to be more similar in their tastes for Sensationspeak, but more diverse in their preferences for more rational discourse. By satisfying everyone, such collective schizophrenia integrates alternative voices, hence neutering them. Third, because we cannot collectively agree upon a moral code, we engage in Sensationspeak to escape the debate, to avoid arguments. Moral relativism seems to flourish when too much information saturates a culture: a simple overabundance of information can guarantee that any assertion can be contradicted. Fourth, in the absence of a generally shared moral code, we have no customs or habits to anchor us when we face the incoherent desires stimulated by media.

The Core of Sensationspeak Must Be Nourished

The core of Sensationspeak is drama and narrative—our most powerful means of learning and understanding the world. Storytellers who craft powerful narratives through verbal and visual representations provide us a way to imagine the actual, as well as the possible. Also, humor in drama and narrative help us relieve tension, as well as distract us from life's pains, large and small, including our own mortality. In fact, we can hardly live without Sensationspeak. However, when our senses and emotions are stroked (or rubbed raw) in pointless ways, devoid of humane values, we are diminished as people. The ever-more engrossing forms of narrative require new ways and structures for us to interpret and deal with them.

RECOMMENDATIONS

Given that media, technology, and the free market's drive for profits are so powerful, the most promising solutions to media violence (the most immediately dangerous form of Sensationspeak) may be those that employ these very forces. Other reasons for these recommendations are that (1) the media industry has not restrained itself, and (2) politicians have been ineffective. Any specific recommendations for providing some counterbalance to something as "organic" as media violence must include recommendations that are broader in scope. First, major social systems—federal and state governments, businesses, schools, the entertainment industry, and others—must understand the problems inherent in Sensationspeak and how they link to education, technology, health, and culture. Second, once these major social systems understand the problems and are ready to act, they must coordinate their efforts. Again, something as organic and pervasive as Sensationspeak can never be effectively addressed in a fragmented or piecemeal way.

Third, the concentration of media ownership must be reduced. Most of America's news and entertainment is owned by a handful of corporations, including Time Warner, General Electric, and Disney (Miller 1996). America's public media is a very private enterprise. With so few media owners, it should not be surprising that program choices are often limited to a few proven formulas, in order to earn fast megabucks—and the formulas of violence and sex have always topped this list. Few dissenting or alternative voices exist. Average people have long felt powerless about matters of public discourse: we feel we shouldn't dare inhibit free speech; we feel lacking in communication expertise and technological savvy. However, public matters belong to the public. Because the public is most affected by media, the public should exert the most control. Yet we have none. Accordingly, the following recommendations focus on the four most important "fronts": consumer activism, litigation, legislation, and education. The more we coordinate these efforts, the better.

Boycott Sponsors of Media Violence

Parents, especially, have the economic power to send potent messages to corporations that sponsor violent and crass media products, especially television shows, popular films, and video games. In an August 1999 letter to Robert Pitofsky (chairman of the Federal Trade Commission), Ralph Nader (consumer activist) and Gary Ruskin (director of Commercial Alert) encouraged the FTC "to tally televised acts of violence by show and sponsor, to assist parents in making choices about whether to buy from companies that support unwholesome entertainment" (Nader and Ruskin 1999). They argue that our free market is based on choice, and that the market does not work when it comes to selling violence to children. Why? Simply because parents don't have the information they need to make healthful selections. Nader and Ruskin also advocate that the FTC tally the "average number of televised violent acts by show and by sponsor, and publish statistics regarding which shows are the most violent, and which companies sponsor the most violent TV shows." Parents, then, could learn which brands of peanut butter and soft drinks, for example, are most associated with violence, and choose accordingly.

Fight Media Violence through the Courts

Lawsuits may eventually prove to be an effective way of curbing media violence. In April 1999, the families of three Paducah, Kentucky, girls killed in a high school shooting filed a $130 million lawsuit alleging that specific media texts (a movie, violent video games, and Internet pornog-

raphy sites) motivated the murderer to kill. This lawsuit was partly inspired by the U.S. Supreme Court's earlier decision to allow a lawsuit to
go forward against the director and producers of the violent film *Natural
Born Killers*. The Kentucky families' attorney, John B. Thompson, pursuing the "law of unintended consequences," successfully prosecuted
three "shock" radio stations in Florida. In 1986, he represented sexually
abused women and children whose attackers were partly inspired by the
pornography they had consumed (Dyson 1999b). In an open letter to
Christine Todd Whitman, governor of New Jersey (dated September 14,
1999), Thompson states that he filed this lawsuit eight days before the
Littleton massacre, naming some of the very media products that
encouraged the Littleton killers, Klebold and Harris (Dyson 1999b).
Therefore, Thompson is not, in his words, an "after-the-fact ambulance
chaser."

Tax Violent Media Products (and Their Advertising)

Why not wage a heavy tax on media violence, one that would eventually be passed on to consumers? Violent media is as harmful as alcohol
and tobacco and should be taxed accordingly. The plan might work
something like this: If guns or other weapons appear in a scene from a
film or TV program, producers would pay a large amount of money. If
that weapon appears again in a later scene, the tax increases. If the
weapon is used, another, higher fine is levied. If the weapon is used
against children, the fine would be extremely high. A scene depicting
the rape of a woman would also require an exorbitant tax. And so on.
What I am suggesting here is a sliding scale—not just for physical violence, but for psychological violence, too. The proceeds from such a
"peace tax" could go to crime victims, media literacy organizations, public safety organizations, and so forth. Also, because the high-voltage ads
for violent media products constitute an especially powerful, compressed
form of media violence, they, too, should be taxed. Finally, I should note
that the taxing of violent media is an idea that seems to be gaining at
least a little ground. The Joint Committee on Domestic Violence in Ontario, Canada, recommended the very same thing in its report called
"Working Toward a Seamless Community and Justice Response to Domestic Violence: A Five Year Plan for Ontario." Almost immediately after
this report was released, the taxation idea was killed by the Ontario
attorney general. Washington state tried, unsuccessfully, to initiate a similar tax in 1998.

Learn about Media

In the long run, the most rational answer to dealing with Sensationspeak, especially media violence, resides in our learning about ourselves

and how we interact with media (see Chapter 2, "Making Sense of MediaSpeak"). "Media literacy" (or "mediacy") means thinking critically about media messages: connecting media content to our actual experiences; analyzing and interpreting media messages for the ideologies and values they communicate, directly or indirectly; and even constructing our own media messages. In the past twenty years, media literacy organizations (such as the National Telemedia Council, Citizens for Media Literacy, and the Assembly on Media Arts of the National Council Teachers of English) have grown. Also promising are umbrella groups, especially, the Cultural Environment Movement, that promote networking among organizations. Further, media education for teachers of all disciplines and levels requires graduate programs in media, as well as funding of media literacy research. Learning about the print and media texts we consume allows us to control them, rather than their controlling us.

Voices Entwined

INTRODUCTION

Of course, more than three voices ring throughout America. A land so sprawling and diverse must include some other dominant forms of discourse. One of these is Culturespeak, the language that surrounds our differences and similarities in how we choose to live, such as the abortion rights and right-to-life debate, the English-only movement, multiculturalism, and other public policy issues, from health care to poverty to immigration laws. Also left out of this book is Cyberspeak, the discourse surrounding technology. And the best of American voices, Heartspeak, occurs whenever we communicate directly and sincerely. However, despite their overlap and for well or ill, Doublespeak, Salespeak, and Sensationspeak represent our most common voices.

In this book, these three voices appear in separate chapters, so that each can be explored in some detail—a mere convenience. In reality, these boundaries don't exist. Instead, these voices merge, diverge, and merge again, in endless cycles. Also, these voices—the products of media—are determined by media processes—how we interact with media, the baggage we bring with us to each encounter. So, too, these voices are shaped by the conduits that deliver them. For example, each communication vessel—TV, film, radio, computer—carries its own biases and strengths. It's not just a matter of the information that is conveyed through them, but also of the channel itself that can dispose us one way or the other. These dominant voices feed, and are in turn nourished by, media and technology, our two most powerful megasystems. Like these voices, media and technology themselves blur, especially as they are filtered through our culture, an act that helps create culture. In fact, media and technology make up two main ingredients of our culture, even though "culture," of course, consists of additional components (see Chapter 7, "Media, Technology, and Culture Entwined").

CONCLUSIONS

This chapter offers conclusions and recommendations that focus, simultaneously, on all three of the voices explored in this book: Doublespeak, Salespeak, and Sensationspeak. These three voices are entwined with one another because, first, this is the way we usually encounter them in everyday life. We don't stop to sort out and label the cascade of messages that fall upon us every day. Second, these voices will continue to entwine themselves with one another. It's not unusual for a Salespeak message to merge with one of Sensationspeak. A TV advertisement for life insurance may include the explosion of a sudden car accident. The development of hybrids is natural in the evolution of most forms of communication. Finally, understanding the collective power of these three dominant voices—as well as their interactions—may help us evaluate and respond to them.

Media Voices Generate Themselves and Each Other

The three voices in this book may result from the self-replicating units of culture known as "memes": icons (the McDonald's arch); images (JFK waving from an open limousine); lines from advertising ("Where's the beef?"), and jingles (DUM, dee, DUM DUM, the opening music of the old *Dragnet* TV series). Jokes, bits of knowledge, catchphrases, tunes, and fashions, also function as memes, which take on lives of their own, with widespread (and imperfect) replication throughout a culture. According to Dawkins, a meme functions like a virus that "infects" the culture, spreading horizontally: "Our cultural life is full of things that seem to propagate virus-like from one mind to another" (Dawkins 1999, 52). In Darwinian terms, just as organic life may be determined by the fittest genes in the gene pool, so, too, may a culture be determined by its most potent memes.

If information technology continues to develop rapidly, these voices will be considerably more prevalent, and, it seems, more than instantaneous. Silicon-chip technology is supposed to reach its limit about the year 2015. The computer chip of the future will reportedly come from a new field of research, "Moletronics" or "Molecular Electronics." Researchers in this field are developing a new chemical process for producing chips as small as a molecule. According to researchers at Hewlett-Packard and the University of California-Los Angeles, computers could then operate "100 billion times faster" than the most powerful ones do now (*New York Times*, July 16, 1999, 8A).

If the past is any indication, in addition to obvious benefits, such technology will also bring increased fragmentation and decontextualization, possibly investing these voices with even more influence than they wield now. Any discussion of memes assumes that media, technology, and culture are interacting in quicksilver ways, sometimes deliberately and sometimes accidentally. Hence, as information (and the production of memes) increases in the future, so, too, will the degree of chaos that is a natural part of such a fast, complex process. In short, our symbolic environment could well become increasingly volatile. In such environments—when things happen so fast and most people don't think they know what is really going on—our society becomes more prone to the juntas of power-plays and exploitation.

When We Don't Develop Our Own Voices, Media Can Fill the Vacuum

It's natural for us to turn toward media voices to help us order our consciousness. This is especially true with Doublespeak, Salespeak, and Sensationspeak. According to Csikszentmihalyi (1991) and others, the "normal" state of our minds is chaos. Without some external object, person, or idea tugging at our attention, most of us don't focus our thoughts for very long periods of time. Csikszentmihalyi believes that we have plenty of socially assigned roles to occupy our attention during daily life (jobs, homes, families, etc.) and that these roles often become routinized, as we sail through our days on "automatic pilot." However, when these demands stop, there is often nothing to structure our attention *for* us. And when this occurs,

the basic order of the mind reveals itself. With nothing to do, it begins to follow random patterns, usually stopping to consider something painful or disturbing. ... To avoid this condition, people are naturally eager to fill their minds with whatever information is readily available, as long as it distracts attention from turning inward and dwelling on negative feelings. This explains why such a huge proportion of time is invested in watching television. ... The better route for avoiding chaos in consciousness, of course, is through the habits that give control over mental processes to the individual, rather than to some external source of stimulation, such as the programs of network TV. (Csikszentmihalyi 1991, 119)

This internal "control" over consciousness is, essentially, the development of your own voice. To have your own voice is to use—and to trust—your own reflective thought processes, made up mainly of language, images, and feelings. Representations of the world that we have meaningfully internalized—not those undigested from the media—more effectively order our consciousness by making it more complex. Of course, media language and images can also develop our voices, especially if they are "processed" or somehow actively explored through our own thinking and language. If we allow most media to wash over us in passive ways, it tends to displace our own voice or merely fill a void. In other words, internalized imagery and language help us to grow as thinkers. Such growth or voice is best developed by focusing on tasks that are unique to the individual, which he or she can interact with more intimately—that is, interaction with people, with ideas through reading and writing, as well as reflection on these people and concepts.

Electronic media, then, can also serve as a source of developing our own voices—if it "gives control over mental processes to the individual." And individuals gain control over their mental processes primarily when they view media actively, discussing and exploring it with other people, and reflecting on how it connects to their own lives, families, and communities. On the other hand, individuals do not develop their own voices, do not develop their own internal symbol systems of imagery and language, gaining control over their own mental processes, if they accept media passively, allowing it to structure their consciousness for them. In short, if individuals do not possess their own voice or internal symbol system, media may fill the vacuum.

In addition to the prevalence of media, the other factor militating against young people establishing their own voices is that schools reward students for *not* developing their own voices. From kindergarten on, students succeed the most if they follow instructions, if they conform, so that order can be maintained. Despite many improvements over the past few decades, schools generally adhere to this three-stage cycle: (1) listen to the teacher lecture; (2) memorize facts from the lecture, and (3) regurgitate them on a multiple-choice test. In a media-saturated environment, this deadening cycle is exactly what we don't need. Memorizing isolated and hence irrelevant facts, filling in work sheets, and completing computerized bubble forms produce students who do not develop their own voices, who seldom rely upon their internal symbol systems. This approach produces only students primed to follow instructions, to absorb media as diversion, and to consume the material items that media promotes.

On the other hand, to cultivate individual voices, students must read widely and deeply—not memorize facts and spit them out on a test and forget them within two hours. Students must also write all the time, talk about their writing with peers, teachers, and others, and reflect upon it and revise it. Again, such reflective thought and action should include media, but it often does not. If we cultivate our individual voices, we will become less dependent upon the external stimulation of electronic media. If we don't develop our own voices, then media voices will fill the vacuum.

Voices That Reflect Our Own Experience Are Difficult to Evaluate

The messages that flow from the three voices described in this book are often shaped in terms of current everyday life. It's widely accepted that most of popular culture and media operate within the bounds of the familiar. Consequently, we often have trouble evaluating media in ways that go beyond our own immediate experience. As Spiegel (1999) observes, "Everything in our society, so saturated with economic imperatives, tells us not to surrender our interests even for a moment, tells us that the only forms of cultural expression we can trust are those that give us instant gratification, useful information, or a reflected image of ourselves" (76). In Spiegel's terms, we fear "surrendering ourselves to the work's strangeness," because doing so may make us seem "vulnerable and naive and intellectually unreliable." For example, Spiegel contends that most major film critics completely missed Stanley Kubrick's message in his last film, *Eyes Wide Shut*, because they were too rooted in their own immediate experience and faulted the film for not accurately portraying it. In this sense, our information environment and especially electronic media keep us fixated on the familiarity of ourselves, resulting in a house of mirrors that seldom allows us to view it from outside or above it.

An Economic System Based on the Arousal of Desire Ensures That Voices Will Thrive

We seem to live in a perpetual state of "If only": If only I could buy that house or car, I would be satisfied. If only I could be someone else, I'd be happier. If only I could live somewhere else. If only I could get what I want. . . . The three voices in this book bark at us to achieve absolute gratification—if we support a new crime policy. If we purchase a Ford Explorer. If we buy a ticket for that Hawaiian cruise. If. Can gratification ever be partial? Of course it can, but we are not conditioned to believe so. Reality in media-fueled capitalism is forever guaranteed to be less than what it delivers. The development and spread of media and technology intensifies the myth of absolute gratification. Accordingly, the ultimate frustration and cynicism that occur when promises don't pan out will also increase, as long as we fail to understand media voices, and fail to focus on the workings of media, technology, and culture.

Media Voices Are Partly Determined by How We Define Information and Communication

Of course, not all messages from the voices described in this book are devoid of meaning—meaning that will help us lead constructive, humane lives. But meaningless messages often dominate, especially when you consider their shallow purposes: to lie, to manipulate, to sell, to shock. Too many messages in our communication landscape are focused exclusively on accomplishing these purposes. Why?

Although the main reason lies in our type of economic system (see the previous section, "An Economic System Based on the Arousal of Desire Ensures that Doublespeak, Salespeak, and Sensationspeak Thrive"), another reason is that, decades ago, the word "information" was appropriated by scientists and technologists to mean something quite different from what it used to—the meaningful content of a message between people. Roszak (1994) describes how a 1950 publication by Claude Shannon of Bell Laboratories ("A Mathematical Theory of Communications") helped to redefine this concept: "In his theory, information is no longer connected with the semantic content of statements. Rather, information comes to be a purely quantitative measure of communicative exchanges . . . through some mechanical channel which requires that messages be encoded and then decoded, say, into electronic impulses. . . . From his point of view, even gibberish might be 'information' if somebody cared to transmit it" (Roszak 1994, 11–12).

Roszak further notes that history is filled with instances when the popular, commonsense meanings of words have been appropriated by science and skewed toward a new definition. For example, the word "intelligence," Roszak notes, "has been reshaped by the psychologists . . . and IQ testers" to instead mean "whatever certain highly eccentric academic tests measure" (1994, 13). Although the appropriation of the word "information" created confusion back then, most people now accept it, just as we accept that the terms "data," "communication," "communications," and "mass communications" have little to do with meaningful content. These shifts in meaning have now become widely accepted. However, the ways in which we agree to define "information" and "communication" and "data" cannot help but influence the nature of whatever symbols are transmitted. When we define meaning as any impulse transmitted over phone wires or via satellites, then anything can be considered a "meaningful" message.

When public messages (and hence public voices) become defined in ways that have nothing to do with meaning, they are tailormade for purposes of garnering profits, because, literally, anything goes. "Let's use this data," a market researcher might say, "and that information on this demographic sector to bolster sales." Never mind what "this data" might actually mean to people beyond its purposes of sales. Never mind that "that information" might communicate to kids that it's okay to laugh after killing another human being. Roszak concludes, "Thanks to the high success of information theory, we live in a time when the technology of human communication has advanced at blinding speed; but what people have to say to one another by way of that technology shows no comparable development" (Roszak 1994, 16).

Media Voices Are Partly Determined by the Vessels That Carry Them

We sometimes fall into the trap of focusing too much on content—or lack of meaningful content—and not enough on the unique characteristics of the electronic vessel that conveys that content. That is, we often ignore the impact of media technologies themselves—how each medium's unique characteristics help shape the meanings we construct. For example, when we focus on issues such as violence in the media, these messages are often communicated and received as violence in all media. This approach assumes that (1) content can be isolated from its technological conduits, and (2) these conduits are neutral vessels for carrying ideas. However, neither of these assumptions is warranted (Chesebro and Bertelsen 1996). Content cannot be separated from the vessel that conveys it. Most of us realize that violence in a Madonna music video significantly differs from violence in a Shakespearean printed text or violence in an old radio episode of *The Shadow*. However, we seldom make the distinctions that each technology demands. And when we do focus on the medium, it's usually only one; we seldom compare several. We need to compare our perceptions of media more systematically, so that we may become more aware of each technology's differences.

Media Voices Can Deplete Social Capital

Most adults, at different times and to varying degrees, are susceptible to the guiles of the voices described in this book. Less-aware adults and especially children and young adults, however, probably constitute those who suffer the most as a result of exposure to such messages. This seems logical. However, when anyone becomes aware of their manipulation by media, or simply grows weary of its continual presence, a kind of distrust and cynicism can take hold. Such distrust seems similar to that described by Putnam (1996), Fukuyama (1999), and others. These analysts cite survey data that portray America's "depletion of social capital"—the decrease in the types of trust that help a culture be cohesive and work. This can be seen in the declining numbers of people who join organizations such as the Kiwanis Club, Boy Scouts of America, Salvation Army, and the American Red Cross. Also fewer voters turn out for elections, and fewer people join social, religious, and recreational groups, such as bowling leagues and churches.

This decline in social capital, along with the rise of an information economy (which is characterized by decentralized authority and the valuing of employees' mental abilities) has led to a kind of egoistic, radical individualism. Such self-interest can become intensified when people learn more about why and how messages work; their newfound cynicism or distrust of media reinforces their radical individualism. As Fukuyama notes, "In societies where individuals enjoy more freedom of choice than at any other time in history, people resent all the more the few remaining ligatures that bind them." The result is an increasing depletion of social capital and a greater hemorrhaging of those ties that make a culture cohere and function on a daily basis. Those people who do not invest in social capital may instead focus on media. And if they perceive that media, too, may disappoint them, then fewer options remain in which they can invest their time and energy. One possible result is that social distrust and egoistic individualism are related to increases in crime and illegitimate births.

Improve Media Voices with a Unified Approach

The problems and inequalities resulting from the major voices of Doublespeak, Salespeak, and Sensationspeak are entwined within the mega-systems of media, technology, and culture, the subject of the following chapter. Therefore, we can most effectively focus on these issues by coordinating our efforts on the four most important "fronts": consumer activism, litigation, legislation, and education. Examples of these approaches range from consumer boycotts of sponsors of violent films, to lawsuits filed against makers of violent media products, to passing laws to protect captive audiences of children from advertising, to enacting legislation that taxes the makers of violent media products, to training teachers in media literacy.

Media, Technology, and Culture Entwined

INTRODUCTION

This chapter explores how media, technology, and culture interact with one another to generate the dominant public voices examined in this book. This chapter also explores how these three megasystems help shape our individual and collective identities. What follows are speculative conclusions and recommendations about these relationships.

MEDIA, TECHNOLOGY, AND CULTURE SHOULD BE VIEWED HOLISTICALLY

For most of us, it's nearly impossible to think of the sprawling, complex megasystems of media, technology, and culture simultaneously. They are too large and our minds are too small. However, so much is at stake, we have little choice but to try. The most obvious reason for keeping these three huge systems "on the same page" is because of the unpredictable ways in which they often interact with one another, not to mention the consequences these interactions have upon individuals, communities, and cultures.

One way to keep these three in mind simultaneously or holistically is to think of them as operating within a figure/ground relationship: what's in the foreground and what's in the background. For most of the 20th century, media commanded center stage in the foreground, whereas technology and culture more often resided in the background. Whatever operates in the foreground demands most of our attention, most of the time. What lies in the background does not, because it is more hidden and submerged. However, what is in the background often has more effect on people's lives and is more important in the long run. Popular media perpetuates itself by *constantly* changing its foreground act: one second it's Madonna, then it's the Versace murder, then it's a threat of war, and so on. This basic positioning of media in the foreground, can change, of course, but it seldom does. Even during those rare times when technology or culture shift to the foreground, as in, say, America's moon landing in 1969, or in the cloning of Dolly, the sheep, those events are sifted and filtered through the media, and hence become largely media events. Therefore, media seldom gives up its center-stage position, and when it does, it does so only briefly. In short, a media frenzy can obscure the technology and culture that produced the media in the first place (and which may be more important in the long run).

However, the technology and culture producing these changes of focus, changes of foreground, deserve far more attention. The main function of the foreground is to distract us from the background. The exotic, shimmering images flashed upon the walls distract us from who makes them, how they are made, why they are made, who is left out and why, what issues are left out and why, and how they may influence us. The late anthropologist Erving Goffman (1959) describes this concept in humans as "front stage" behavior and "back stage" behavior. What happens in front of the curtain is what we see, what we focus on. But what happens back stage—who produces and directs the action, and why and how—has more impact on our lives than the front stage (or big screen) representations and other shadows that dance before us.

MEDIA, TECHNOLOGY, AND CULTURE—ABOUT EQUAL IN POWER—INTERACT WITH ONE ANOTHER

Postman (1993) worries that one megasystem, technology, will subsume another megasystem, culture. Although I agree with this stance, I worry in a different way. In the past decade, media, technology, and culture have become increasingly unstable, even volatile at times. The main reason for this is that the three megasystems of media, technology, and culture are now coexisting and shifting entities. They are becoming too equal in power. Consequently, they are prone to jockeying with one another for a kind of dominance. Sometimes one overshadows the others. For instance, in HyperDramas (see the following section), media and technology can jointly militate against culture, against community, by isolating us from each other, simultaneously creating the illusion that they are unifying us. What's most important, then, are the dynamics and relations among these three megasystems.

What is true of our media culture itself—a terrain in which many social groups and ideologies constantly compete with each other for dominance—also holds true, I believe, for these three megasystems. In other words, if skirmishes occur in the media over representations of race, age, gender, class, religion, and political affiliation, then it seems similarly true that these three megasystems would also interact. The interactions among these megasystems usually do not result in one becoming stronger or weaker than another. On the contrary, their interactions ultimately end up nourishing one another. This seems especially true when "HyperDramas" erupt.

HYPERDRAMAS ERUPT WHEN MEDIA, TECHNOLOGY, AND CULTURE INTERACT

Decades of television and other media have defined us as audiences who view an endless series of personality-driven dramas strutted across the national stage. Unlike other countries, since the rise of television, the United States has had no ongoing debates between economic classes. We are too distracted by a parade of HyperDramas, which seem to erupt when the three powerful megasystems of media, culture, and technology interact with each other in complex, quicksilver, unpredictable ways. Like Charles Dickens's serialized sagas of old, HyperDramas seize, then keep, our attention for extended periods of time, taking on lives of their own. Following is a list of some of these dramas from the 1990s:

- Monica Lewinski and the impeachment trial of then-President Bill Clinton
- Susan Smith and the murder of her children
- Anita Hill and the Clarence Thomas confirmation hearings
- Andrew Cunanan and the Versace murder
- The Jon Benet Ramsey murder
- Louise Woodward, the British au pair accused of killing a child
- The death of Princess Diana
- The O. J. Simpson trials
- The Lyle and Eric Menendez murder trial
- The Columbine School shootings in Littleton, Colorado

Literally, HyperDramas consist of celebrities and people striving to become celebrities, as well as several (or all) forms of media. Hyper-Dramas combine Doublespeak, Salespeak, and Sensationspeak, with one voice sometimes dominating the others. Also, HyperDramas fuse many traditional genres, including the TV soap opera, Western, talk show, commercial, mystery, adventure, news, romance, press conference, cop show, documentary, docudrama, courtroom drama, and Super Bowl. Also, of course, HyperDramas require communication technology, a participating public, some effective timing, and serendipity.

Why and When Do HyperDramas Occur?

It's possible that the sudden eruption of a HyperDrama cannot be predicted any more than we can identify the precise time at which we come down with a case of the flu. That is, a HyperDrama may result from the self-replicating units of culture known as "memes"—images, jokes, bits of knowledge, jingles, and so forth, which take on lives of their own. Memes spread quickly throughout a culture, sometimes changing form along the way.

In the case of HyperDramas, the meme "evolves" (or mutates or transforms) as it is quickly sifted through multiple layers of "gatekeepers," or those who modify the messages. This process can alter the meme in intentional, as well as accidental ways. Also in HyperDramas, different memes appear to fuse and create new memes. That is, a number of "subplot" memes may develop and surround the central meme. For example, during the Clinton-Lewinsky impeachment HyperDrama, the cigar and blue dress memes seemed to take on lives of their own, as they also fed the central meme of the Clinton-Lewinsky relationship.

Also, HyperDramas may occur when media seizes an opportunity to fill a void in the cultural landscape. And voids quickly filled by media could change the larger figure/ground relationship discussed earlier in this chapter. That is, if fiction (usually presented up front, as fabrication) becomes the foreground, then it reproduces itself more quickly. For example, one HyperDrama starred an ensemble cast of former President Bill Clinton, Kenneth Starr, Monica Lewinsky, Paula Jones, Vernon Jordan, and Betty Currie. This production ("The Boyfriend") was much like previous extravaganzas. However, the main difference—and it's an important one—is that this situation broke new Doublespeak ground. That is, until the end of Clinton's impeachment trial, for the first time in history, we knew more about the fiction of the event, than we did about the facts. We knew more rumor and speculation and hypothesis and scenarios (from Clinton jokes circulating on the Web, to the TV and radio talk shows, to the films *Primary Colors* and *Wag the Dog*) than we did about *actual occurrences*.

In previous HyperDramas, it was the other way around: reality was in the foreground and the alleged or hypothetical was in the background. For instance, we knew for sure that Nicole Brown Simpson and Ronald Goldman had been murdered. At the beginning, these looming facts were the foreground, and the suspicion and speculation about Brown Simpson's husband, O. J. Simpson, were in the background (although this circumstance later changed). However, with the Clinton-Lewinsky scandal, the usual foreground and background somehow reversed themselves. There were few hard facts to constitute a foreground. Hence, the surrounding speculations and fictions slid right into the foreground to take the place of facts—to fill a vacuum, as only media can do so well.

Psychically, HyperDramas are volatile mixtures of Doublespeak, Salespeak, and Sensationspeak, sometimes with one voice outshouting the others. They synthesize elements of religion by enabling us to feel "large," as we identify with heroes within the small, intimate medium TV. They can also help us feel "equal," as we see ourselves and our egos in the pageant before us. HyperDramas are also part newscast (our excuse for following the story) and part porno flick, in its voyeuristic overtones. HyperDramas also function as our town square, providing us safe but titillating topics for social interaction—a definite need in a society of isolated individuals. HyperDramas increasingly blur distinctions between fact and fiction; real and imaginary; present, past, and future; local, national, and global; public and private; race, gender, age, class, religion, and political affiliation; good and evil.

According to one study (Lewis, Morgan, and Jhally 1998), Americans knew many details about the Clinton-Lewinsky impeachment Hyper-Drama (e.g., 75 percent of respondents identified Linda Tripp's role in the Monica Lewinsky incident). However, the study also found that Americans know precious little about Clinton's policies: only 13 percent knew that Clinton signed the welfare reform bill. Only 38.5 percent of respondents knew that Independent Counsel Kenneth Starr is a Republican. Such findings should not surprise us. As Shakespeare said, "The play's the thing." And these days, HyperDramas are big plays. One question is, How long will we be the audience?

IF MEDIA, TECHNOLOGY, AND CULTURE SHAPE OUR IDENTITIES, WHY ABANDON THEM TO OTHERS?

Much of our individual and collective identities are formed by the culture that surrounds us—a culture increasingly driven by media and technology. Our identity is often our primary means for making sense of the world around us. Our identity is a construct, created from the social roles available to us, and many of these social roles are now found in media representations. If we grow up taking for granted that technology and media are best left to "techies" and experts in the entertainment industry, then we abandon our own culture as well as our own identity shaping. This merely perpetuates a system that controls us, rather than the other way around. When we consider that media, technology, and culture are powerful forces in shaping identities, we must first be aware that the lion's share of media and technology (and hence much of culture) is controlled by a few corporations (Miller 1996; McChesney 1997). It's terrible to abandon much of our identity building to others; it's unconscionable to abandon it to only a few others, whose goal is profit.

Second, we must remember that these owners of our identity wield power in increasingly random and idiosyncratic ways, blurring and reconfiguring not just race, gender, class, politics, and age, but also fact and fiction; the real and the imaginary; the present, past, and future; the local and global; the public and private. We are far from understanding how media, technology, culture, and identity interact within an individual over time.

Groups such as the Cultural Environment Movement grasp some of the intricate ways in which media, technology, culture, and identity—both personal and social—are entwined. So do other countries, such as France, which employs a Ministry of Culture—not because the French are a controlling people and not because they are "cultural snobs," but because they recognize the importance of the complexities inherent in an information-rich society. If we have little understanding of these megasystems, we have little understanding of ourselves.

MEDIA AND TECHNOLOGY MAKE UP MUCH OF CULTURE— AND CULTURE BELONGS TO EVERYONE

Because technology (especially the Internet) and media are massively huge, complex megasystems, we don't think about them as part of our everyday lives. We don't think of them as workaday realities within our control or our expertise. This is partly because of how diffuse media and technology are. Nonetheless, perceiving media and technology as irrelevant or incomprehensible is still a problem. We should perceive media and technology the same way we view other large systems, such as religion, education, or political affiliation—areas in which we're more likely to voice our opinions. It is wrong to surrender technology and media to the "experts" and a handful of media owners. In 1999, the largest media merger in history occurred when CBS combined with Viacom in a $37 billion deal. As you might expect, the coverage of this event by organizations that serve the few other big media outlets (e.g., the Associated Press, the *New York Times*, the *Washington Post*) gushingly praised it as "a good deal for everybody" (Solomon 1999c). Nobody mentioned that allowing the few to control the many was miserable for democracy.

In leaving media and technology to the "experts," we abandon our own culture to others. The only technology we should abandon to the experts is true, hard-core technology—the design and manufacture of silicon chips, electrical circuitry—that kind of thing. However, when we get to such questions as who uses technology and for what purposes, and how media and technology represent and do not represent public issues, then this agenda becomes public—very public. When the technology creates and controls representations of life, then the agenda becomes everyone's responsibility. That is, media and technology *are* our culture and therefore our responsibility. To abandon this duty is to desert the most important things in life: humane values, teaching and learning, safety, physical and environmental health. The list goes on.

AMERICA'S TRADITIONS OF INDIVIDUALISM CREATE PROBLEMS IN A MEDIA CULTURE

We often fail to realize that our history of "rugged individualism" and independence has flourished only because it's always been supported by interdependence—by community. Throughout American history, individualistic, unique, successful Americans, contrary to myth, have seldom made it alone. They had husbands, wives, families, friends, and all manner of support networks. Today, whether male or female, the "rugged individual" is no different. Today, we will still need that sense of community with other people, but we have much less of it. According to Putnam (1996), Fukuyama (1999), and others, our "social capital" is in sharp decline. Participation in community organizations and events, from PTAs to bowling leagues, has dropped dramatically in past decades.

To compound the situation, we live in a "do your own thing" environment in which individualism (the term here is used loosely) is glorified in the media, from Clint Eastwood to Arnold Schwarzenegger to Dennis Rodman, to the TV kids of *South Park*. Fukuyama (1999) and others argue that our information economy breeds extreme individualism—people who look out for themselves more than for others. Decades ago, historians Will and Ariel Durant (1968) wrote, "Caught in the relaxing interval between one moral code and the next, an unmoored generation surrenders itself to luxury, corruption, and a restless disorder of family and morals." Since neither religion, nor art, nor any other social force seems able to counter the extreme individualism nourished by media, technology, and consumption, we may well exist "between one moral code and the next." With our traditions of extreme individualism firmly rooted in our nation's birth, and further solidified by taming the wild West, we were ripe for advancements in media, technology, and culture to take it further, as described in the following section.

MEDIA, TECHNOLOGY, AND CULTURE HELP US FEEL LIKE LITTLE GODS

Shenk (1997) and others have said that too much information (what he calls "data smog") creates problems for us—with our bodies, our brains, our relationships, and our culture. One of Shenk's "laws" is that "Cyberspace breeds libertarianism." I agree, but I think cyberspace—and all of electronic media—breeds tendencies that go beyond this. Roszak (1994) describes a vision which he finds "deeply embedded in the cult of information. . . . One sits before a brightly lit screen, stroking keys, watching remarkable things flash by on the screen at the speed of light. Words, pictures, images appear out of nowhere. Like a child, one begins to believe in magic all over again. And because one is making the magic happen, an intoxicating sense of power comes with the act. One has the culture of the entire planet there at one's fingertips!" (Roszak 1994, 186).

Media and technology position the individual at the center of the universe. They make us feel that we can control and consume everything around us—that we are, in effect, little gods. (This little god syndrome greatly differs from the development of an individual's voice, discussed in the previous chapter.) Some of us can feel like little gods when advertising and other forms of media present consumption as a natural and pleasurable way of life. With profit behind the wheel, the material and natural worlds are presented to us only as things to use up. In fact, what becomes communicated most powerfully through media is not so much the individual products or messages, but the idea that consumption (of all types) is glamorous, erotic, gorgeous, healthy. Products, people, and nature are presented as infinite resources, when this cannot be true. For example, when we are urged to buy fast food, no connection is made to the environmental consequences of all that packaging, all that paper, Styrofoam, plastic. No one mentions the exhaust from millions of cars lined up at the little window.

Media and technology can also make us believe we are little gods in more subtle ways. We increasingly focus on the purely symbolic, of course, because that's what an information society does. Most of us don't move around piles of bricks or boxes of nails as much as we manipulate text and other symbols. And when we become immersed in a film or TV program, or when we focus intently on making a home video or even writing an e-mail message, we are, in effect, entering into worlds other than this one. Media and technology seem to have replaced religion and art as the medium that most often allows us to enter into worlds other than this earthly one. However, there are definite differences. Simply put, entering into another world of religion or even art usually makes us feel smaller and less significant, as though we are all in our smallness together. Among other things, the traditional symbolic worlds of religion and art teach us humility, humanity, and the importance of connection with others. On the other hand, immersion in electronic and symbolic worlds may have the opposite effect.

Often, immersion in electronic and symbolic worlds helps us devalue our own bodies, our own real world, each other. Why? Mainly through simple displacement, through benign neglect. When we are absorbed in the virtual, whatever is ignored or displaced becomes diminished in slow and subtle ways. Consider an analogous situation. Feminist critics (e.g., Kilbourne 1997) have long argued that saturation advertising helps turn people into objects. It's broadly true that reproducing infinite images of beautiful people puts them right next to us, makes us long to be like them. At the same time, it has another effect: it helps isolate them from us. In addition, advertisers' frequent focus on body parts, such as a women's legs or breasts, displaces the fact that this person is a whole human being, complete with all the baggage and glories that everyone bears. Seeing people as objects, then, is the first step in devaluing people, the first step toward violence, whether we commit it or condone it.

Another way in which media and technology help us to feel like little gods is that it helps us feel empowered when we create our own little worlds. Although our creative impulse is as old as the human race, what has changed is that great numbers of people now engage in it fairly routinely, at varying levels. Technology, media, and culture have enabled more people to write books, compose music, sculpt, design Web sites, create houses, clothes, and quilts. No longer is imagining and composing the avocation of only the rich, talented, or idle. Imagining and making things has always bestowed a sense of empowerment upon those who create, because, among other reasons, we find pleasure (and often, intoxication) in designing and manipulating materials and symbols. And if we're at all successful, our feelings of empowerment cannot operate in a vacuum: they naturally spill over into our dealings with others and with the world around us.

Consequently, we now have more little gods running around than ever before in our history—people who, emboldened by their experiences in "other worlds," too often feel above or distanced from other people, including their family, friends, and colleagues. Also, in some people, this false self-esteem can lead to risk taking and law breaking. Ultimately, little gods become frustrated when their false self-esteem is threatened, or when they realize that they cannot reign supreme over others, especially in open societies. This results in conflicts of all kinds. With the help of a bucketful of other social factors, the stage is set for factionalism, gridlock, and even culture wars. These are a few of the ways in which technology and media encourage us to dominate the world and people around us. If too many of us are feeling superior, our ability to listen, to understand, and to cooperate is diminished.

MEDIA, TECHNOLOGY, AND CULTURE REQUIRE NEW FORMS OF STEWARDSHIP

These three megasystems must be considered together. At best, in the past we have usually focused on just one megasystem, or on one medium, or one type of technology. As overwhelming as it can be, viewing these three megasystems together helps us see how they connect to one another. This is important because such relationships and interactions exert a strong influence on our lives—on how we define ourselves and our world. Also, viewing media, technology, and culture simultaneously helps us to better understand who controls the messages around us. Especially in free-market economies, "following the money" throughout these megasystems can help us see how the main parts of the whole organism are put together. Following the money trails, though, requires more expertise, time, support, and commitment than average people possess. However, the economics of cultural production is not on the agenda of America's media literacy movement: "Almost no one wants to look at key questions of who owns and controls the media. There is little attention to the profit-driven nature of our economy and how that gives rise to a commercially driven media. With the exception of organized religion, most of the media literacy movement emphasizes awareness over social change, and places responsibility for mediating the media squarely on the shoulders of parents and teachers, and the children themselves" (Peters 1998, 1).

However, a few people already understand many of the ways in which media, technology, and culture work in tandem, as well as against each other. In the main, they are marketers in the business world, as well as pollsters and other media professionals who run large political campaigns. In Noam Chomsky's terms, they are people who "manufacture consent" (Herman and Chomsky 1998). To survive, though, we must determine it ourselves.

DISTRUST MEDIA IN THE SHORT RUN, BUT TRUST IT IN THE LONG RUN

First, I don't believe that media functions like a mirror held up to society, reflecting exactly what's there. Media messages are tinkered with and filtered and mediated by far too many layers of people and ideologies. The "media as mirror" analogy has been cracked from the beginning. However, we must remember that media cannot help but reflect culture, cannot help but echo, to some extent, what average people say and do and think. It seems natural and logical that at least some deep patterns of culture could never remain divorced from media (and to a lesser extent, technology). This is a complex, curious phenomenon. Consider the issue of stereotypes communicated in popular media.

It's easy to see that today's kids suffer a bum rap at the hands of the popular media. American youth is stereotyped as sex crazed, illiterate, drug-headed, stupid, and materialistic. They are depicted as Bart Simpson (who grows up to be Homer), Beavis, Butthead, Erkle, Screech, Dumb, Dumber, and the kids of *South Park*. (Note that more than half of these representations are cartoons.) These stereotypes change, of course. My oldest sister belonged to the 1950s rebel-without-a-cause-or-clue generation, courtesy of Marlon Brando and James Dean. In the early '70s, members of my generation were branded as hippies and politically radical insurgents (both national security threats, of course). The '80s kids (with help from TV programs such as *Family Ties*) were portrayed as conservative, shallow, and materialistic—kids whose genetic code was stamped with the word "Republican." Next came Generation X. These kids were supposed to be confused and fragmented slackers.

These are the stereotypes because they do not apply to most or even many people, especially at the time they are communicated. However, in this case, the deeper pattern that may remain—and hence become reflected in later media—is the opposition to such stereotypes. If TV's Beaver Cleaver was the stereotypical good kid of several decades ago, he was eventually replaced by his polar opposites, the stereotypical bad kids of the '90s, Beavis and Butthead and the *South Park* gang. In short, we have to remember that media eventually reflects certain deep patterns of culture, mainly its oppositions or tensions. Like other art forms, media is easier to trust in the long run than it is in the short run.

NEVER FEAR MEDIA, TECHNOLOGY, AND CULTURE

Many people will argue that more communication among people would lessen feelings of distrust and fear. Indeed, sometimes this is true. Through television, America was able to collectively experience shock, grief, and solace, at the death of President John F. Kennedy, and, more recently, at the death of Princess Diana of Great Britain. On the other hand, more communication, easier to access by more people, sets more brushfires of fear. The greater the technology and the larger the number of people communicating, the more smoke and mirrors we have to navigate through. In fact, at no other time in our history have these three megasystems been in alignment to generate more distrust and fear among people than they are today.

Because of such rapid and extensive changes in media, technology, and culture—and because of the often volatile ways in which these changes are communicated—it's easy to fear them. Such fears may naturally focus on the voices described in this book and especially upon the people—particularly the youth—who embrace these voices, technologies, and subcultures. But young people, especially, have no choice. They have to forge their identities and perceptions by working with whatever raw materials are available. For a young Abe Lincoln, these materials may have been an axe and borrowed books. But for the people in our lives right now, especially kids, what's available to them is media and technology. It is natural for them to embrace these materials to figure out themselves and their world. This is why, throughout these pages, I have tried to articulate some reasons for not trusting media, technology, and culture. More and more, these megasystems provide the raw materials with which we construct our identities, relationships, and ways of defining the world. This book, though, advocates nothing more than a robust, critical frame of mind. It's a serious mistake to generalize from this stance and distrust media, technology, and culture. After all, these cannot be—should not be—separated from you and me and everything else.

Works Cited

Aaker, David, & D. Stayman. 1990. "A Micro Approach to Studying Feeling Responses to Advertising: The Case of Warmth." In *Emotion in Advertising: Theoretical and Practical Explorations*, edited by Stuart Agres, Tony Dubitsky, & Julie A. Edell, 53–68. Westport, CT: Quorum.

Aaker, David, D. M. Stayman, & M. R. Hagerty. 1986. "Warmth in Advertising: Measurement, Impact, and Sequence Effects." *Journal of Consumer Research* 12, no. 4: 365–381.

Abrams, Bill. 1982. "National Enquirer Starts Drive to Lure Big-Time Advertisers." *Wall Street Journal*, March 18: Western edition, sec. 2, pp. 27, 29.

Aitken, P., D. Leather, & A. Scott. 1988. "Ten- to Sixteen-Year-Olds' Perceptions of Advertisements for Alcoholic Drinks." *Alcohol and Alcoholism* 23, no. 6: 491–500.

American Psychological Association. 1993. Summary Report of the American Psychological Association Commission on Violence and Youth, vol. 1. Washington, DC: American Psychological Association.

American Psychological Association. September 30, 1999. "The Use of Psychology to Exploit and Influence Children for Commercial Purposes," Open letter to Richard Suinn.

Arnheim, Rudolph. 1986. *New Essays on the Psychology of Art*. Berkeley, CA: University of California Press.

Atlanta Quick City Guide. 1990. Guest Informant, a subsidiary of LIN Broadcasting Corp., New York.

Baker, C. Edwin. 1994. *Advertising and a Democratic Press*. Princeton, NJ: Princeton University Press.

Barsamian, David. 1991. *Chronicler of Dissent: Interviews with Noam Chomsky, 1984–1991*. Monroe, ME: Common Courage Press.

Benton, Thomas Hart. 1983. *An Artist in America*. 4th ed. Columbia, MO: University of Missouri Press.

Bingham, Janet. 1998. "Today's Topic: Soft Drink Flavors." *Denver Post*, June 12: p. 1A.

Bloland, Sue Erikson. 1999. "Fame: The Power and Cost of a Fantasy." *The Atlantic Monthly*, November: 52–62.

Blum, Alan. 1983. "Using Athletes to Push Tobacco to Children." *New York State Journal of Medicine* 83, no. 13: 1365–1367.

Boihem, Harold, & Chris Emmanouilides. 1997. "The Ad and the Ego." Video. San Francisco, CA: California Newsreel.

Bowen, Wally. 1995. "Ads, Ads Everywhere! Are There Any Limits?" *New Citizen* 2, no. 2:1.

Bradford, William. 1995. *Bradford's History "Of Plymouth Plantation."* First edition in 1901. Boston: Wright & Potter.

Brent, Harry, ed. 1997. "Environment." *Quarterly Review of Doublespeak* 24, no. 1:4.

Buckingham, David, & J. Seftan-Green. 1997. "From Regulation to Education? Sex, Violence, & Censorship." *The English & Media Magazine*, no. 36: 28–32.

Bushey, John. 1998. "District 11's Coke Problem." September 23, 1998, letter sent to School District 11 in Colorado Springs, Colorado, and reprinted in *Harper's Magazine*, February 1999: 26–27.

Cabbage, Michael. 1997. "Out There." *Columbia* (Missouri) *Daily Tribune*, July 6: p. 1D.

"Cause Celebs." 1999. *People* (November).

Center for Commercial Free Education, November 16, 1998: http://www.commercialfree.org/channelonetext.html.

Chesebro, James W., & Dale A. Bertelsen. 1996. *Analyzing Media: Communication Technologies as Symbolic and Cognitive Systems*. New York: Guilford Press.

Chmielewski, Dawn C. 1998. "ZapMe! Follows Channel One's Lead." *Orange County Register*, November 19: http://www.ocregister.com/education/zapme19w.htm/.

Commercial Alert, Washington, DC. October 29, 1998. "ZapMe! A New Corporate Predator in the Schools." Press release.

Considine, David. 1993. "Media Literacy and Human Health." *Telemedium: The Journal of Media Literacy* 39, nos. 3–4: 8–9.

Considine, David, & G. E. Haley. 1992. *Visual Messages: Integrating Imagery into Instruction*. Eaglewood, CO: Teacher Ideas Press.

Cookson, Peter W. 1998. "The Forgotten Issue: Education's Intrinsic Worth." *Education Week*, March 4: 46.

Corliss, Richard. 1995. "Autopsy or Fraud-Topsy?" *Time*, November 27: 105.

———. 1998. "True Colors." *Time*, March 16: 66.

———. 1999. "The X Phones." *Time*, August 9: 64–66.

"Corporate Curriculums." 1994. *Columbia* (Missouri) *Daily Tribune*, April 12: 8A.

Csikszentmihalyi, Mihaly. 1991. *Flow: The Psychology of Optimal Experience*. New York: HarperPerennial.

Dawkins, Richard. 1999. "The Selfish Meme." *Time* (April 19): 52–53.

Dawson, Brenda, J. Balfour, and J. Walsh. 1988. "Television Food Commercials' Effect on Children's Resistance to Temptation." *Journal of Applied Social Psychology* 18, pt. 2 (December): 1353–1360.

de Graaf, John, and Vivia Boe. 1997. *Affluenza*. Video recording. KCTS/Seattle and Oregon Public Broadcasting.

DeVaney, Ann. 1994. "Reading the Ads: The Bacchanalian Adolescence." In *Watching Channel One: The Convergence of Students, Technology, and Private Business*, edited by Ann DeVaney. Albany, NY: State University of New York Press.

Doheny-Farina, Stephen. 1999. Personal correspondence (March 17).

Doherty, Thomas. 1997. "Seamless Matching: Film, History, and JFK." *Phi Kappa Phi Journal* 77, no. 3: 39–42.

Donelson, Kenneth, and Aleen Nilsen. 1997. *Literature for Today's Young Adults*, 5th ed. New York: Longman.

Dyson, Rose. 1999a. "Violent Films Like 'American Psycho' Could Become High-Risk Investment." News release: Canadians Concerned About Violence in Entertainment. Posting to Cultural Environment Movement Listserv (March 20).

———. 1999b. "Governor Whitman, Howard Stern, and Columbine." Posting to Cultural Environment Movement Listserv (September 14).

Eco, Umberto. 1976. *A Theory of Semiotics*. Bloomington: Indiana University Press.

Edell, Julie A. 1990. "Emotion and Advertising: A Timely Union." In *Emotion in Advertising: Theoretical and Practical Explorations*, edited by Stuart Agres, Tony Dubitsky, & Julie A. Edell, xiii-xviii. New York: Quorum Books.

"Effects of TV Advertisements on Black Children: Fifth Annual Cross-Cultural Conference: Crises, Changes, and a Holistic Approach to Survival, 1983, Myrtle Beach, S. C." 1984. *Psychiatric Forum* 12, no. 2: 72–81.

Elbow, Peter, ed. 1994. *Landmark Essays on Voice and Writing*. Davis, CA: Hermagoras Press.

Erikson Bloland, Sue. 1999. "Fame: The Power and Cost of a Fantasy." *Atlantic Monthly* (November): 51–62.

Fariello, Griffin. 1995. *Red Scare*, 23. New York: W. W. Norton.

Fenton, Brian. December, 1998. "Media Monsters." *Stereo Review* 63, no. 12: 9.

Firmage, Joseph. The Truth. http://www.thewordisthetruth.org.

Fiske, John. 1993. *Television Culture*. New York: Routledge.

Fleckenstein, Kristie S. 1996. "Images, Words, and Narrative Epistemology." *College English* 58, no. 8:914–933.

Fox, Roy F. 1989. "Sensationspeak in America. In *Beyond 1984: Doublespeak in a Post-Orwellian Age*, edited by William Lutz. Urbana, IL: National Council Teachers of English.

———, ed. 1994. "Where We Live." In *Images in Language, Media, and Mind*, edited by Roy F. Fox. Urbana, IL: National Council Teachers of English.

———. 1996. *Harvesting Minds: How TV Commercials Control Kids*. Westport, CT: Praeger Press.

———, ed. In press. *UpDrafts: Case Studies in Teacher Renewal*. Urbana: National Council Teachers of English.

Franck, Peter. 1998. "Jonesboro, So What!" Posting to Cultural Environment Movement Listserv (April 5).

Frank, Thomas. 1999. "Brand You: Better Selling through Anthropology." *Harper's Magazine* (July): 74–79.

Fukuyama, Francis. 1999. "The Great Disruption: Human Nature and the Reconstitution of Social Order." *Atlantic Monthly* (May).

Gerbner, George. 1994. "Instant History, Image History: Lessons from the Persian Gulf War." In *Images in Language, Media, and Mind*, edited by Roy F. Fox, 123–141. Urbana, IL: National Council Teachers of English.

———. 1998. "New Weapon Against TV Commercials?" Posting to Cultural Environment Listserv (August 10).

———. 1999. "Media Violence." Reprint of a policy statement by the Academy of Pediatrics re media violence, in *Pediatrics 95*, no. 6 (June 1995): 949–951. Posting to Cultural Environment Movement List Serve.

Gerbner, George, & John Cones. 1998. "Moviegoers Beware." Posting to Cultural Environment Movement Listserv.

Gibbs, Nancy, & T. Roche. 1999. "The Columbine Tapes." *Time*. December 20. Posting to Cultural Environment Movement Listserv (October 24).

Gibson, Walker. 1966. *Tough, Sweet, and Stuffy: An Essay on Modern American Prose Style*. Bloomington, IN: Indiana University Press.

Gibson, Walker, & William Lutz. 1991. *Doublespeak: A Brief History, Definition, and Bibliography*. NCTE Concept Paper Series, no. 2. Urbana, IL: National Council Teachers of English.

Gitlin, Todd. 1994. "Imagebusters: The Hollow Crusade Against TV Violence." *The American Prospect* 16 (Winter): http://www.prospect.org/archives/index.html.

Gleick, James. 1997. "Addicted to Speed." *New York Times Magazine* (September 28): 55–61.

Glionna, John. 1999. "Slot Machine Designers Use Controversial Spin." *Los Angeles Times*. (October 25): p. 4A.

Goffman, Erving. 1959. *The Presentation of Self in Everyday Life*. Garden City, NY: Doubleday.

Goodman, Ellen. 1997. "Sojourner is Proof that We Romanticize High-Tech World." *Columbia Daily Tribune*, July 10: p. 6A.

Grant, Martin. August 9, 1995. Press Release. Channel One Television.

Greenberg, Bradley, & J. E. Brand. 1982. "Television and Role Socialization: An Overview." In *Television and Behavior: Ten Years of Scientific Progress and Implications for the Eighties*, edited by D. Perl et al. Rockville, MD: National Institute of Mental Health.

Greenfield, Patricia M. 1984. *Mind and Media: The Effects of Television, Video Games, and Computers*. Cambridge, MA: Harvard University Press.

Greenstein, Jennifer. 1999. "Plotting a Revolution—Again." *Brill's Content* (February): 104–105.

Grossman, Mary Ann, & Chris Hewitt. 1997. "Chicshocks." *Columbia* (Missouri) *Daily Tribune*, May 4: p. 1E.

"Group Culls Disney Films, Finds More Scenes Offensive." 1995. *Columbia* (Missouri) *Daily Tribune*, September 2: p. 8A.

Gup, Ted. 1998. "Technology and the End of Serendipity." *Education Digest* (March): 49–50.

Harrison, Albert A. 1997. *After Contact: The Human Response to Extraterrestrial Life*. New York: Plenum Press.

Hayakawa, S. I., ed. 1962. *The Use and Misuse of Language*. Greenwich, CT: Fawcett Publications.

Hays, Constance L. 1999. "Math Books Salted with Brand Names Raises New Alarm." *New York Times*, March 21: p. 1A, 22A.

Herman, Edward S., & Noam Chomsky. 1998. *Manufacturing Consent: The Political Economy of the Mass Media*. New York: Pantheon Books.

Hilgartner, Stephen, R. C. Bell, & R. O'Connor. 1983. *Nukespeak: The Selling of Nuclear Technology in America*. New York: Penguin Books.

Hite, R., & R. Eck. 1987. "Advertising to Children: Attitudes of Business vs. Consumers." *Journal of Advertising* (October/November): 40–53.

Holbrook, Morris, & Barbara B. Stern. 1997. "The Paco Man and What Is Remembered: New Readings of a Hybrid Language." In *Undressing the Ad: Reading Culture in Advertising*, edited by Katherine Frith. New York: Peter Lang.

Honan, William H. 1997. "Scholars Attack Public School TV Program." *New York Times Educational Supplement* (January 22): B7.

Horovitz, Bruce, & Melanie Wells. 1997. "Ads for Adult Vices Big Hit with Teens." *USA Today*, January 31-February 2: pp. 1A–2A.

Hoynes, William. 1997. "News for a Captive Audience: An Analysis of Channel One." *EXTRA!* (May/June): 11.

Huston, A. C., et al. 1992. *Big World, Small Screen: The Role of Television in American Society*. Lincoln, NE: University of Nebraska Press.

Kaplan, Justin. 1980. *Walt Whitman: A Life*. New York: Simon and Schuster.

Karl, Herb. 1994. "The Image Is Not the Thing." In *Images in Language, Media, and Mind*, edited by Roy F. Fox. Urbana, IL: National Council Teachers of English.

Karpatkin, Rhoda, & A. Holmes. 1995. "Making Schools Ad-Free Zones." *Educational Leadership* 53, no. 1: 72–76.

Kaul, Donald. 1999. "Bad Taste Replaces Dignity as Today's Social Norm." *Columbia* (Missouri) *Daily Tribune*, March 15: p. 4A.

Kehl, D. G. 1988. "Doublespeak: Its Meaning and Its Menace." *Quarterly Review of Doublespeak* XIV, no. 2: 8.

Kelly, Kevin. 1994. "Embrace It." *Harper's Magazine* (May): 20.

Key, Wilson Bryan. 1976. *Media Sexploitation*. New York: Prentice-Hall.

Kieger, Dale. 1994. "The Dark World of Park Dietz." *Johns Hopkins Magazine* (November): 18–19.

Kilbourne, Jeane. 1997. In *The Ad and the Ego*. Newsreel, directed by Harold Boihem. San Francisco, CA: California Newsreel.

Kline, Stephen. 1993. *Out of the Garden: Toys and Children's Culture in the Age of TV Marketing*. New York: Verso.

Korzybski, Alfred. 1933. *Science and Sanity*. Lancaster, PA: Science Press.

Kozol, Jonathan. 1992. "Corporate Raid on Education: Whittle and the Privateers." *Nation* (September 21): 273–278.

Kunkel, Dale, & Donald Roberts. 1991. "Young Minds and Marketplace Values: Issues in Children's Television Advertising." *Journal of Social Issues* 47, no. 1: 57–72.

Labi, Nadya. 1999. "Classrooms for Sale." *Time* (April 19).

Landay, Jerry M. 1998. "Speed-Up Victims, Unite." Posting to Cultural Environ-
    ment Movement Listserv (March 10).
Lanham, Richard. 1992. *Revising Prose*, 3d ed. New York: Macmillan.
Lapham, Lewis H. 1997. "In the Garden of Tabloid Delight." *Harper's Magazine*
    (August): 35–43.
Lewis, Justin, Michael Morgan, & Sut Jhally. 1998. "Libertine or Liberal? The
    Real Scandal of What People Know about President Clinton." Unpub-
    lished research report (February 10). Amherst, MA: Department of Com-
    munications, University of Massachusetts.
" 'Lion King' Sex Scene Has Christian Group Seeing Red." 1995. *Columbia* (Mis-
    souri) *Daily Tribune*, August 31: p. 14A.
Lippmann, Walter. 1962. In *Sinclair Lewis: A Collection of Critical Essays*, edited by
    Mark Schorer. Englewood Cliffs, NJ: Prentice-Hall.
Liu, Eric. 1999. "Remember When Public Spaces Didn't Carry Brand Names?"
    USA Today, March 25: p. 15A.
Lokeman, Rhonda Chriss. 1998. "Crazy Chain." *Columbia* (Missouri) *Daily Trib-
    une*, June 2: p. 7A.
Lutz, William. 1989. *Beyond 1984: Doublespeak in a Post-Orwellian Age*. Urbana, IL:
    National Council Teachers of English.
———. 1996. *The New Doublespeak: Why No One Knows What Anyone's Saying
    Anymore*. New York: HarperCollins
Maddock, Richard, & R. Fulton. 1996. *Marketing to the Mind: Right Brain Strategies
    for Advertising and Marketing*. Westport, CT: Greenwood Publishing Group.
McCafferty, Dennis. 1999. "www.hate.comes to your home." *USA Weekend*
    (March 26–28).
McCannon, Bob. 1999. "Censorship 1999: The Problem & A Solution." *The New
    Mexico Media Literacy Project Newsletter* (Fall/Winter): 8–9.
McCarthy, Colman. 1993. "Channel One Whittles Away Education in U.S." *Co-
    lumbia* (Missouri) *Daily Tribune*, November 6: p. 4A.
McChesney, Robert W. 1997. "Rise of the Media Giants." *Extra! The Magazine of
    Fair (Fairness and Accuracy in Reporting)* 10, no. 6:11–19.
McKibben, Bill. 1990. *The End of Nature*. New York: Anchor.
McLaren, Carrie, ed. 1997. "The Babysitter's Club." *Stay Free!* (Spring): 9.
———. 1997b. "Toy Stories." *Stay Free!* 23 (Spring): 8–16.
———. 1998. "World View." *Stay Free!* (January): 4–5.
———. 1999. "How Advertising Can Wreck Your Health." *Stay Free!* 16 (Fall/
    Winter): 30–36.
McLuhan, Marshall. 1964. *Understanding Media: The Extensions of Man*, 2d ed.
    New York: McGraw-Hill.
"Media Mash XIII." 1998. Media Culture Review (June 4): http://www.
    mediademocracy.org.
Miller, Mark Crispin. 1996. "Free the Media." *The Nation* (June 3): 9–15.
Minow, Newton N., & Craig L. Lamay. 1996. *Abandoned in the Wasteland: Children,
    Television and the First Amendment*, 8. New York: Hill and Wang.
Mitchell, Arnold. 1983. *The Nine American Lifestyles*. New York: Macmillan.
"Monsters Next Door." 1999. *Time* (May 3): 270.
Moog, Carol. 1994. "Ad Images and the Stunting of Sexuality." In *Images in Lan-*

guage, Media, and Mind, edited by Roy F. Fox. Urbana, IL: National Council Teachers of English.

"Movie Most Foul." 1999. *Harper's Magazine* (September): 28.

Mueller, Barbara, & K. Wulfemeyer. 1991. "A Framework for the Analysis of Commercials in the Classroom: The Decoding of Channel One." *The High School Journal* (February/March): 138–159.

Naureckas, Jim, ed. 1997. "Hate Talk & Politics." *EXTRA!Update* (August): 3.

Nelson, Richard A. 1981. "Propaganda." In *Handbook of American Culture*, vol. 3, edited by M. Thomas Inge, 353. Westport, CT: Greenwood Press.

New York State Department of Education memo to the New York State Assembly, May 23, 1995. Obligation, Inc.: http://www.obligation.org/channelonequotes.html#anchor60064.

Perrin, Tom. 1997. "Pop Quiz: Who's Paying Schools Big Bucks to Advertise?" *Kansas City Star*, October 18: p. 1A.

PeTA: People for the Ethical Treatment of Animals. n.d. "PeTA Factsheet, Wildlife #8." Norfolk, VA.

Peters, Cynthia. 1998. "Media Literacy." *Z Magazine* (February): http://www.lol.shareworld.com/zmag/articles/feb98peters.htm.

Peterson, R. C., & L. L. Thurstone. 1933. *Motion Pictures and the Social Attitudes of Children*. New York: Macmillan.

Pipher, Mary. 1994. *Reviving Ophelia: Saving the Selves of Adolescent Girls*. New York: Ballantine Books.

"Poll Shows Tolerance for Violence in Films." 1999. *Columbia* (Missouri) *Daily Tribune*, July 3: p. 2A.

Postman, Neil. 1985. *Amusing Ourselves to Death: Public Discourse in the Age of Show Business*. New York: Viking.

———. 1993. *Technopoly: The Surrender of Culture to Technology*. New York: Alfred A. Knopf.

Proulx, E. Annie. 1997. "Dead Stuff." *Aperture* (Fall). Reprinted, "Returning Death's Gaze" in *Harper's Magazine* (April 1998): 31–34.

Putnam, Robert D. 1996. "The Strange Disappearance of Civic America." *The American Prospect* 24 (Winter): 1–16.

Rank, Hugh. 1976. "Teaching About Public Persuasion: Rationale and a Schema." In *Teaching About Doublespeak*, edited by Daniel Dieterich, 3–19. Urbana, IL: National Council of Teachers of English.

Ray, Michael. 1982. *Advertising and Communication Management*, x. Englewood Cliffs, NJ: Prentice-Hall.

Reese, Charley. 1997. "Internet Is No More than a Bunch of Filing Cabinets." *Columbia* (Missouri) *Daily Tribune*, July 7: p. 6A.

"Report Says U.S. Is 'Nation of Speakers.' " 1998. *Columbia* (Missouri) *Daily Tribune*, June 24: p. 11A.

Report to the Legislature on Commercialism in Schools. January 1991. Olympia: Washington Office of the State Superintendent of Public Instruction. Eric Document #EA332301.

Ressner, Jeffrey. 1998. "The People's Choice." *Time* (March 16): 71.

Richards, I. A. 1921. *Practical Criticism: A Study of Literary Judgment*. New York: Harcourt Brace Jovanovich.

Ritchin, Fred. 1990. *In Our Own Image: The Coming Revolution in Photography*. New York: Aperture Foundation.

Robertson, Heather-jane. 1999. "Hyenas at the Oasis: Corporate Marketing to Captive Students." Reprinted with permissions from Our School, Our Selves Education Foundation. Media Awareness: http://www.media-awareness.ca/eng/med/class/edissue/hyenas.htm.

Robertson, Linda R. 1994. "From War Propaganda to Sound Bites: The Poster Mentality of Politics in the Age of Television. In *Images in Language, Media, and Mind*, edited by Roy F. Fox, 92–108. Urbana, IL: National Council Teachers of English.

Robischon, Noah. 1999. "Commercial Interruption." *Brill's Content* (February): 64, 66.

"Rock-A-Buy Baby." 1994. *Harper's Magazine* (April): 22.

Ross, R. et al. n.d. "When Celebrities Talk, Children Listen: An Experimental Analysis of Children's Responses to TV Ads with Celebrity Endorsements." Unpublished paper, Center for Research on the Influences of Television on Children, University of Kansas.

Rossiter, J. 1980. "Source Effects and Self-Concept Appeals in Children's Television Advertising." In *The Effects of Television Advertising on Children*, 61–94. Lexington, MA: D. C. Heath & Co.

Roszak, Theodore. 1994. *The Cult of Information*. Berkeley, CA: The University of California Press.

Ruskin, Gary. 1999. "Slot Machines for Children." Personal correspondence, coalition letter to Senator John McCain, Representative Thomas Bliley, et al. (November 19). Commercial Alert: http://www.essential.org/alert.

Ryan, Chris. 1997. Letter to the Editor. *Harper's Magazine* 295, no. 1767: 7.

San Francisco Chronicle. 1998 (March 26). In "Radio in the USA" by David Cone. Posting to Cultural Environment Listserv (March 26, 1998).

Schlosser, Eric. 1997. "The Business of Pornography." *U.S. News and World Report* (February 10): 42–53.

Schwed, Mark. 1995. "TV Commercials and Your Kids." *TV Guide* (February 18): 19.

Seagal, Debra. 1993. "Tales from the Cutting-Room Floor." *Harper's Magazine* 287, no. 1722: 50–57.

"Selling to School Kids." 1995. *Consumer Reports* (May): 327–329.

Shalek, Nancy. September 21, 1999. Qtd. in Ralph Nader and G. Ruskin, "Protecting Children from Exploitive Advertising." Memo to U.S. Congressional Leaders, Commercial Alert, Washington, DC: http://www.essential.org/alert.

Shalit, Ruth. 1999. "Return of the Hidden Persuaders." Salon Media: http://www.salon.com/media/col/shal/1999/09/27/persuaders/.

Shenk, David. 1997. *Data Smog: Surviving the Information Glut*. New York: HarperCollins.

———. 1999. "Why You Feel the Way You Do?" *INC*. (January): 56–70.

"Sleep." 1998. *Quarterly Review of Doublespeak*, no. 4: 12.

Smith, Jeff. n.d. "The Battle for Kids Minds: How to Kombat Corporate Control of Fantasy." Grand Rapids Institute for Information Democracy: http://www.grcmc.org/griid/articles.htm.

Solomon, Norman. 1998a. "When All the World's a Stage—For Cashing In." Posting to Cultural Environment Movement Listserv (April 20).

———. 1998b. "Is the V-Chip a Stealth Weapon Against Commercials?" Posting to Cultural Environment Movement Listserv (December 30).

———. 1999a. "The Performance Art of American Politics." Posting to Cultural Environment Movement Listserv (February 10).

———. 1999b. "And Now . . . Another Episode of Media Jeopardy." Posting to Cultural Environment Listserv (February 18).

———. 1999c. "Think of All We'd Miss Without Commercials." Posting to Cultural Environment Listserv (August 27).

———. 1999d. "Big Media Applaud Big Media Merger." Posting to Cultural Environment Movement Listserv (September 9).

Solomon, Rainbow, & Brian Quigg. 1999. "Advertising on MTV: A Sociological Study." http://it.stlawu.edu/~advertiz/mtv/advertis.htm.

Spiegel, Lee. 1999. "Eyes Wide Shut: What the Critics Failed to See in Kubrick's Last Film." *Harper's Magazine* (October): 76–84.

Stein, Joel, & Jeanne McDowell. 1999. "When Good Networks GO BAD." *Time* (February 1): 60–61.

Steinbeck, John. 1996. *America and Americans*. New York: The Viking Press, 29–34.

Stone, Brad. 1998. "An Icon from Our Sponsor." *Newsweek* (November 23): 71.

Stossel, Scott. 1997. "The Man Who Counts the Killings." *The Atlantic Monthly* (May). http://www.TheAtlantic.com/atlantic/issue/97/May/gerbner.htm.

"Strange New World." 1994. *Time* (July 25).

Stringfield, Leonard H. 1980. "The UFO Crash/Retrieva Syndrome (Status Report II: new Sources, New Data)." Sequin, TX: Mutual UFO Network Inc.

Strong, Morgan. 1992. "Portions of the Gulf War Were Brought to You by . . . the Folks at Hill and Knowlton." *TV Guide* (February 22): 11–13.

"Systems." 1997. *Quarterly Review of Doublespeak* 23, no. 4: 5.

"Targeting the Stoned Cyberpunk." 1994. *Harper's Magazine* (December): 26–27.

"Technology." 1998. *Quarterly Review of Doublespeak*, no. 3 (April): 11.

"The Ticker." 1999. *Brill's Content* (January): 140.

"This School Is Brought to You By: Cola? Sneakers?" 1998. *USA Today*, March 27: p. 11A.

Thomas, Karen. 1999. "Wannabes Are Mimicking Sport's Racier, Uhm, Moves." *USA Today*, February 26–28: p. 1A.

"Tobacco Firms Studied Smokers' Reasons." 1998. *Columbia* (Missouri) *Daily Tribune*, February 27: p. 5B.

Tough, Allen. 1998. "After Contact and Before, Too." *Contemporary Psychology* 43, no. 9: 625–626.

"TV Station Broadcasts Suicide." 1994. *Columbia* (Missouri) *Daily Tribune*, October 30: p. 15A.

Weinberg, Lawerence. 1988. *What Was It Like? George Washington*. Stamford, CT: Longmeadow Press.

Wells, Melanie. 1997a. "Absolut's Eye-Catching Ads Command Teens' Attention." *USA Today*, January 31–February 2: p. 5B.

———. 1997b. "Kids Know Joe Camel, But They Follow Marlboro Man." *USA Today*, January 31–February 2: p. 5B.

"What You Need to Know about Television and Violence." 1998. *Center for Parent and Youth Understanding Summer 1998 Newsletter*: http://www.cpyu.org/news/98Summerm.htm.

White, Walter. 1951. "Negro Leader Looks at TV Race Problem. *Printer's Ink* (August 24): 31.

Whitman, Walt. 1965. "Leaves of Grass." In *The Collected Writings of Walt Whitman—Comprehensive Reader's Edition*. New York University Press edition, edited by Harold W. Blodgett and Sculley Bradley, 714–715.

Will, George. 1997. "Advertisers Are in The Business to 'Rent' Our Attention." *Columbia* (Missouri) *Daily Tribune*, July 9: p. 6A.

World Opinion, November 11, 1998. "Quick Facts." http://www.worldopinion.com/latenews.

Wright, Robert. 1998. "Sin in the Global Village." *Time* (October 19): 130.

Zachary, G. Pascal. 1997. "Male Order: Boys Used to Be Boys, But Do Some Now See Boyhood as a Malady?" *Wall Street Journal Internet Edition* (May 2).

Zakia, Richard D. 1976. "MaMa Media: An Introduction." In *Media Sexploitation*, by Wilson Bryan Key. New York: Prentice-Hall.

Zinn, Howard. 1995. *A People's History of the United States*. New York: The New Press.

Index

About the Author

ROY F. FOX teaches courses in language, literacy, and culture at the University of Missouri-Columbia, where he also directs the Missouri Writing Project. He is the author of *Harvesting Minds* (Greenwood, 1996).